WORKING WITH ASIAN AMERICANS

WORKING WITH ASIAN AMERICANS
A Guide For Clinicians

EVELYN LEE, Editor

Foreword by STANLEY SUE

THE GUILFORD PRESS
New York   London

© 1997 The Guilford Press
A Division of Guilford Publications, Inc.
72 Spring Street, New York, NY 10012
www.guilford.com

Printed in the United States of America

This book is printed on acid-free paper.

Last digit is print number: 9 8 7 6 5 4 3 2 1

Library of Congress Cataloging-in-Publication Data

Working with Asian Americans: a guide for clinicians / Evelyn Lee,
   editor.
      p.   cm.
   Includes bibliographical references and index.
   ISBN 1-57230-244-5
   1. Asian Americans—Mental health.   2. Asian Americans—Mental
health services.   I. Lee, Evelyn.
RC451.5.A75W67   1997
616.89′008995—dc21   97–25930
                                                              CIP

To my mother, Isabel Choi Lum, who gave me
the roots *to be proud of who I am*
and the wings *to fly where I want to be.*

Contributors

Phillip D. Akutsu, PhD, Assistant Professor, Pacific Graduate School of Psychology, Palo Alto, California

Bart K. Aoki, PhD, Social Science Research Analyst, University-Wide AIDS Research Program, Office of the President, University of California

Evelyn F. Balancio, LCSW, Assistant Clinical Professor, Department of Psychiatry, University of California, San Francisco, California; Director, MOST Team, South of Market Mental Health Clinic, San Francisco, California

James K. Boehnlein, MD, MSc, Associate Professor, Department of Psychiatry, Oregon Health Sciences University, Portland, Oregon

Loo Hang Chao, BA, Research Assistant, Department of Psychiatry, Oregon Health Sciences University, Portland, Oregon

Freda Cheung, PhD, Associate Clinical Professor, Department of Psychiatry, Harbor-UCLA Medical Center, Torrance, California; Clinical Psychologist, Evangelist County Department of Mental Health, Los Angeles, California; Research Associate, Research Center on the Psychobiology of Ethnicity, Harbor-UCLA Medical Center, Torrance, California

Wai Chung, LCSW, Psychiatric Social Worker, Department of Psychiatry, Kaiser Permanente Medical Center, San Francisco, California

Joel Crohn, PhD, private practice, Kensington and San Rafael, California; Adjunct Faculty, California School of Professional Psychology, Alameda, California

Nang Du, MD, Assistant Clinical Professor, Department of Psychiatry, University of California, San Francisco, California; Department of Psychiatry, San Francisco General Hospital, San Francisco, California

Albert Eng, PhD, Assistant Director, Children, Adolescent, and Family Section, Division of Mental Health Services, Department of Public Health, San Francisco, California

Kenneth K. Gee, MD, Assistant Clinical Professor, Department of Psychiatry, University of California, San Francisco, California; Unit Chief, Asian Focus Unit, Department of Psychiatry, San Francisco General Hospital, San Francisco, California

Reiko Homma-True, PhD, Assistant Clinical Professor, Department of Psychiatry, University of California, San Francisco; Fulbright Fellow, Kobe University School of Medicine, Kobe, Japan

Shiao-Ling Judy Hsieh, PhD, Visiting Professor, Department of Psychology, Beijing University, Beijing, China; Consultant Psychologist, International Medical Center, Beijing, China

Larke Nahme Huang, PhD, Consulting Psychologist, National Technical Assistance Center for Children's Mental Health, Georgetown University, Washington, DC

Mutsumi M. Ishii, MD, Department of Psychiatry, Dean Medical Center, Madison, Wisconsin

Davis Ja, PhD, California School of Professional Psychology, Alameda, California

Rudolf Sing-Kee Kao, LCSW, Senior Psychiatric Social Worker, Chinatown/North Beach Community Mental Health Services, San Francisco, California

Kham-One Keopraseuth, MSW, Research Assistant, Department of Psychiatry, Oregon Health Sciences University, Portland, Oregon

Sung C. Kim, PhD, private practice, San Francisco, California

J. David Kinzie, MD, Professor, Department of Psychiatry, Oregon Health Sciences University, Portland, Oregon

Mary Leong Lam, LCSW, Psychiatric Social Worker, Chinatown/North Beach Community Mental Health Services, San Francisco, California

Godwin Lau, PhD, private practice, Toronto, Ontario, Canada

Evelyn Lee, EdD, LCSW, Associate Clinical Professor, Department of Psychiatry, University of California, San Francisco, California; Executive Director, Richmond Area Multi-Services, Inc., San Francisco, California

Paul K. Leung, MD, Associate Professor, Department of Psychiatry, Oregon Health Sciences University, Portland, Oregon

Keh-Ming Lin, MD, MPH, Professor and Director, Research Center on the Psychobiology of Ethnicity and Department of Psychiatry, Harbor-UCLA Medical Center, Torrance, California

Hung-Tat Lo, MBBS, FRCPC, private practice, Scarborough, Ontario, Canada

Francis G. Lu, MD, Clinical Professor, Department of Psychiatry, University of California, San Francisco, California; Director, Cultural Competency and Diversity Program, Department of Psychiatry, San Francisco General Hospital, San Francisco, California

Beckie Masaki, MSW, Executive Director, Asian Women's Shelter, San Francisco, California

Matthew R. Mock, PhD, Program Supervisor, Family, Youth and Children's Service, City of Berkeley Mental Health Division, Berkeley, California; Director and Associate Professor, Cross-Cultural Program, Graduate School of Professional Psychology, John F. Kennedy University, Orinda, California; private practice, Berkeley, California

Laurie Jo Moore, MD, private practice, Portland, Oregon

Russell E. Poland, PhD, Professor and Associate Director, Research Center on the Psychobiology of Ethnicity and Department of Psychiatry, Harbor-UCLA Medical Center, Torrance, California

Sudha Prathikanti, MD, Clinical Instructor, Department of Psychiatry, University of California, San Francisco, California; Department of Psychiatry, San Francisco General Hospital, San Francisco, California

Michael Smith, MD, Assistant Professor, Research Center on the Psychobiology of Ethnicity and Department of Psychiatry, Harbor-UCLA Medical Center, Torrance, California

Juliana Sustento-Seneriches, MD, private practice, Pleasanton, California

Nadine M. Tang, LCSW, private practice, Berkeley, California

Philip Tsui, LCSW, Program Director, Richmond Area Multi-Services, Inc., San Francisco, California

Lorena Wong, LCSW, private practice, San Francisco, California; Student Health Services, City College, San Francisco, California; Women's Resource Center, University of California, San Francisco, California

Jennie Yee, PhD, Clinical Psychologist, Chinatown/North Beach Community Mental Health Services, San Francisco, California

Wing H. Yeung, MD, Assistant Clinical Professor, Department of Psychiatry, University of California, San Francisco, California; Staff Psychiatrist, Richmond Area Multi-Services, Inc., San Francisco, California

Yu-Wen Ying, PhD, Associate Professor, School of Social Welfare, University of California, Berkeley, California

Francis K. Yuen, DSW, Assistant Professor, School of Social Work, Southwest Missouri State University, Springfield, Missouri

Foreword

Over the years, much knowledge has accumulated about mental health problems and the means to treat them in various Asian American groups. Much of this knowledge has been vested in practitioners or clinicians who work with Asian American clients and families. Unfortunately, the insights of practitioners have not been widely distributed because practitioners are often not in a position to conduct research or to publish papers. This is especially unfortunate because practitioners are in a direct position to know the kinds of problems exhibited by clients, to test different kinds of interventions, to translate research findings into assessment and therapeutic strategies, and to deal with the practical and cultural dilemmas posed by clients. For years, those of us in the field of Asian American mental health have lamented the fact that a practice-oriented handbook on clinical issues cannot be found.

Working with Asian Americans: A Guide for Clinicians is a highly important contribution toward addressing these clinical issues. Practical guidelines for assessment and treatment are given, which should be of interest to psychologists, psychiatrists, social workers, counselors, and psychiatric nurses. The edited book is comprehensive, organized into various sections that deal with family dynamics, developmental issues, therapeutic interventions, and different kinds of treatment modalities. In addition to these topics, issues pertinent to specific Asian groups (e.g., Chinese, Filipino, Japanese, Korean, Cambodian, and East Indian), special populations (e.g., gays and lesbians and women), and particular disorders (e.g., schizophrenia, depression, suicide, substance abuse, etc.) are examined. Thus, the book will appeal to those readers who may have very specific interests as well as to those who want to know about Asian Americans in general, and the commonalities and differences in their status and background. The insights provided by the chapter contributors are quite profound.

While this book focuses on Asian Americans, there are aspects of it that have significance for minority groups in general, namely, that attention must be given to cultural values and practices within an ethnic group, to the specific experiences of individuals as part of that minority group, and to interventions that are tailored to the cultural lifestyles of clients. How do we take into account the cultural values of our clients? Are there practical guidelines for working with Asian American clients? What kinds of questions are important to ask in order to ascertain how acculturated a client is? Are there ethnic differences in responses to psychotropic medications? These are but a few of the interesting and important questions that are of concern to a broad audience. Researchers should also find the book very helpful. Many of the contributions provide testable hypotheses, and, although the book deals primarily with clinical practice issues, a number of researchers also share their experiences from their work with Asian Americans.

Given the numerous issues and topics that are covered by the book, one can easily appreciate the complexities in the field of Asian American mental health. This book makes an important contribution by bringing out these complexities, by offering suggestions on how to deal with cultural–interpersonal issues in treatment, and by sharing the thoughts of those who directly work with Asian Americans in clinical practice.

STANLEY SUE, PhD
University of California, Davis

Preface

Putting together this book has proved to be exciting and challenging. The excitement has been the unique opportunity to share years of clinical experience working with Asian American families. More importantly, the book has brought together a group of culturally competent clinicians and researchers who have tremendous experience and knowledge in their areas of specialization. The first challenge was to present complex clinical issues for very diverse Asian American groups, which led us to decide to cover only those groups with the largest populations. The second challenge was to present cultural characteristics of a particular group without reinforcing stereotypes. Finally, we wanted to offer practical suggestions for clinical interventions without suggesting that there was one answer with any client. We hope that we have met these challenges and that this book shows our respect for each Asian American as an individual within his or her cultural context.

We attempted to produce a comprehensive handbook exploring many important topics. Part I gives an overview of Asian American families and presents chapters on each major Asian group, highlighting the diversity among Asian American family systems. Part II addresses special developmental and life cycle issues, with implications for the treatment of children, adolescents, adults, and the elderly. Part III discusses therapeutic issues and focuses on DSM-IV diagnoses, including schizophrenia, depressive disorders, posttraumatic stress disorder, substance abuse, and anxiety disorders. Part IV presents different treatment modalities and discusses their relevance for Asian Americans. Part V covers special topics such as gays and lesbians, intermarriage, domestic violence, and cross-cultural communication.

A recurring theme throughout the book is the importance of ethnic and cultural dimensions in the assessment and treatment of Asian American families. As a bilingual clinician for over thirty years, I have developed an appreciation for the integration of cultural, racial, political, and spiritual dimensions in understanding individuals and families. In addition, I have learned much from my clients' cultural strengths and survival spirit, and I am constantly exploring new ways to mobilize these positive traits in therapy.

My interests in the role of culture in counseling also stems from my own background. Having grown up in Hong Kong, I remember the joy of being raised by my aunt and grandmothers, with their unconditional love, colorful festivals, and strong sense of family and community. I also recall the pain caused by my family's uprooting and relocation, separation and losses, and sexism in traditional Chinese culture. My early career in Hong Kong and Vietnam exposed me to human suffering caused by war and poverty. I was also the first member of my family to come to the United States, where I underwent many typical immigrant experiences such as culture shock, language difficulty, racism, and acculturation stress. Through my life experiences, I have a heightened understanding of the forces of ethnicity and culture in my own personal development. In my professional practice, I am continually challenged to integrate those factors in my own clinical work.

As a Buddhist, I appreciate the *karma* to have the opportunity to edit this book, with wonderful support from many individuals. In particular, I want to acknowledge all of the authors, without whose contributions this book would not have been possible.

EVELYN LEE

Contents

Part V   **Special Issues**

Part I

Asian American Families

1

Overview: The Assessment and Treatment of Asian American Families

EVELYN LEE

The aim of this chapter is to present a conceptual framework in assessing and treating Asian American families, with special emphasis on immigrants and refugees. The first objective is to expand clinicians' knowledge of Asian American family structure and dynamics. The second is to provide clinicians with culturally competent clinical skills in working with this population. This overview discusses Asian Americans as a group; subsequent chapters examine each Asian group's individual characteristics.

This chapter is organized around four major subject areas:

1. Demographics and background information on cultural diversity among various Asian American groups.
2. Common characteristics among Asian families.
3. Assessment guidelines incorporating unique Asian American cultural backgrounds and life experiences.
4. Effective treatment strategies to guide clinicians to produce optimal treatment outcomes.

DEMOGRAPHICS AND CULTURAL DIVERSITY

Asian Americans are not a homogeneous group. It must be emphasized at the outset that no one single set of Asian American family characteristics applies to all groups. There is tremendous cultural diversity within and among Asian American communities. In fact, the term "Asian Pacific American," which has been in common use since the 1960s, applies to 43 ethnic groups, including 28 Asian groups and 15 Pacific Islander groups (Asian American Health Forum, 1990). This population has increased from less than 1 million in the United States in 1960 to more than 7 million by 1990 and represents the fastest growing ethnic community in the United States today.

Asian American groups differ in terms of population, immigration history, language, foreign-born population, educational level, family income, residential preference, religion, and exposure to war trauma. The following discussion is drawn largely from the U.S. Bureau of the Census 1990 statistics and population statistics analysis by the Asian American Health Forum (1990). I describe the major Asian American ethnic groups: Asian Pacific Islanders have their own unique characteristics and are not included.

Population

According to the 1990 U.S. Census, the seven largest Asian American groups are Chinese (22.6% of the Asian American population), Filipino (19.3%), Japanese (11.7%), Asian Indian (11.2%), Korean (11.0%), Vietnamese (8.5%), and Cambodian (5.8%). Groups with less than 3% include Thai, Lao, and Hmong (see Table 1.1).

Immigration History

Each Asian American group has a complex migration history in the United States. Individual chapters discuss these histories in detail. In summary, Chinese Americans were the first Asians to immigrate to the United States in large numbers and have arrived over a 150-year period. The 1965 Immigration Act brought a large number of Chinese, as well as Koreans and Filipinos. Most Japanese Americans today are the descendants of Japanese who migrated to Hawaii or the U.S. mainland before 1924. After the Vietnam War ended in 1975, a large number of Southeast Asian refugees arrived. Those who came were mostly educated Vietnamese. Since 1978, a second wave has come to the United States to escape persecution, including Vietnamese, Chinese–Vietnamese, Cambodians, Lao, Hmong, and Mien. Future waves of Asian immigrants will depend

TABLE 1.1. Asian American Pacific Islander Population Based on 1990 Census Estimates

Ethnic group	Percentage of Asian American population	Population in United States	Percentage of population foreign-born
Chinese	22.60%	1,645,472	56%
Filipino	19.30%	1,406,770	64%
Japanese	11.70%	847,562	33%
Asian Indian	11.20%	815,447	57%
Korean	11.00%	798,849	71%
Vietnamese	8.50%	614,547	92%
Cambodian	5.80%	417,411	80%
Hawailan	2.90%	211,014	n/a
Lao	2.10%	149,014	n/a
Thai	1.30%	91,275	n/a
Hmong	1.20%	90,082	n/a
Samoan	0.90%	62,964	n/a
Guamanian	0.70%	49,345	n/a

Note. Data from U.S. Bureau of the Census.

largely on the political situation in each country and the ever-changing U.S. immigration policies.

Foreign-Born Population and Acculturation Rate

In 1960, most Asian Americans were descendants of early Japanese and Chinese immigrants. Now, more than half of Asian Americans are foreign-born. The 1990 U.S. Census revealed the following foreign-born percentages: Vietnamese (92%), Cambodian (80%), Korean (71%), Filipino (64%), Asian Indian (57%), and Chinese (56%) (Table 1.1).

Language

Among Asian American groups, at least 32 different primary languages are spoken. Within each group (e.g., Chinese and Filipino), there may be many dialects. Proficiency in English varies greatly among the different groups. Most American-born Asians speak English fluently, with no accent, but often they do not speak their mother tongue at all. The majority of foreign-born Asians struggle with the English language and continue to speak their primary language at home. As a result of many years of foreign occupation and/or migration history, some groups have developed multilingual capabilities (e.g., the ethnic Chinese from Vietnam, who typically speak Vietnamese, French, English, and several Chinese dialects; the Chinese who migrated to Brazil, who speak Portuguese, English, and several Chinese dialects).

Education Attainment

As compared to the overall American population, several Asian American groups stand out in their college graduation rates and postgraduate training, such as Asian Indians, Chinese, and Japanese. On the other hand, only 27% of Laotians and 38% of Cambodians are high school graduates.

Family Income

Although data suggest that Asian Americans as a group have the highest average family income in the United States, Southeast Asians are among the poorest. Those living below the poverty level include 66% of the Laotians, 49% of Cambodians, and 34% of Vietnamese.

Residential Preference

Except for isolated communities of Southeast Asian refugees settled throughout the United States, Asian American communities are scattered throughout the West and East coasts. About 70% of the total population resides in five states: California (35%), Hawaii (16%), New York (9%), Illinois (5%), and Texas (4%). Honolulu, Los Angeles, San Francisco, New York, Chicago, and San Jose have the highest concentrations of Asian Americans.

Religion

Among the Chinese Americans, the most popular religions include Buddhism, ancestor worship, and Christianity. Filipinos, under past Spanish influence, are heavily Catholic. More than 70% of Korean Americans are Protestant Christians; some are Buddhists. Japanese Americans follow Shintoism, Buddhism (especially the Zen sect), and Christianity. Vietnamese practice Buddhism and, from their French colonial past, Catholicism. The Cambodians and Laotian religions are strongly influenced by the Brahmanism of the Hindus as well as by Buddhism. The Hmong and the Mien are usually animistic and believe strongly in supernatural causes. It is important to note that in many Asian countries under communist rule, religion was essentially abolished. Consequently, many immigrants from those countries may not practice any religion.

Exposure to War Trauma

One common theme among Asian countries is that all suffered war and political turmoil. Consequently, many immigrants have undergone torture, psychological and physical trauma, separation, and loss of family members. Another fact is that immigrants come from Asian countries that have long fought each other, sometimes for many generations. This historical background profoundly affects many immigrants' feelings about other Asian groups.

Asian Americans are thus a diverse group. Although some groups have been here for generations (e.g., Chinese and Japanese) and have attained higher economic status, most recent Asian immigrant and refugee groups (e.g., Vietnamese, Cambodian, and Lao) are still struggling with language and cultural barriers and often face economic difficulties. The so-called model minority image of Asian Americans is a myth.

TRADITIONS AND CHANGES IN ASIAN FAMILIES

This section discusses traditional characteristics of Asian families and their contrast with Western families and socioeconomic changes that affect contemporary Asian families.

Traditional Characteristics of Asian Families

Although it is necessary to emphasize the heterogeneity of Asian groups, it is equally important to acknowledge a certain level of cultural similarity among them. Historically, the agricultural background and the teachings of Confucianism and Buddhism have had a profound influence on Eastern philosophical approaches to life and family interactions. Traditional Asian families place a high value on the family unit—rather than the individual. The individual is seen as the product of all the generations of his or her family. Such rituals and customs as ancestor worship, family celebrations, funeral rites, and genealogy records reinforce this concept. Because of this continuum, an individual's personal action reflects not only on himself but also on his extended family and ancestors (Shon & Ja, 1982). An individual is expected to function in his or her clearly defined roles and positions in the family hierarchy, based on age, gender, and social class. Obligations and shame are the mechanisms that traditionally help to reinforce societal expectations and proper behavior. There is an emphasis on harmonious interpersonal relationships, interdependence, and mutual obligations or loyalty for achieving a state of psychological homeostasis or peaceful coexistence with family or other fellow beings (Hsu, 1971).

Marital Subsystem

In traditional Asian families, it was common for three or four generations of family members to live in the same household. In an agricultural society, this arrangement was economical, practical, and one way to ensure the continuity of the family line (on the husband's side). Marriages are arranged by parents or grandparents. The dominant relationship is more likely to be placed on the parent–child dyad rather than the husband–wife dyad. The husband assumes the role of leadership and authority and is the provider and protector of the family. The wife assumes the role of homemaker and childbearer. Physical and verbal expressions of love are uncommon. When things go wrong, the difficulties may be repaired by other adult mediators or confidantes. Divorce is not a common practice. The wife is usually dominated by the authority of her husband, her father, her in-laws, and, sometimes, her son.

Parent–Child Subsystem

The traditional role of a mother is to provide nutrients and support. The father's role is to discipline. The father's and mother's functions tend to be complementary rather than symmetrical. The strongest emotional attachment for a woman is sometimes not her husband but her children (especially her sons). Most parents demand respect and obedience from their children. In many extended families, children are not solely raised by their parents but are cared for by a wide range of adults (grandparents, uncles, aunts, cousins, wet nurses). The social norm built on the Confucian teaching of filial piety required that children not only provide food and shelter for their elderly parents but also pay them respect and loyalty.

Sibling Subsystem

Because of the large number of children in many Asian families, the parents usually delegate child-care functions to older siblings (especially the eldest daughter). Cooperation and sharing among siblings are expected. The emotional ties among the siblings are especially strong for those who survived war and escapes. Due to historical practices of sexism, sons are favored. Sibling rivalry is not uncommon.

Cultural Differences: East versus West

Family values are strongly influenced by the socioeconomic structure of society. Whereas Eastern cultures are based on agricultural origins, modern Western culture is largely derived from the Industrial Revolution. Table 1.2 highlights some of these differences. It is beyond the scope of this chapter

TABLE 1.2. Comparison of Eastern and Western Cultural Values

Eastern agricultural system: Traditional society values	Western industrialized system: Modern society values
1. Family/group-oriented	1. Individual-oriented
2. Extended family	2. Nuclear/blended family
3. Multiple parenting	3. Couple parenting
4. Primary relationship— parent–child bond	4. Primary relationship—marital bond
5. Emphasis on interpersonal relationships	5. Emphasis on self-fulfillment and self-development
6. Status and relationships determined by age and role in family	6. Status achieved by individual's efforts
7. Well-defined family members' roles	7. Flexible family members' roles
8. Favoritism toward males	8. Increasing opportunities for females
9. Authoritarian orientation	9. Democratic orientation
10. Suppression of emotions	10. Expression of emotions
11. Fatalism/karma	11. Personal control over the environment
12. Harmony with nature	12. Mastery over nature
13. Cooperative orientation	13. Competition orientation
14. Spiritualism	14. Materialism/consumerism
15. Past, present, and future orientation	15. Present, future orientation

to describe these differences in detail. The following family-related examples merely point out some these differences (Steinhoff, 1994).

Family Goals

In many Asian countries, there is a general cultural assumption that the family exists as the basic unit of society. Individual family members can be called on to make personal sacrifices for the sake of the family. In contrast, in the United States, there is a general assumption that the family exists for the development and protection of individual family members. Unlike the extended family in Eastern cultures, the nuclear family in the West stresses independence and autonomy among family members. A Western family life cycle begins when two individuals meet, fall in love, marry, and have children. They raise their children to be self-sufficient, ultimately to leave and repeat the process.

Internal Family Structure

In Eastern cultures, a well-defined hierarchy of authority exists depending on age, role, sex, and birth order. The head of household (usually the father) makes important family decisions. However, in the West, equality tends to exist among family members and each individual's opinion is valued. Decision making is more democratic.

Family Conflicts

Traditional Asian cultures avoid open conflict. Family conflict is frequently managed by role segregation, indirect communication, and polite inattention. The strong hierarchy within the family defines who may voice an opinion and who must suppress it. In the West, open conflict is relatively common and normal and is part of family communication and dynamics.

Attitude toward the Elderly

A striking contrast exists in the East-versus-West attitude toward the elderly. For example, a 1988 National Family Survey in Japan found that more than 70% of adult respondents desired to live with a parent when he or she became old or ill. Recent family surveys in the United States indicated that fewer than 5% of Americans have such desires (Cho & Yada, 1994).

Note that the East–West cultural differences in Table 1.2 do not apply to *all* individuals in each culture, because most people fall somewhere within this continuum. An acculturated person from the Eastern culture may possibly identify more with Western culture, or vice versa. Within one particular family, the likelihood is that various family members (depending on age and acculturation rate) may identify with different elements within the continuum.

Changes in Contemporary Asian Countries

In the past two decades, Asian countries have changed rapidly in many aspects as a result of the forces of modernization, urbanization, and industrialization. The socioeconomic revolution and consequent rapid widespread migration from villages to cities and towns began to have a major impact on the form, structure, and functions of the family. The most notable change was the transformation of the family's function from production to consumption, as people began to work away from home. In addition, the transition from high to low fertility led to the decrease of traditional extended families and the emergence of nuclear families as a predominant form.

These changes are more obvious in modern industrialized Asian countries such as Taiwan, Japan, Hong Kong, Singapore, and Korea. For example, in Taiwan, the per capita gross national product rose from US$250 in 1967 to more than US$6,000 by 1986 (Sun & Liu, 1994). The proportion of couples living with the husband's parents decreased from 60% in 1967 to 41% in 1986. In Japan, the average number of household members has decreased from 4.89 in 1920 to 2.99 in 1990 (Kuroda, 1994).

It is important for clinicians to remember that an Asian country, as it evolves from these recent socioeconomic forces, may take on dramatically different characteristics which affect their people and family systems. For instance, a family from the mountaintop in Laos is very different in family values, Westernization, education, and outlook from an urban family in Hong Kong or Singapore.

ASIAN AMERICAN FAMILIES IN TRANSITION

The different Asian American groups came to the United States at different times and exhibit varying degrees of acculturation. They represent a wide range of cultural values, from very traditional to very "Americanized." Within this continuum, there are numerous variations. Generally speaking, five types of Asian American families are described in the succeeding paragraphs. These five family types are hypothetical constructs for the purposes of discussing and understanding the complexity of Asian American families.

Type 1: The Traditional Family

Such families usually consist of all family members who are born and raised in Asian countries. These include families from agricultural backgrounds, families recently arrived with limited exposure to Western culture, unacculturated immigrants who are older at time of immigration, and families living in ethnic Asian communities (e.g., Chinatown or Koreatown) with limited contact with mainstream U.S. society. Family members hold strong beliefs in traditional values as described previously and speak in their native languages and dialects. They practice traditional customs and belong to family associations and other social clubs consisting of people with a similar heritage.

Type 2: The "Cultural Conflict" Family

In these families, members usually hold different cultural values. A typical family consists of parents and grandparents with strong traditional beliefs who live with a more acculturated and Westernized younger generation. This type of family experiences a great deal of family stress caused by intergenerational conflicts. These conflicts are usually caused by the disparity between the children's and the parents' values and expectations. Traditional parents expect the children to be obedient, hardworking, and respectful to authority. Such value orientation is not only different but opposite to American values, which place a strong emphasis on independence, self-reliance, autonomy, assertiveness, open communication, and competition. The family members frequently argue over dating, marriage, educational goals, and career choice. Role reversal occurs because the children speak better English and the monolingual parents/grandparents depend on them as the "cultural brokers" to deal with the outside world. Such dependence can evoke anger and resentment in both parties and may lead to prolonged family stress.

Another type of "cultural conflict" occurs one when one spouse is more acculturated than the other. For example, a husband may have lived in the United States for many years and then gone home and brought back a wife who is not familiar with American culture. Cultural conflicts may be caused not only by different degrees of acculturation rate of family members but also by religious, philosophical, or political differences.

Type 3: The Bicultural Family

A majority of these families consist of well-acculturated parents who came to the United States many years ago and are quite familiar with American culture. Many of them grew up in major Asian cities and were exposed to urbanization, industrialization, and Western influences. Some are American-born who were raised in traditional families. These parents often hold professional jobs and come from middle- or upper-class family backgrounds. They are bilingual and bicultural and are familiar with both Eastern and Western cultures. In such families, the power structure has moved from a patriarchal to an egalitarian relationship between parents. Decision making is not solely the father's responsibility; family discussions are allowed between parents and children. Such families typically do not live in the Chinatowns, Japantowns, Koreatowns, or Little Saigons but in the suburbs. The nuclear family members usually visit their extended family members (e.g., the grandparents) on weekends and holidays.

Type 4: The "Americanized" Family

Most of these families consist of parents and children who are both born and raised in the United States. As generations pass, the roots of the traditional Asian cultures begin to disappear and individual members tend not to maintain their ethnic identities. Family members communicate in English only and adopt a more individualistic and egalitarian orientation.

Type 5: The Interracial Family

Interracial marriages for Asian Americans are increasing rapidly, with an estimated 10% to 15% of all marriages. Japanese Americans lead in this trend, with more than half marrying outside their group, followed by Filipino, Chinese, Vietnamese, and Korean Americans (Karnow & Yoshihara, 1992). Some interracial families are able to integrate both cultures with a high degree of success. However, others, for example, often experience conflicts in values, religious beliefs, communication style, and childrearing issues and in-law problems.

MANIFESTATIONS OF PSYCHOPATHOLOGY

No large-scale prevalence studies on psychopathology have been conducted on Asian Americans. Available research strongly implies that major mental health problems exist among various Asian American groups, contrary to the widespread belief that Asian Americans are well adjusted. Research also suggests that Asian Americans have a rate of psychopathology equal to or higher than that of European-Americans. If, indeed, Asian Americans do have higher rates of psychopathology than other Americans, it is reasonable to attribute such differences to additional psychosocial stressors resulting from their minority status and migration experiences (Uba, 1994).

The most common mental health problems among Asian Americans are depression, somatization, anxiety disorder, adjustment disorder, and suicide. Chinese Americans and Japanese Americans have reported more somatic complaints than European-Americans on the Minnesota Multiphasic Personality Inventory (Sue & Sue, 1974). Kuo and Tsai (1986) found that Asian Americans have higher average scores on the Epidemiological Studies Depression Scale measure than do whites. In a study of anxiety levels, Chinese American males and females expressed significantly more discomfort than their control counterparts. This study also revealed that recent immigrants were more likely to experience anxiety than those immigrants who have been in the United States longer (Sue & Zane, 1987). The rate of suicide among Japanese Americans and Chinese Americans is generally lower than among European-Americans. However, the suicide rate is higher than that of European-Americans for Chinese Americans after the age of 64, and for Japanese Americans after the age of 74. The foreign-born Chinese Americans and Japanese Americans have higher suicide rates than do their American-born counterparts (Yu, Chang, Liu, & Fernandez, 1989).

The mental health problems of Southeast Asian refugees require special attention. Researchers have found that this group has a very high rate of psychiatric disorder (Berry & Blondel, 1982; Gong-Guy, 1987; Kinzie, 1989; Lin, 1986). They have displayed a variety of disorders, including posttraumatic stress disorder, dissociative disorders, organic brain syndromes, schizophrenia, conversion disorders, and paranoia (Uba, 1994).

Another area of special interest is culture-bound syndromes. Certain illnesses, known by their indigenous names, have been reported in many countries in Asia, such as *amok, koro,* and *qi-gong* psychotic reaction. With the increase in the Asian immigrant and refugee population, some of these rather dramatic and rarer forms of mental disorder are increasingly found in the United States (Gaw, 1993).

In comparing the severity of psychopathology of Asian Americans with other ethnic groups, research studies also revealed some interesting interracial differences. For example, studies have found that Asian Americans who use mental health services are more severely disturbed than their non-Asian American counterparts (Sue & McKinney, 1975; Sue & Sue, 1974). An extensive study in Los Angeles found that the proportion of Asian Americans diagnosed as psychotic was larger than that of European-American clients. Asian Americans were found to have major affective disorders at a proportionally higher rate than African Americans or Latino Americans (Flaskerud & Hu, 1992). There is also some evidence of interethnic differences among Asian American groups. Southeast Asians refugees, given the traumas and hardships many of them have experienced, apparently have the most severe problems, whereas Japanese American have the least severe problems (Gim, Atkinson, & Whitely, 1990).

HELP-SEEKING PATTERNS

Most Asian Americans attempt to deal with their psychological problems without seeking professional services. Many tend to rely on the family in dealing with their problems. Traditional families often treat mental disorders by urging the disturbed family members to change their behavior. They believe that self-control, will power, avoidance of unpleasant thoughts, keeping busy, and trying not to think too much about problems can help individuals to deal with their troubles. Each family member, including the extended family members, may offer his or her recommended treatment. When the troubled person and his or her family are not able to resolve the problem, they often turn to resources available in their community, such as elders, spiritual healers, ministers, monks, herbalists, fortune tellers, or physicians. Many come to mental health professionals as the last resort, while others are forced to receive counseling by the courts, hospitals, schools, and other social services agencies.

Acculturated Asian Americans have a more positive attitude toward receiving professional counseling. Unlike newly arrived immigrants and refugees, who come to agencies with specific, concrete problems that require assistance, their presenting problems are commonly associated with intrapsychic difficulties or relationship-related issues. They may even opt for long-term psychotherapy. A survey of Asian American therapists revealed that depression, low self-concept, and relationship conflicts affected at least 50% of Asian American clients. Between 40% and 50%

of the clients were affected by problems with parent–child relationships, acculturation, somatic complaints, and isolation (Matsushima & Tashima, 1982).

MAJOR FAMILY THERAPY APPROACHES AND RELEVANCE TO TREATMENT

In working with Asian groups, the clinician must be flexible and able to draw from the work of many schools of family therapy. Whereas some acculturated Asian Americans can benefit from Western psychotherapy, such therapy may not be effective in working with the majority of immigrant and refugee Asians. Some traditional Western psychotherapeutic approaches are designed based on the assumptions of individuation, independence, self-disclosure, and verbal expression of feelings. These may be contrary to Asian values, which focus on interdependence, self-control, and repression of feelings. However, some therapeutic approaches in the field of family therapy have been found to be useful.

- The *structural family therapy model* provides a method for assessing the structure of a family, identifying the areas of difficulties, and restructuring the family system to produce change. The roles of the grandparents and the parental child in the three-generation family are quite applicable to Asian American families (Minuchin, 1974).
- The *problem-solving approach* is particularly helpful in engaging many immigrant, multiproblem families. It is focused, concise, and directive. This approach provides a sense of empowerment and accomplishment as each problem is resolved (Haley, 1976).
- The *Bowenian approach* provides strategies for exploring extended family dynamics. The use of a family tree to help families map their genealogy is helpful (Bowen, 1976). However, given the resistance of Asian families in initial therapy sessions, this history-based approach may raise suspicion and tends to be more helpful in the midphase of therapy—after trust is established.

In the past two decades, several family therapy books have been published with special focus on ethnic minorities (McGoldrick, Pearce, & Giordano, 1982; Hansen & Falicov, 1983; Ho, 1987; Comas-Díaz & Griffith, 1988; Paniagua, 1994). In addition, some authors focused on specific groups (Sue & Zane, 1987; Kim, 1985; Boyd-Franklin, 1989). In addition to contributions from authors in the field, national organizations of mental health professionals have also developed cultural competence criteria or cultural formulation guidelines. In 1991, The American Psychological Association published *Guidelines for Providers of Psychological*

Services to Ethnic, Linguistic, and Culturally Diverse Populations. In 1994, the *Diagnostic and Statistical Manual of Mental Disorders* provided an outline for cultural formulation designed to assist the clinician in systematic evaluation and reporting of the impact of an individual's cultural context. A glossary of culture-bound syndromes is also included. All these contributions have created a new impetus and immense excitement in the field.

ASSESSMENT GUIDELINES

The family is a complex institution which can be investigated and understood from various dimensions. The proposed assessment guidelines emphasize two perspectives:

1. *Assessment of the family dynamics based on system theory.* The family is examined and understood within the network of each system inwardly and outwardly in ecological and dynamic ways (Tseng & Hsu, 1991). The clinician needs to assess (a) the *internal* family system, which includes understanding individual members, family subsystems, family life cycle, family hierarchy, leadership, communication, behavioral styles and norms, and role patterns; and (2) the *external* factors, which include the impact of war, migration, racism, housing, and other environmental stressors. Clinicians must also recognize available support systems.

2. *Assessment of mental health problems based on a holistic concept of health and illness.* In addition to Western psychological and biological understanding of emotional difficulties, we need to appreciate the Eastern holistic way of thinking and incorporate it into clinical practice.

Based on these two perspectives, I recommend a model that takes into account the psychological, social, biological, spiritual, cultural, and political influences on the lives of families. The evaluation and assessment of Asian American families should include additional information beyond traditional intake data, as discussed next (Lee, 1989, 1996).

Assessment of the Family's Ethnocultural Heritage

The clinician should obtain information on the family's past background, including culture of origin for both maternal and paternal lines of the client's family and delineation of ethnic heritage. A simple statement of parental geographical origin is not sufficient for a complete understanding of a client's often complex multicultural–multiethnic background. Unfortunately, it is far too common for a single, readily identifiable attitude of an individual or family (e.g., name or native language spoken) to be simply accepted as implying a vast assortment of stereotyped cultural characteristics (Jacobsen, 1988). For example, a Cantonese-speaking young woman who was raised by her grandparents in Mexico experiences very different cultural influences in comparison with a Chinese woman who grew up in China during the Cultural Revolution.

Assessment of Migration Stress

Sluzki (1979) provides an excellent framework in his article on migration and family conflict. He describes a five-stage model: (1) preparatory stage, (2) migration, (3) period of overcompensation, (4) period of crisis decompensation, and (5) transgeneration phenomena. Each state requires assessment and interventions geared for the specific phase the family is experiencing. In family assessment, the clinician should be aware of which stage of development the family is in and its impact on the family dynamic.

For many Asian American families, especially immigrants and refugees, the stress of migration can result in psychological strain, which in turn jeopardizes mental health. With few exceptions, a majority of Asian countries have suffered years of war and political turmoil. Many immigrants and refugees experienced unwilling separations and exposure to trauma, both in their home country and in their search for sanctuary. Caught in varying degrees of unpreparedness, many suffered personal losses in many aspects of their lives. A systematic and longitudinal understanding of the refugee experiences is crucial and should be included as part of the assessment of all Asian refugee families. When taking a thorough migration history, the clinician can apply the following chronological approach focusing on two major aspects of the family migration history: premigration history and immigration history.

Family premigration history. History includes the following: country of origin, cities or villages where the family previously lived, relocation experiences, family composition, educational level of each member, employment status, level of support from other extended family members and community, religious beliefs, social and economic status of the family, major political changes, and experiences of war and traumatic events.

Family immigration history. History includes the reasons for leaving, who decided, who left first and who was left behind, and who was the sponsor, as well as hardships endured during the trip. Working with refugee families, it is very important to explore the family's experiences of trauma, such as starvation, rape, torture, and imprisonment. Clinicians also need to explore the extent of loss.

Five types of losses are associated with refugee status: (1) material losses, such as properties, business, career, and investment; (2) physical losses, such as disfigurement, physical injuries, hunger, and malnutrition;

(3) spiritual losses, such as freedom to practice religion and support from religious community; (4) loss of community support and cultural milieu; and (5) loss of family members, other relatives, and friends. Such losses are particularly traumatic for the Southeast Asian refugees, to whom the family, community, and religion are exceedingly important (Lee, 1990).

Clinicians sometimes fall into two extremes in the exploration of premigration and migration history. Some fail to ask for the information with the belief that the former life data is not relevant to current problems. Others may not be ready to deal with the trauma stories. The reasons the victimized refugee clients often do not report these events spontaneously are numerous: guilt, shame, wanting to deny and forget, fear of reprisal, emotional distress in recalling and discussing the events, and lack of the "psychological mindedness" that these events may be related to the current clinical problems (Westermeyer, 1989). At the other extreme, some clinicians are too eager to explore the past traumatic events and force the family members to deal with their psychological trauma prematurely. Skillful assessment of the family members' readiness to share their migration history is very important. Before the establishment of trust, the clinician should try to avoid questions or commentaries dealing with traumatic events. Also, clients should not be pressured to say more than what they want to (Paniagua, 1994).

Assessment of Postmigration Experience and Cultural Shock

In discussing the family's postmigration experiences, it is essential to assess the degree of cultural shock and its impact on the family. Many new Asian immigrants are placed in a strange and unpredictable environment. In addition to language barriers and homesickness, they have to adjust to physical changes (new city to live, different type of housing arrangement, increased population density, etc.), economic changes (new forms of employment, downward social mobility, etc.), cultural changes (religious, educational, and value orientation of the host country), political changes, and social relationship changes. For many immigrant and refugee families, there is a sudden lack of extended family support when it is most needed. The new isolated family unit is, for the first time, responsible for making and maintaining its own set of rules and adjusting to a new environment with its strange demands. When the stresses are extreme and the support system is insufficient, the family may become isolated, enmeshed, and disengaged (Landau, 1982).

Assessment of the Impact of Migration on Individual and Family Life Cycle

The adjustment to a new culture is a prolonged developmental process that will affect family members differently, depending on the individual and family life cycle phase they are in at the time of transition (McGoldrick, 1982). For example, a Chinese teenager who migrates during adolescent years is confronted by not only migration and acculturation stresses but also the special developmental tasks such as identity and sexual role formation, separation, and individuation (Lee, 1988). An elderly Korean who lost his family members and business has to deal with the physical and psychological impact of growing old, particularly in a youth-oriented society.

The impact of the migration experience on the family life cycle may be different at every stage. For example, families that migrate with young children are perhaps strengthened by having each other, but they are vulnerable to the parental reversal of hierarchies. Families migrating when their children are adolescents may have more difficulty because they will have less time together as a unit before the children move out on their own. Thus, the family must struggle with multiple transitions and generational conflicts at once (McGoldrick, 1982). When families migrate in the launching phase, it is very difficult for the parents to break into new jobs, find new friends, and deal with "empty nest" syndrome.

Assessment of Acculturation Level of Each Family Member

Several researchers have made significant contributions in the area of acculturation. Lin, Matsuda, and Tazuma (1982) proposed five adjustment patterns: (1) neurotic marginality (develops high levels of anxiety while trying to comply with expectations of both cultures), (2) deviant marginality (becomes isolated due to ignoring norms of both cultures after being unable to satisfy both simultaneously), (3) traditionalism (withdraws into the old culture to escape loss and confusion), (4) overacculturation (abandons former culture, loses traditional supports), and (5) biculturation (integrates both cultures with the best possible compromises). Berry (1990) suggested that the greater the cultural dissimilarity across two cultures, the greater the acculturation stress.

The acculturation rate of each individual depends on the following factors: (1) age at the time of migration—the younger, the easier; (2) language; (3) past and present exposure to Western culture; (4) ethnic and cultural pride; (5) ethnic density of the neighborhood; (6) socioeconomic status and profession; and (7) immigration status—temporary or permanent. Each family member may have a different acculturation within the same family. Intergenerational conflict may be caused by the disparity between grandparents, parents, and children, who have different acculturation rates.

According to my experiences, traditional views of acculturation need to be adapted to our contemporary multicultural society:

1. Acculturation is not totally a linear process. An individual does not necessarily have to give up his or her own culture to become

Americanized. For example, a highly acculturated Chinese American can still hold on to some traditional Chinese values with minimum conflict.

2. Acculturation to the mainstream culture may not be all positive. For many immigrant and refugee youths, giving up their own cultures and identifying with the new culture (e.g., drugs, alcoholism, and gangs) may have negative effects.

3. In a multicultural society, one can become acculturated not only to the mainstream American culture but also to other cultures of ethnic groups, such as Latino and African American.

4. A higher acculturation rate does not necessarily imply better mental health. Maintaining a positive identification with one's ethnic group as well as the mainstream culture provides a more solid base for positive self-esteem.

Assessment of Work and Financial Stresses

Research studies have found that clinical depression was significantly associated with unemployment (Yamamoto, Lam, Fung, Tan, & Iga, 1977). For Asian Americans, two common types of stress related to employment exist. Among immigrants, many experience unemployment and underemployment. "Downward mobility" leads to low self-esteem, insecurity, and role reversal in families. For acculturated and professional Asian Americans, a "glass ceiling" (a term that refers to a barrier to promotions and success because of one's ethnicity or gender) and subtle discrimination at work sites often lead to frustrations and job dissatisfaction.

The parents' type of work and work hours often influence the family dynamics. At one extreme, a typical Asian American small business owner (e.g., laundry or grocery store) requires the whole family to spend long hours together, sometimes resulting in relationships that are intense and too close. At the other extreme, parents may work extremely long hours away from home (e.g., restaurant or engineering/research office). Family members seldom have sufficient time together to communicate. One recent phenomenon is the so-called astronaut family, where the family resides in the United States and one parent still maintains a business in the home country. Such families maintain their relationships by telephone, fax, and "frequent flyer" trips.

Assessment of the Family's Place of Residence and Community Influence

Whether or not the family lives in an ethnic neighborhood will influence the impact of the family cultural heritage on their lives (McGoldrick, 1982). For those Asians who live in their ethnic communities, such as Chinatowns and Japantowns, the community support systems provide a cushion against the stresses of migration. Unfortunately, due to housing shortages, many recent immigrants and refugees have to live in poor neighborhoods, where they feel isolated from their ethnic communities and encounter problems of crime, violence, drugs, racism, and inadequate housing. Those who live in areas with relatively small Asian populations, such as small towns and rural areas, generally have more trouble adjusting and are pressured to assimilate more rapidly.

Assessment of Family Stresses Caused by Role Reversal

In many Asian American families, conflict may be caused by role reversal among grandparents, parents, and children. Many monolingual adults depend on the English-speaking children as cultural brokers and interpreters. Such dependence can cause anger and resentment. Role reversal may also occur between husband and wife. Husbands who are accustomed to male-dominated Asian cultures find it difficult to accept wives who may find work more easily and become more independent and assertive.

The issue of family loyalty is another source of stress. Such stress may be caused by the fact that many immigrants and refugees are raised by someone other than their biological parents, because of the extended family system and separation from family members. Family reunions in the United States after years of separation may trigger many unresolved family conflicts and resentment.

Assessment of Stress Caused by Legal Problems and Sponsor Relationship

Because of language difficulties and unfamiliarity with immigration law, many immigrants depend on their sponsors for legal, financial, and emotional support, especially when they first arrive in this country. The legal sponsor is often given a great deal of power in many family decisions, including where to live, which school to attend, and even which family members back home will be sponsored. Sometimes the sponsor may object to the family's receiving assistance from a social services or mental health agency because he or she fears that doing so may jeopardize future sponsorships and bring shame to the family name. The family may simultaneously feel gratitude as well as resentment toward a sponsor's exercise of power. A hostile–dependent relationship may result.

Assessment of Family's Experiences with Racism, Prejudice, and Discrimination

As a visible minority with distinctive physical characteristics and accents, Asian Americans find it impossible to hide their ethnic heritage to achieve total acceptance. Historically, Asians have been subjected to many forms of racism and discrimination in the United States. For example, from the 1880s through World War II, Chinese men who immigrated to this country to work in the gold mines and railroads were prohibited from bringing their wives with them. Many Japanese families suffered immensely due to their internment experience during the war. Despite significant improvement in the life of minority groups in this country as a result of the civil rights movement, racism and discrimination still persist against Asian Americans. Many clients encounter racial discrimination in their workplaces, schools, and communities. Not only recent immigrants but also well-educated and highly trained professionals face such discrimination. Clinicians should be sensitive to the impact of immigration policies on the Asian family system and should encourage the family members to share their frustration and anger caused by their minority status in this society.

Assessment of Family's Religious and Spiritual Beliefs

Asian Americans come from a variety of religious backgrounds (e.g., Christian, Buddhist, Shintoism, or Muslim). Family behavior is governed to a great extent by religious beliefs. In many Asian countries, religious organizations are highly respected. The priest, minister, or Buddhist monk is a key figure in the process of understanding and solving family problems. The clinician should assess whether the family is a member of a particular church or temple and the availability of emotional support or counseling from the particular organization. In many Asian American households, beliefs shared by the grandparents or parents may be in conflict with and challenged by the beliefs of the younger generation, who are typically exposed to Western religions. The clinician should encourage family members to share their religious beliefs in relation to the presenting problem and problem-solving strategies.

Assessment of Family's Physical Health and Medication History

The exploration of physical health is important for three major reasons. First, Asian clients tend to express their emotional problems in somatic terms. They usually come to treatment with many physical complaints. Second, many Asians, especially refugees, are in need of medical attention as a result of physical injuries, malnutrition, and lack of adequate medical treatment during war. It is important to request information on the client's physical condition and family medical history. Third, many Asians who are not familiar with Western medicine may become confused by drug names, dosages, and effects. Furthermore, for many Asian Americans, concurrent use of Western and traditional medicine is quite common. A clinician's concern over these health and medication matters is often appreciated.

Assessment of Culturally Specific Responses to Mental Health Problems

When trying to understand the causes of emotional problems or mental illness, many traditional Asians do not accept Western biopsychological explanations. A mental health problem may be conceptualized as a manifestation of organic disorders, hereditary weakness, imbalance between *yin* and *yang,* disturbance of *qi* energy, supernatural intervention, or emotional exhaustion caused by external environmental factors (Lee, 1982). In the assessment process, it is essential for the clinician to encourage the client and his or her family members to openly discuss their cultural and religious viewpoints on the cause of the problem, their past coping style, their health-seeking behavior, and their treatment expectation. The discussion can be based on the following questions (Lee, 1990):

> What are the symptoms and problems as perceived by each family member?
> What would be the diagnostic label given in the client's home country?
> What are the family's cultural explanations of the causes of the problem?
> What kind of treatment would the family get if they were back in their home country?
> Where did the family go for help before they came to see the clinician?
> What is the family's experience with herbal medicine and indigenous healers?
> What was the family's previous experience with Western health and mental health care systems?
> What are the family's treatment expectations?

Assessment of Cultural Strengths and Community Support Network

In addition to the assessment of family stress and pathologies, an assessment is necessary with respect to individual and family strengths in past adaptation, coping, and problem solving. The Asian family usually arrives in the United States with many problems. At the same time, the family also brings along highly developed cultures, religions, and philosophies. For instance, these strengths may include the Confucian teaching of the "middle way," the Buddhist teaching of karma and compassion, the strong focus on the importance of family harmony and interpersonal relationships, and the high value of education and hard work. Asian cultures emphasize family, friends, and ethnic community. During a crisis, Asian families can usually count on support from extended family members, friends, and ethnic community network and organizations. The clinician should explore and recognize such support systems.

Special Issues in Family Assessment

The previous assessment guidelines provide a comprehensive and holistic view of Asian American families. However, in the evaluation process, the clinician may encounter several potential difficulties.

First, Asian American families may be very discreet about family secrets and problems. Family members feel loyal and protective of each other and will not readily offer information before trust is established.

Second, many Asian Americans do not comprehend the significance and sometimes lengthy procedures of evaluation. Either they are not used to detailed history taking or they do not understand the relationship between the questions and the presenting problems. Some may even suspect that such information will be put to political use, thus jeopardizing their immigration status.

Third, there is a lack of bilingual and culturally competent assessment tools. Many psychological testing and mental status examination questions are irrelevant to the Asians' world views and may lead to over- or underdiagnosis.

Fourth, Asian families may not be accustomed to verbal expressions of emotion to outsiders. Therefore, data collection on Asian American families may require more than the usual question-and-answer mode of interaction. Effective techniques include the use of family genograms (McGoldrick, 1985), photographs and albums, sharing of trauma stories, paintings, songs, and philosophical discussions.

TREATMENT RECOMMENDATIONS: STRUCTURE AND STRATEGIES

Structural Aspects of Family Therapy

Assessing Readiness for Family Therapy

Even though family therapy can be highly effectively as a treatment modality in working with Asian American families—due to the strong family orientation—Asian American clients generally are quite reluctant to seek family treatment. The following reasons highlight some of the possible difficulties:

1. Asian American clients are mostly unfamiliar with the concept of family therapy or the role of the family therapist. Traditionally, family members consult family elders, village chiefs, a trusted member of the clan, monks or ministers, or indigenous healers in case of family crises.

2. Asian family members usually do not see individual problems as family related. They are unfamiliar with "family system" or "family communication" theories and usually do not understand the need for family therapy as a way to improve the individual's pathological symptoms. They rarely agree to the suggestion that the problem is the group's instead of the identified client's.

3. Because of the traditional hierarchical and vertical structure of Asian American families, which prohibits free verbal expression of emotions, especially true thoughts and negative feelings, family members may not be equipped with the communication skills to discuss problems and to express themselves openly in a family group setting. For example, for parents to discuss their "adult" problems or to express their sadness in front of the children is considered culturally inappropriate and is viewed as losing control.

4. In view of the long years of separation among the family members of immigrant and refugees families, there are many family secrets and unresolved grief that members are not ready to share openly with each other. Family therapy may bring out the "ghosts" in the past and can be very overwhelming and at times damaging to family relationships.

5. Traditional Asian husbands or fathers are quite resistant to attending family sessions or allowing the therapist to enter into the family system. Many traditional Asian men may interpret the admission of emotional problems and receiving help from outside the family network as a sign of weakness and losing face. In the event that their children are in trouble and the parents are forced to receive treatment, they usually send their wives to be the family representative to deal with service agencies. It is very difficult to conduct family therapy without the cooperation and participation of the male adult figures.

6. Many immigrant and refugee Asian families do not have all the family members living in the same country or city. Sometimes, family members do not reside in the United States or in the same city.

7. The great discrepancy in the degree or level of acculturation among family members may discourage individual members to accept family therapy as the means to resolve family problems. In those families with severe intergenerational conflicts and very different value orientations and communication styles, family sessions can be overwhelming not only to the family members but to the therapist as well.

Prior to determining family therapy as the treatment of choice, the clinician needs to assess the previously mentioned factors and the readiness of family members to work together as a group. For some families, family therapy sometimes is neither the feasible nor the desired treatment modality. However, if the clinician believes in his or her best clinical judgment that family therapy is the most effective treatment strategy, the family members (especially the decision makers) should be educated on the benefits and rationales of such decision. This can be done by making the initial appointment with the head of the family (e.g., the father) and soliciting his (or her) assistance.

Involving Family Members in Therapy

The definition of "family" in traditional Asian cultures may include a wide network of kinship. For example, a Vietnamese teenager who left his homeland with his aunt when he was an infant may have many more emotional ties with his aunt and her family than with his own biological parents. In many Filipino families, trusted friends and allies serve as godparents to children and play an important role in their growth and development. If appropriate, the clinician can ask the identified client to define his or her own concept of family members and discuss who should be included in therapy. In many cases, it is advisable to encourage all family members to come to the first session so that the family dynamic can be observed. However, in many instances, family members are either emotionally not ready or physically unavailable to participate in treatment.

Family therapy for Asian families does not always require all-encompassing family involvement. A *flexible family subsystem* approach in the establishment of therapeutic relationships with family members at the beginning phase can be very helpful. For example, an effective method is for a clinician to interview the parents first, then the identified client, and then the sibling group. The parents can discuss their adult concerns or express their emotions freely when the children are absent. The children, usually more acculturated and more fluent in English, can negotiate issues they might not bring up with their parents present. When all parties feel safe and have more control over what may be discussed in the family group, they will be more willing and ready to accept family therapy. This "staging" process requires skills in establishing trust and credibility with each family member at the initial phase of treatment.

Setting Client-Centered Goals

Many Asian Americans find it difficult to admit having family problems or psychological difficulties. They usually present themselves as victims of some unfortunate environmental events or physical discomfort. The clinician should take their presenting problem seriously and respond immediately to the concrete needs of the clients. A *problem-focused, goal-oriented, and symptom-relieving approach* is highly recommended in the beginning phases of treatment. Rather than defining goals in abstract, emotional terms, goals may be best stated in terms of external resolution or symptom reduction. Many clients find loosely targeted and emotionally oriented goals as incomprehensible, unreachable, and impractical (Ho, 1987). Long-term goals may best be broken down into a series of easy-to-understand, achievable, measurable short-term goals. Once the family is engaged in the therapeutic relationship and gains a sense of success, the therapist can introduce other more insight-oriented goals and renegotiate with the family members.

Deciding on Language Used in Therapy

There is a lack of common language spoken in many Asian American households, especially families with "Westernized" adolescents who do not speak their parents' and grandparents' native dialects. It is quite difficult to conduct therapy in two or three different dialects and different communication styles. Ideally, the clinician is fluent in the languages spoken by the family members and has a good understanding of the variability in linguistic expressions. When family members are bilingual in both English and their native dialect, the therapist can discuss with them which language they prefer to use in therapy. English-speaking clinicians should avoid the use of bilingual children as interpreters, particularly when the presenting problem involves parent–child issues. The bilingualism of a child could reinforce the problem of role reversal and the monolingual parents' sense of helplessness. Also, clinicians should avoid the use of relatives and friends as interpreters. They are often not objective and tend to minimize or maximize family pathology, depending on their own issues with the family. If interpreters are used, clinicians should try to use interpreters who match the Asian dialects and cultural background (see Lee, Chapter 32, this volume, for more details).

Determining Duration of Therapy and Number of Sessions

It is not uncommon for Asian American families to ask for mental health assistance only in times of crisis. The first session is usually the most crucial one and may determine whether the family will stay in treatment. The clinician should take advantage of the family energy mobilized by the presenting family crisis to conduct an extensive evaluation and offer immediate help if possible. An extended amount of time for the first session is often necessary. In the beginning phases of therapy, the traditional 1-hour, once-a-week session may not be sufficient. Appointments should be made at the convenience of the family. Most Asian families expect a short-term treatment period, no more than 2 to 3 months. Asians who seek help for chronic psychiatric disorders should be informed that an immediate recovery may be unrealistic and that treatment may require a longer period.

Conducting Office Interviews versus Home Visits

For family members who are motivated to engage in treatment, office interviews can be very therapeutic and cost-effective. Although travel to the home increases the expense of therapy, use of the home offers many unique benefits. Family members are more relaxed. Therapy can be "delivered" to resistant members who are less motivated to join the family sessions. Family members can reenact family disputes and rehearse more effective communication and problem solving. The clinician also has the opportunity to observe the community and neighborhood in which the family resides. Furthermore, the home visits may enhance the therapeutic alliance. Family members may see such visits as symbols of the clinician's caring and commitment to help.

Treatment Strategies

The following guidelines summarize treatment strategies I have found to be effective in working with Asian American families.

Forming a Social and Cultural Connection with the Family during the First Session

The most important process in working with Asian American families is "joining," that is, initiating therapeutic intervention by building a relationship with the family. Many Asian American families are often new to therapy, and they need to be prepared and "coached." During the first session, the clinician should address the family in a polite and formal manner. Giving the Asian cultures' emphasis on interpersonal relationships, the family may expect the clinician to disclose a certain amount of personal information regarding his or her family, country of origin, academic, and professional background. Appropriate self-disclosure may facilitate positive cultural alliance and a level of trust and confidence. Asking nonthreatening personal questions can put the family at ease. It is also important to avoid direct confrontation, to demand greater emotional disclosure, or to discuss such culturally taboo subjects as sex or death. There is a need for caution in the use of paradoxical approaches. This technique is particularly problematic in the initial stage of treatment.

Acknowledging the Family's Sense of Shame

For many Asians, public admission of mental health problems can bring intense shame and humiliation. The clinician may counter those emotions by empathizing with them and encouraging them to verbalize this feeling. It is important to reassure family members about confidentiality and anonymity. One helpful technique is to reframe their courage in seeking help as love and concern for family members. If appropriate, the mobilization of the family's sense of obligation to receive help to achieve family harmony or for the sake of the children can be very effective.

Establishing Expertise, Power, Credibility, and Authority

Many Asian clients come to their first session believing that the clinician is an authority who can tell them what is wrong and how to solve their problems. It is helpful for the clinician to establish credibility right away, to ensure that the client will return. An air of confidence, empathic understanding, maturity, and professional mannerism are all important ingredients. Other ways to establish credibility and authority include (1) using professional titles when making introductions; (2) displaying diplomas, awards, and licenses in the office; (3) obtaining sufficient information about clients and their families before seeing them for the first time; (4) offering some possible explanation for the cause of the problem; (5) showing familiarity with the family's cultural background; (6) providing a set of cues that will help the family to judge the clinician's expertise (e.g., "according to my experience working with Asian families during the past 20 years . . . "); and (7) utilizing the crisis intervention approach to offer some immediate solutions to the problems. It is important for family members to feel that they are in good hands and there is a sense of hope before they leave the first session.

Defining the Problem

A *problem-focused* family therapy approach with Asian American families appears to be very effective. The clinician should focus on the immediate crisis or problem that brought the family to the agency. In most instances, family members ask for professional help because of the difficulties they encounter with one particular family member (the identified patient). Family members are either unaware of their roles in contributing to the problem or are unwilling to discuss it openly in front of others, particularly the children. For many families, working on the parent–child issue at the beginning is safer than working on marital problems that may exist.

To engage the family in therapy, it is important for the clinician to (1) acknowledge the family's feeling that the identified patient has problems, (2) verbalize the family pain caused by the difficulties, (3) assist the family to shift from a person-focused orientation to a problem-focused orientation to minimize scapegoating, (4) focus on the effect of the problem on each family member, and (5) reinforce the sense of family obligation and the significance of solving the problem together. At times, it may be helpful to encourage family members to elaborate on previous attempts in dealing with the problem. Acknowledging their failure to cope and the unpleasant consequences if the problem remains uncorrected may motivate the family to continue in treatment. In some instances, the clinician may use the family's sense of guilt to induce them to participate in treatment for the sake of the family name (Lee, 1990).

Applying a Family Psychoeducational Approach

Asian cultures value education highly. The psychoeducational approach based on social learning principles may be compatible with Asian values and beliefs. Such intervention focuses on four major areas: (1) education about the illness (or problem)—printed educational materials in the patient's primary language are helpful; (2) communication training; (3) problem-solving training; and (4) behavioral management strategies (McGill & Lee, 1986). Family education about the U.S. legal system (child-abuse laws, patients' rights, etc.) may be necessary. In addition to providing education on individual and family levels, psychoeducational programs dedicated to multiple families in the Asian community can be very effective.

Building Alliance with Members with Power

An accurate assessment of the power structure of the family is essential. Generally speaking, there are two types of power in the family system: "role-prescribed power" (usually given to the grandfather, father, eldest son, or sponsor) and "psychological power" (usually maintained by the grandmother or the mother). Treatment will not be effective without permission of the leader(s). Clinicians should acknowledge and respect their power in decision making, avoid competition, and use all possible means to build a therapeutic alliance.

Employing Reframing Techniques

The technique of reframing can be helpful to build rapport with family members with power. For example, the clinician can reframe the mother's overprotectiveness as "loving too much" and the father's overly excessive working hours as "sacrificing for the economic well-being of the family."

Assuming Multiple Helping Roles

Flexibility and willingness to assume multiple helping roles enhance the therapeutic relationship, especially when working with multiproblem families. In addition to being the counselor, the clinician should be comfortable with playing the role of teacher, advocate, interpreter, and the like. Acting as a "cultural mediator" or using a family intermediary can be an effective tool in dealing with family conflicts. Show caring by *doing* and *being there* when the family needs help.

Restructuring Social Support System

Asian American families usually consist of strong and close-knit extended families and support systems. However, many families isolate themselves when they encounter problems. As soon as possible, the clinician should assist the family to establish a social support network whereby the family or the individual can form friendships, ventilate frustrations, and learn social and problem-solving skills.

Integrating Eastern–Western Health Approaches

Clinicians should take advantage of the holistic model of health in Eastern cultures and integrate its elements with the best Western medical and psychological practices. For example, in the treatment of a depressive Chinese patient, it can be helpful to educate the patient on the Western biological and psychological perspectives of the illness. It is also important to explore the Eastern approaches of treatment (e.g., Chinese herbal medicine, acupuncture, and *qi gong*). It is my belief that such treatments will benefit not only Asian patients but also mainstream American society.

Mobilizing the Family's Cultural Strength

One of the functions of therapy is to mobilize the family's cultural strength. Strengths include support from the extended family, the strong sense of obligation and family loyalty, parental sacrifice for the children's future, filial piety, strong focus on educational achievement, the work ethic, and the support from their ethnic communities. In many circumstances, especially when family members are coping with death, losses, and unpredictable changes, discussions of religious stories or philosophical teachings in the Asian culture can be very therapeutic.

Employing the Concept of Empowerment as a Treatment Goal

Empowerment is the process whereby the clinician mobilizes the family's ability to interact successfully with external systems. It is particularly important in working with immigrant women who have victimized by years of sexism, loss of power due to language barriers, role reversal, and racism in the new country.

Understanding the Family's Communication Style

In addition to determining the preferred language and dialect used in therapy, the clinician must understand a family's communication style. Shon and Ja (1982) discussed the communication process with Asian American families in three areas: the revelation of information, the expression of feelings, and the process of disagreement in therapy. Traditionally, Asian Americans have been taught to employ indirect styles of communicating and to avoid direct confrontations. The clinician is expected to read between the lines to grasp the major issue. On the other hand, the family may perceive the clinician to be too blunt, pushy, and insensitive.

If Asian clients discuss emotional difficulties, they are often expressed in an oblique, understated way with little obvious emotion, implying that the problem is less serious than it really is (Hong, 1989). Negative emotions such as anger, grief, and depression may be expressed in an indirect way. A culturally naive clinician may mistake this style for denial, lack of affect, lack of awareness of the client's own feelings, deceptiveness, or resistance on the part of the client (Sue, 1990). Even positive feelings (e.g., love) are frequently not expressed in an open manner. Asian parents may be misunderstood as unloving and uncaring. To overcome this communication barrier, it is quite helpful to introduce the structural family therapy model (Minuchin, 1974) because of its emphasis on actively restructuring the interaction in the family to create change rather than relying on direct, open expression of feelings (Shon & Ja, 1982).

Acknowledging Countertransference and Racial Stereotypes

Clinicians should explore their own stereotypes, both positive and negative, about Asian American families. Many non-Asian clinicians who have been exposed to the "model minority" myth may tend to minimize a family's pathology. On the other hand, a clinician who has worked with poor, traumatized refugee families may adopt a missionary zeal and may not recognize the many family strengths. In addition, a clinician with a superficial or stereotypical understanding of Asian American cultural values might overemphasize cultural similarities in all people of a particular ethnic group. Such a clinician might unconsciously assume that the cultural values and behavioral patterns of a client's ethnic group coincide with the values and behaviors of a particular Asian American client (Sue & Zane, 1987). Such stereotyping can have a negative impact on clinician–client relationship.

For Asian American clinicians, special issues include overidentification with the family and guilt for "having made it" in mainstream America. For those who still have their own identity issues (denial or rejection of one's racial identity), working with Asian American families may evoke unresolved pain and emotions. An Asian American clinician who works in mainstream settings as a token expert may feel undue pressure to succeed. He or she should receive supervision or consultation on countertransference issues that may exist.

CONCLUSIONS

Most Western family therapy approaches have been limited in their application to families with an Eastern value orientation. This chapter offers an alternative assessment and treatment model that takes into account the physical, psychological, social, spiritual, and cultural background of Asian American families. The proposed framework is intended to be a stimulus for the future development of a systematic approach more compatible with Asian Americans' world view and family characteristics.

Asian Americans are a heterogeneous group reflecting a diversity of educational, political, socioeconomic, and religious backgrounds, as well as different migration histories. The scope of this chapter does not allow for an in-depth discussion of each group, and readers are encouraged to examine the following chapters for more in-depth discussions.

REFERENCES

American Psychiatric Association. (1994). *Diagnostic and statistical manual of mental disorders* (4th ed.). Washington, DC: Author.

American Psychological Association. (1991). *Guidelines for providers of psychological services to ethnic and culturally diverse populations.* Washington, DC: Author.

Asian American Health Forum. (1990). *Asian and Pacific Islander American population statistics* (Monograph Series No. 1). San Francisco: Author.

Berry, J. W. (1990). Acculturation and adaptation: A general framework. In W. H. Holtzman & T. H. Bornemann (Eds.), *Mental health of immigrants and refugees* (pp. 91–102). Austin, TX: Hogg Foundation for Mental Health.

Berry, J. W., & Blondel, T. (1982). Psychological adaptation of Vietnamese refugees in Canada. *Canadian Journal of Community Mental Health, 21,* 81–88.

Bowen, M. (1976). Theory in the practice of psychotherapy. In P. J. Guerin (Ed.), *Family therapy: Theory and practice.* New York: Gardner Press.

Boyd-Franklin, N. (1989). *Black families in therapy: A multisystems approach.* New York: Guilford Press.

Cho, L. J., & Yada, M. (1994). *Tradition and change in the Asian family.* Honolulu: East–West Center.

Comas-Díaz, L., & Griffith, E. H. (1988). *Clinical guidelines in cross-cultural mental health.* New York: Wiley.

Flaskerud, J., & Hu, L. T. (1992). Relationship of ethnicity to psychiatric diagnosis. *Journal of Nervous and Mental Disease, 180*(5), 296–303.

Gaw, A. C. (Ed.). (1993). *Culture, ethnicity, and mental illness.* Washington, DC: American Psychiatric Press.

Gim, R., Atkinson, D., & Whiteley, S. (1990). Asian American acculturation, severity of concerns, and willingness to see a counselor. *Journal of Counseling Psychology, 37*(3), 281–285.

Gong-Guy, E. (1987). *California Southeast Asian mental health needs assessment.* Oakland, CA: Asian Community Mental Health Services.

Haley, J. (1976). *Problem-solving therapy.* San Francisco: Jossey-Bass.

Hansen, J. C., & Falicov, C. J. (1983). *Cultural perspectives in family therapy.* Rockville, MD: Aspen Systems.

Ho, M. K. (1987). *Family therapy with ethnic minorities.* Newbury Park, CA: Sage.

Hong, G. (1989). Application of cultural and environmental issues in family therapy with immigrant Chinese Americans. *Journal of Strategic and System Therapies, 8,* 14–21.

Hsu, F. L. K. (1971). *Under the ancestor's shadow: Kinship, personality, and social mobility in China.* Stanford, CA: Stanford University Press.

Jacobsen, F. M. (1988). Ethnocultural assessment. In L. Comas-Díaz & E. E. H. Griffith (Eds.), *Clinical guidelines in cross-cultural mental health* (pp. 135–147). New York: Wiley.

Karnow, S., & Yoshihara, N. (1992). *Asian Americans in transition.* New York: Asia Society.

Kim, S. (1985). Family therapy for Asian Americans: A strategic–structural framework. *Psychotherapy, 22*(2), 342–348.

Kinzie, J. D. (1989). Therapeutic approaches to traumatized Cambodian refugees. *Journal of Traumatic Stress, 2,* 75–91.

Kuo, W. H., & Tsai, Y. (1986). Social networking hardiness and immigrants' mental health. *Journal of Health and Social Behavior, 27,* 133–149.

Kuroda, T. (1994). Family structure and social change: Implications of fertility changes in Japan and China. In L. J. Cho & M. Yada (Eds.), *Traditions and change in the Asian family* (pp. 45–55). Honolulu: East–West Center.

Landau, J. (1982). Therapy with families in cultural transition. In M. McGoldrick, J. K. Pearce, & J. Giordano (Eds.), *Ethnicity and family therapy* (pp. 552–572). New York: Guilford Press.

Lee, E. (1982). A social systems approach to assessment and treatment for Chinese American families. In M. McGoldrick, J. K. Pearce, & J. Giordano (Eds.), *Ethnicity and family therapy* (pp. 527–551). New York: Guilford Press.

Lee, E. (1988). Cultural factors in working with Southeast Asian refugee adolescents. *Journal of Adolescence, 11,* 167–179.

Lee, E. (1989). Assessment and treatment of Chinese-American immigrant families. *Journal of Psychotherapy and the Family, 6*(1/2), 99–122.

Lee, E. (1990). Family therapy with Southeast Asian refugees. In M. P. Mirkin (Ed.), *The social and political contexts of family therapy* (pp. 331–354). Needham Heights, MA: Allyn & Bacon.

Lee, E. (1996). Asian American families: an overview. In M. McGoldrick, J. Giordano, & J. K. Pearce (Eds.), *Ethnicity and family therapy* (2nd ed., pp. 227–248). New York: Guilford Press.

Lin, K. M. (1986). Psychopathology and social disruption in refugees. In C. L. Williams & J. Westermeyer (Eds.), *Refugees and mental health* (pp. 61–73). Washington, DC: Hemisphere Press.

Lin, K. M., Masuda, M., & Tazuma, L. (1982). Adaptational problems of Vietnamese refugees: III. Case studies in clinic and field—Adaptive and maladaptive. *Psychiatric Journal of the University of Ottawa, 7,* 173–183.

Matsushima, N. M., & Tashima, N. (1982). *Mental health treatment modalities of Pacific/Asian American practitioners.* San Francisco: Pacific Asian Mental Health Research Project.

McGill, C., & Lee, E. (1986). Family psychoeducation intervention in the treatment of schizophrenia. *Bulletin of the Menninger Clinic, 50*(3), 269–286.

McGoldrick, M. (1982). Ethnicity and family therapy: An overview. In M. McGoldrick, J. K. Pearce, & J. Giordano (Eds.), *Ethnicity and family therapy* (pp. 3–30). New York: Guilford Press.

McGoldrick, M. (1985). *Genograms in family assessment.* New York: W. W. Norton.

McGoldrick, M., Pearce, J. K., & Giordano, J. (Eds.). (1982). *Ethnicity and family therapy.* New York: Guilford Press.

Minuchin, S. (1974). *Families and family therapy.* Cambridge, MA: Harvard University Press.

Paniagua, F. A. (1994). *Assessing and treating culturally diverse clients.* Thousand Oaks, CA: Sage.

Shon, S., & Ja, D. (1982). Asian families. In M. McGoldrick, J. K. Pearce, & J. Giordano (Eds.), *Ethnicity and family therapy* (pp. 208–228). New York: Guilford Press.

Sluzki, C. E. (1979). Migration and family conflict. *Family Process, 18,* 378–390.

Steinhoff, P. G. (1994). A cultural approach to the family in Japan and the United States. In L. J. Cho & M. Yada (Eds.), *Tradition and change in the Asian family* (pp. 29–44). Honolulu: East–West Center.

Sue, D. W. (1990). Culture-specific strategies in counseling: A conceptual framework. *Professional Psychology: Research and Practice, 21*(6), 424–433.

Sue, S., & McKinney, H. (1975). Asian Americans in the community mental health care system. *American Journal of Orthopsychiatry, 45,* 111–118.

Sue, S., & Sue, D. W. (1974). MMPI comparisons between Asian American and non-Asian students utilizing a student health psychiatric clinic. *Journal of Counseling Psychology, 21,* 423–427.

Sue, S., & Zane, N. (1987). The role of culture and cultural techniques in psychotherapy: A critique and reformulation. *American Psychologist, 42,* 37–45.

Sun, T. H., & Liu, Y. H. (1994). Changes in intergenerational relations in the Chinese family: Taiwan's experience. In L. J. Cho & M. Yada (Eds.), *Tradition and change in the Asian family* (pp. 319–361). Honolulu: East–West Center.

Tseng, W. S., & Hsu, J. (1991). *Culture and family: Problems and therapy.* Binghamton, NY: Haworth Press.

Uba, L. (1994). *Asian Americans: Personality patterns, identity, and mental health.* New York: Guilford Press.

U.S. Bureau of the Census. (1990). *1990 census of population.* Washington, DC: U.S. Government Printing Office.

Yamamoto, J., Lam, J., Fung, D., Tan, F., & Iga, M. (1977). Chinese-speaking Vietnamese refugees in Los Angeles: A preliminary investigation. In E. F.

Foulks, R. M. Wintrob, J. Westermeyer, & A. R. Favazza (Eds.), *Current perspectives in cultural psychiatry* (pp. 113–118). New York: Spectrum.

Yu, E., Chang, C. F., Liu, W., & Fernandez, M. (1989). Suicide among Asian American youth. In M. Feinleib (Ed.), *Report of the secretaries task force on youth suicide* (pp. 157–176). Washington, DC: U.S. Department of Health and Human Services.

Westermeyer, J. (1989). *Psychiatric care of migrants: A clinical guide.* Washington, DC: American Psychiatric Press.

2

Cambodian American Families

JAMES K. BOEHNLEIN
PAUL K. LEUNG
J. DAVID KINZIE

HISTORICAL BACKGROUND

From 1975 to 1979, millions of Cambodians were traumatized in prisons and work camps during the Pol Pot regime, through torture, witnessing executions of family and friends, and disease and starvation. After the genocidal Pol Pot government was overthrown in 1979, waves of refugees escaped to Thailand, where they spent difficult years awaiting resettlement in host countries. Hundreds of thousands have remained there, awaiting repatriation. However, more than 200,000 became refugees throughout the world, with about two-thirds of those settling in the United States.

Prior to the onset of war, Cambodia was a relatively stable and prosperous country, able to feed its people from rich agricultural land and bountiful water resources. Most people lived in small villages in rural areas, farming or fishing. Merchants, teachers, clergy, soldiers, and other professionals lived in towns or in the capital, Phnom Penh. The middle and upper classes were educated in Buddhist monasteries or schools run by the French colonial government.

Despite economic prosperity, the government was continuously unstable and embroiled in centuries-old tension with its more powerful and populous neighbors, Thailand and Vietnam. The alliance with the French was also tenuous; thus, French colonial influence on traditional Cambo-dian culture was significantly less than the French influence in Vietnam.

The traumas of war and resettlement have had profound effects upon Cambodian refugees who have been resettled. They have been found to have particularly high rates of depression and posttraumatic stress disor-der (PTSD) (Kinzie, Fredrickson, Rath, Fleck, & Karls, 1984; Boehnlein, Kinzie, Rath, & Fleck, 1985; Mollica, Wyshak, & Lavelle, 1987; Kinzie et al., 1990). The effects of depression and PTSD reach beyond the individ-ual who experienced the original trauma, also disrupting the person's family life and social network (Boehnlein et al., 1995; Clarke, Sack, & Goff, 1993; Sack et al., 1993; Sack et al., 1994).

Migration and acculturation place additional stress on refugees, who have already experienced many years of trauma and multiple losses, including family members, economic status, cultural traditions, and coun-try of birth. The refugee's journey from Southeast Asia to the United States often takes many years and involves lengthy stays in refugee camps. Upon arrival in the host country, refugees face additional challenges such as language barriers, unemployment, and fragmentation of social supports (Boehnlein, 1987b).

TRADITIONAL ORGANIZATION AND VALUE ORIENTATION OF CAMBODIAN FAMILIES

Traditional Cambodian values include a strong family identity, which also provides the basis for personal identity and self-worth. Elders assume authority roles and are treated with respect because of their age and experience. Children are considered to be independent at birth and then are wooed into a sense of interdependency by attentive, indulgent childrearing from multiple-parenting persons, who then become increas-ingly strict in their expectations as the children mature (Sack, Angell, Kinzie, & Rath, 1986). Parental and grandparental decisions go unques-tioned, and traditionally it is the child's, even the adult child's, duty to follow the wishes of the parents. Older family members are the first consultants or "healers" when a family member becomes ill. Also, people are considered to be elders at a younger age (40s or 50s) than in Western cultures, and adult children begin supporting elders financially at a relatively early age.

General cultural values and expectations are also important in understanding the Cambodian family. These values include (1) an orien-tation to the past, including great respect for ancestors; (2) the tolerance of multiple belief systems in regard to religion and cosmology; and (3) the acceptance of life as it is rather than what it could be (Kinzie, 1978, 1981).

For Cambodians, an orientation to the past, along with a fatalistic approach to one's present life, is primarily related to the central Theravada Buddhist belief in reincarnation, along with the Buddhist teachings that a person controls his or her own destiny through free will and cannot escape present suffering in this world (Boehnlein, 1987a). Religious symbols, beliefs, and rituals enable individuals and groups to deal with the ultimate conditions of existence (DeCraemer, Vansina, & Fox, 1976). Religion also serves as a source of conceptions of the world, the self, and the relations between them (Geertz, 1973).

Eight-five percent of Cambodians traditionally follow the Buddhist religion (Edmonds, 1970). Buddhist rituals during significant life transitions such as birth and death have been at the center of Cambodian life since the 13th century, reinforcing social ties in families and communities (Ebihara, 1979). Important precepts of Buddhism include a correct understanding of the sources of unhappiness, correct intent for specific actions, honest speech, good conduct, honest effort, alertness, and concentration (Zadrozny, 1955). These precepts strongly influence both familial and social norms of communication and behavior. In addition, elements of Brahmanism are still evident in Cambodian life cycle ceremonies (Lebar, Hickey, & Musgrave, 1964), and folk religious traditions beliefs, based on belief in a variety of animistic, ancestral, guardian, or demonic spirits are prominent (Ebihara, 1979; Eisenbruch, 1984).

It is important to keep these basic religious concepts in mind when attempting to understand the frequent chronic grief of Cambodian families. For example, ritual mourning of the loss of family members and friends has not been possible for many refugees (Boehnlein, 1987a). During the Pol Pot era, the majority of Buddhist monks were executed by the Khmer Rouge because they represented a tie to traditional beliefs. The performance of traditional mourning rituals was punishable by death. Moreover, refugees who lost parents, siblings, or children to violence, disease, or starvation during the war are frequently haunted by chronic guilt because they perceive a lack of personal responsibility in ensuring a proper Buddhist burial for family members, although in reality that could have resulted in their own execution.

EFFECTS OF CULTURAL TRANSITION

The process of acculturation may challenge the long-standing traditions and values that enable families to solve problems throughout the life cycle.

The pressures of acculturation have numerous effects on traditional generational and sex roles in refugee families. Acculturation is highly influenced by culturally mandated roles determined by age and social class. It is important to remember that individual psychosocial development is affected by both family life cycle transitions and the ongoing stressors of ethnic–group acculturation (Boehnlein, 1987b).

For example, after migration to Western countries, elderly refugees have had to withstand a diminished status both within the family and in the majority society because of lack of language proficiency, little or no formal education, and lack of employment opportunities. This situation is further complicated by cultural differences in what is considered to be retirement age. Also in many cases women have become the primary wage earners, and men have become the primary care providers for children.

Another source of great conflict for refugee families is the relationship between parents and their adolescents or young children. Due to the carnage of the Pol Pot era, there is a high prevalence of single female heads of household among Cambodian refugees. Women in single-parent families who have lost their husbands during the war are required to function as both father and mother. The normal developmental struggles of adolescence are heightened by the mother's diminished authoritative role; this situation is further exacerbated if the parent is emotionally disconnected from the child because of symptoms of chronic depression or PTSD. The child's greater proficiency with the host country's language often leads to a reversal of generational roles. Particularly as the child becomes older he or she becomes the communication facilitator between the family and the majority society.

The normal life cycle separation of the young adult from the family presents unique conflicts for refugee families. Both parents and children often have suffered numerous serious losses of other family members during the Pol Pot era and during migration, including other parents, grandparents, spouses, and siblings. It is not uncommon for parents to have lost several children as a result of wartime violence, disease, or starvation. The survivors have needed to stay close to each other for physical and emotional survival and have forged a particularly strong family bond. Any threat to that closeness will reawaken memories of prior losses and will be seen as a threat to survival. Parents frequently suffer worsening depression and PTSD at times of significant family life cycle transitions (e.g., a child attending school out of town or contemplating marriage).

For Cambodian women, dating and marriage present further acculturation conflicts, as many parents continue to expect that their approval of the marriage partner (as to ethnic group or social class) will be required no matter what the age of their child.

Young refugees separating from their families to seek educational or work opportunities have frequent conflicts with the pull toward their family and community and their desire for maximizing their own potential. This conflict is particularly difficult for young women who have been the primary care providers for their younger siblings when the single parent was impaired by chronic depression or PTSD. The child of either sex often feels the emotional pressure of enormous expectations placed on him or her, particularly if the family was successful in their homeland. The prevailing style of communication in most Cambodian families, which includes an avoidance of intergeneration conflict, also contributes to a frequent lack of resolution of disagreements and continuing anxiety for parents and children. Optimal family functioning is further complicated by the high rate of PTSD among Cambodian adolescent children (Sack et al., 1986; Kinzie, Sack, Angell, Manson, & Rath, 1986; Kinzie, Sack, Angell, & Rath, 1989).

CASE EXAMPLE

The following case example illustrates the multiple intergenerational stresses and problems that exist in refugee Cambodian families. As indicated earlier, the stresses are ongoing and make resolution or treatment of various disorders complicated and often incomplete.

The patient, a 56-year-old Cambodian woman, was seen in the clinic for 7 years. When first seen, she reported a history of poor sleep, trembling, startle reactions, and numbness in her leg up to the knee to the extent that she was unable to feel any pain. She had nightmares and dreams about ghosts, spirits, and actual traumatic events in Cambodia. She had poor concentration, poor appetite, and decreased interest in her environment, although she had some suicidal thoughts, she was prevented from acting on them by her Buddhist beliefs.

Her family had been poor, and she and her husband, who had joined the military, had a difficult time trying to support their nine children. When Pol Pot took power in 1975, her husband was killed and later she saw his corpse with bullet wounds and his legs cut off. Her oldest son was also killed, and she saw his decapitated body as well. Two children died of starvation. She suffered many hard times, often seeing corpses and being threatened with execution.

Eventually she made it out of Cambodia to Thailand. Ultimately she came to the United States, accompanied by her aged mother and two children, who at that time were 10 and 14. She left five children in Cambodia, several of whom were unaccounted for. The patient had markedly pressured speech and was almost incoherent and unable to remember much of her story. She wore thick glasses and had poorly combed hair and several missing front teeth. She appeared visibly depressed and shaken and showed much anxiety. She did have anesthesia in the lower parts of both legs, which was similar to her description of seeing her husband's body with the legs cut off.

Originally she was diagnosed with PTSD, major depression, and a conversion disorder. She was started on an antidepressant and clonidine and treated in our clinic with regular psychotherapy and a Cambodian socialization group experience. During the therapy, she reported that several of her children were in refugee camps in Cambodia and having a difficult time. She was unable to support them as they requested, which created much stress for her. Slowly her appetite, interest, and depression improved and her nightmares decreased; however, she had multiple somatic symptoms. The conversion symptoms showed much improvement during treatment.

Several years into treatment, it became apparent that her mother also was suffering from severe PTSD and depression. Much of the treatment was then focused on her mother, who responded very well to therapy and improved greatly. The patient's mother often accompanied her to the clinic, and both of them were in therapy together.

Unfortunately, the mother developed lung cancer. When she stopped eating and couldn't move, she went to a nursing home, where she died in a relatively short time.

After her mother died, the patient's symptoms—PTSD as well as depression—recurred. The patient frequently talked about missing her mother a great deal and dreaming about her. She performed the appropriate Buddhist ceremonies and gradually, over a 6-month period, began to accept the death of her mother.

Although she had said very little about her difficulty in raising two children alone, it gradually became apparent that her own family in the United States was changing. When her son was to be married at age 23, the bride requested money for the marriage, which the patient felt unprepared to pay. In addition, only her young daughter remained at home, and she keenly felt the loss of her son moving out on his own.

At age 17, her daughter began a complicated relationship with a man who moved in with them. This man was involved in gangs and the situation was somewhat dangerous for the patient and the daughter. The patient felt embarrassed and shamed in the eyes of the Cambodian community and became more isolated. She also developed hypertension at this time.

Finally, she performed a Buddhist ceremony with her daughter and boyfriend at home, which she felt would symbolize a proper marriage in the eyes of the community. Although her relationship with her daughter improved, she still felt pressure from the community. Furthermore, she received news that a son and a daughter in a refugee camp, both with a large number of children, needed money. She and her family found some money to send them but she felt very sad and pressured that she was unable to help more.

Her daughter's boyfriend left when the daughter was 6 months pregnant. This caused greater community and internal pressure. The patient realized that her daughter was so young that the patient herself would have to take care of the baby. The daughter, who was seen in therapy several times, seemed quite Americanized and moderately realistic about the problems she was facing. Once the daughter and the patient began to talk more directly, both felt relieved, and the patient accepted the situation and her role in helping her daughter and soon-to-be-born grandchild.

FAMILY THERAPY WITH CAMBODIAN FAMILIES

Ishisaka, Nguyen, and Okimoto (1982, 1985) feel that a therapist's store of cultural knowledge should serve as a general template against which an individual or family is assessed. They note that knowledge of basic cultural norms, values, and ideas is important, but there is a danger of ethnic stereotyping if the therapist does not appropriately recognize the immense variability of behavior among cultures. It should also be noted that the stressors of migration can disrupt and change previously normative behavior within families.

Family therapy with Cambodian families involves restoring cultural identity, which was lost or weakened by the years of trauma and migration, and also resolving the pressures of acculturation that were noted previously. This latter task may include helping each generation to understand and accept each other's new beliefs and roles as the family evolves through the life cycle. The therapist's personal style cross-culturally is important in effecting this change. The therapist must communicate a sense of genuineness and competence by being direct yet empathic, by being active in the recommendation of treatment options yet responsive to conflicting cultural concepts of family roles, and finally, by allowing families to report difficult historical information or to express intense emotions without a sense of shame. Finally, the therapist can be a greatly respected and trusted figure for refugee families if he or she approaches the family with respect for the strengths that allowed all members to survive individually and as a unit. The therapist can help the family members to use those strengths to confront the present and future challenges of acculturation.

In the Cambodian culture, traditional healing places a great emphasis on the broader social context of illness and treatment. When socially sanctioned traditional healers are consulted, the healing ritual often takes place with other family members present. Cambodians expect a structured and pragmatic approach to treatment, which includes both individual and family therapy.

Besides dealing with depression and the stresses of acculturation during treatment, many Cambodians are also struggling with the existential concerns that most trauma survivors face. They struggle with doubts about personal and social identities, which affect interpersonal functioning, and conflicts about traditional cultural and religious values. They also face the difficult task of creating meaning for their experiences while structuring a hopeful future for their families.

The therapist can assist patients in slowly rebuilding connections to the altered cultural foundations in life that contribute to self-identity and meaning. This approach includes psychotherapy and medication in individual treatment, family therapy, and encouragement to participate in traditional Buddhist celebrations and life cycle ceremonies. The therapist can become a catalyst to allow individuals and families to reassert control and direction in their lives.

REFERENCES

Boehnlein, J. K. (1987a). Clinical relevance of grief and mourning among Cambodian refugees. *Social Science and Medicine, 25,* 765–772.

Boehnlein, J. K. (1987b). A review of mental health services for refugees between 1975 and 1985 and a proposal for future services. *Hospital and Community Psychiatry, 38,* 764–768.

Boehnlein, J. K., Kinzie, J. D., Rath, B., & Fleck, J. (1985). One year follow-up study of posttraumatic stress disorder among survivors of Cambodian concentration camps. *American Journal of Psychiatry, 142,* 956–959.

Boehnlein, J. K., Tran, H. D., Riley, C., Tan, S., Vu, K. C., & Leung, P. K. (1995). A comparative study of family functioning among Vietnamese and Cambodian refugees. *Journal of Nervous and Mental Disease, 183,* 510–515.

Clarke, G., Sack, W. H., & Goff, B. (1993). Three forms of stress in Cambodian adolescent refugees. *Journal of Abnormal Child Psychology, 21,* 65–77.

DeCraemer, W., Vansina, J., & Fox, R. C. (1976). Religious movements in Central Africa. *Comparative Studies in Society and History, 18,* 458–475.

Ebihara, M. (1979). *Svay, a Khmer village in Cambodia.* Ann Arbor, MI: University Microfilms International.

Edmonds, I. G. (1970). *The Khmers of Cambodia.* Indianapolis, IN: Bobbs-Merrill.

Eisenbruch, M. (1984). Cross-cultural aspects of bereavement: I. A conceptual framework for comparative analysis. *Culture, Medicine, and Psychiatry, 8,* 283–309.

Geertz, C. (1973). *The interpretation of cultures.* New York: Basic Books.

Ishisaka, H., Nguyen, Q. T., & Okimoto, J. T. (1982). Individual functioning and mental health. In Y. B. Rhee (Ed.), *Refugee mental health: Summary of Conference Proceedings.* Kansas City, MO: U.S. Department of Health and Human Services.

Ishisaka, H. S., Nguyen, Q. T., & Okimoto, J. T. (1985). The role of culture in the mental health treatment of Indochinese refugees. In T. C. Owan (Ed.), *Southeast Asian mental health: Treatment, prevention, services, training and research.* Washington, DC: National Institute of Mental Health.

Kinzie, J. D. (1978). Lessons from cross-cultural psychotherapy. *American Journal of Psychotherapy, 32,* 510–520.

Kinzie, J. D. (1981). Evaluation and psychotherapy of Indochinese refugee patients. *American Journal of Psychotherapy, 35,* 251–261.

Kinzie, J. D., Boehnlein, J. K., Leung, P. K., Moore, L. J., Riley, C., & Smith, D. (1990). The high prevalence rate of PTSD and its clinical significance among Southeast Asian refugees. *American Journal of Psychiatry, 147,* 813–917.

Kinzie, J. D., Fredrickson, R. H., Rath, B., Fleck, J., & Karls, W. (1984). Posttraumatic stress disorder among survivors of Cambodian concentration camps. *American Journal of Psychiatry, 141,* 645–650.

Kinzie, J. D., Sack, W. H., Angell, R. H., Manson, S., & Rath, B. (1986). The psychiatric effects of massive trauma on Cambodian children: I. The children. *Journal of the American Academy of Child Psychiatry, 25,* 370–376.

Kinzie, J. D., Sack, W. H., Angell, R., & Rath, B. (1989). A three-year follow-up of Cambodian young people traumatized as children. *Journal of the American Academy of Child and Adolescent Psychiatry, 28,* 501–504.

Lebar, F. M., Hickey, G. C., & Musgrave, J. K. (1964). *Thenic groups of mainland Southeast Asia.* New Haven, CT: Human Relations Area Files Press.

Mollica, R. F., Wyshak, G., & Lavelle, J. (1987). The psychosocial impact of war trauma and torture on Southeast Asian refugees. *American Journal of Psychiatry, 144,* 1567–1572.

Sack, W. H., Angell, R. H., Kinzie, J. D., & Rath, B. (1986). The psychiatric effects of massive trauma on Cambodian children: II. The family, the home, and the school. *Journal of the American Academy of Child Psychiatry, 25,* 377–383.

Sack, W. H., Clarke, G., Him, C., Dickason, D., Goff, B., Lanham, K., & Kinzie, J. D. (1993). A 6-year follow-up study of Cambodian refugee adolescents traumatized as children. *Journal of the American Academy of Child and Adolescent Psychiatry, 32,* 431–437.

Sack, W. H., McSharry, S., Clarke, G. N., Kinney, R., Seeley, J., & Lewinsohn, P. (1994). The Khmer Adolescent Project: I. Epidemiologic findings in two generations of Cambodian refugees. *Journal of Nervous and Mental Disease, 182,* 387–395.

Zadrozny, M. G. (Ed.). (1955). *A handbook on Cambodia.* New Haven, CT: Human Relations Area Files Press.

3

Chinese American Families

EVELYN LEE

In the past three decades, there has been a tremendous influx of Chinese immigrants and refugees in the United States. As the largest Asian Pacific American ethnic group, Chinese Americans share many of the same characteristics and values of other Asian Americans, but they also possess their own unique migration history, political background, linguistic styles, and cultural and religious beliefs. This chapter attempts to sensitize clinicians to the complexities and diversity of major Chinese American subcultures, reviews relevant clinical considerations in the treatment of psychological problems, and recommends effective assessment and treatment strategies.

HISTORICAL BACKGROUND

The Chinese characters for China mean the Middle Kingdom. It has a land mass about 9.6 million square kilometers, which is more than 300,000 square miles larger than the United States. In 1994, the Chinese population in China was 1.192 billion, with a projection of 1.504 billion by the year 2025. The Chinese constitute about one-fifth of all the people on earth. More than 95% of the population live on approximately 40% of the land (Bunge & Shinn, 1981).

China has the world's oldest continuous history and culture. (Although there have been earlier civilizations elsewhere, they have flourished and then become extinct.) China's traditional value system is a complex amalgam of ideas that evolved over centuries from the philo-sophical teachings and religious beliefs of Confucianism, Taoism, Bud-dhism, and other influences. Social values emphasize the importance of family solidarity, friendship, morality, and conformity of prescribed roles. When the Chinese communists came to power in 1949, the political revolution also brought along social revolution. Many aspects of tradi-tional social life–social relations, family organization, women's roles, personal values, and so forth experienced fundamental changes. The industrialization of China in recent years has created another wave of economic and social changes.

MIGRATION HISTORY

The Chinese migration history to the United States tells a complex yet fascinating story of change, adaptation, and survival. Their experience also reveals how the Chinese family system has been affected by the immense power of political, legal, social and economic forces in the United States and in China (see Table 3.1). The Chinese have been residing in this country in significant numbers for more than 150 years. Major national immigration policies and economic upheavals in the U.S. and in Asian countries have resulted in different waves of immigration and different types of family systems.

The First Wave: The Pioneer Family (1850–1919)

Although there were Chinese residing in the United States as early as 1785, the impetus for large-scale immigration to this country did not take place until the discovery of gold in California in 1848 and the need for manual labor for the construction of railroads. Many Chinese migrants, mostly peasant farmers, left their village in China to pursue their dreams in *Gam Saan,* the "Gold Mountain." In addition to employment opportu-nities, many sought sanctuary from intense conflicts in China caused by the British Opium War and the harsh economic conditions. From their arrival in the 1850s until the 1920s, the overwhelming majority of the early Chinese immigrants were men. More than half of the arriving men were single, and those who were not often were separated from their wives and condemned to live as bachelors in Chinese communities. Racial and ethnic antagonism, coupled with xenophobia against early Chinese immi-grants, succeeded in the passage of the Chinese Exclusion Act of 1882. This act barred Chinese laborers and their relatives (including their wives) from entering the United States.

The early Chinese pioneers lived in a virtually womanless world without family life. In 1900, of the 89,863 Chinese on the U.S. mainland,

TABLE 3.1. United States–China Chronology: Significant Events in Chinese Immigration History in the United States and Political Events in China

Year	Events in the United States	Events in China
1850–1860	California "Gold Rush." Male sojourner immigration from southern China to California.	Chinese immigrants came to the United States seeking sanctuary from internal conflicts in China caused by the Opium War with Great Britain; peasant uprisings; Western imperialism; economic and political turmoil; heavy peasant taxation; flooding and starvation.
1864	Central Pacific Railroad recruited Chinese laborers from Canton.	
1866	*Civil Rights Act*: Gave persons of "every race and color, citizenship and all privileges, to hold property and to testify in Court." The law did not apply to the Chinese.	
1869	*Burlingame Treaty*: Unrestricted Chinese immigration was allowed primarily to supply cheap labor to build the railroad.	
1871	Anti-Chinese riots in Los Angeles.	
1877	Anti-Chinese riots in San Francisco.	
1879	California Constitution adopted with anti-Chinese provisions.	
1882	*Chinese Exclusion Act* Suspended immigration of Chinese laborers for 10 years. Barred Chinese naturalization. Provided for deportation of Chinese illegally in the United States.	
1882–1920	Declining immigration; decline of agriculture, mining, and railroad occupations; rise of urban service occupations; immigration of "paper sons" and "treaty merchants."	
1891	*Immigration Act* First comprehensive law for national control of immigration. Established Bureau of Immigration under U.S. Treasury Department. Directed deportation of aliens unlawfully in country.	
1892	*Geary Act*: Extended exclusion for 10 more years.	

TABLE 3.1 *(cont.)*

Year	Events in the United States	Events in China
1898	U.S. Supreme Court recognized children born in the United States with Chinese parents as citizens.	
1900–1930	Rise of "family associations" and "tongs" (secret societies).	
1911		Birth of Republic of China. End of the Ching Dynasty. Sun Yat-Sen became the president.
1924	*Immigration and Naturalization Act* Imposed first permanent numerical limit on immigration. Established the national origins quota system, which resulted in biased admissions favoring northern and western Europeans.	
1927		Kuomintang Party unified most of China.
1929–1939	Great Depression.	
1931		Japan invaded Manchukuo.
1932		"Manchukuo" established under Pu Yi.
1934–1935		The Long March: Communists to Yen'an.
1937		Japanese attacked across China; Communist–Kuomintang alliance.
1940–1946	16,000 Chinese Americans served in Armed Forces in World War II.	
1943	*Repeal of all 15 Chinese Exclusion Acts*: Quota set at 105 per year.	
1945	*War Brides Act*: Facilitated the entry of wives of men in the U.S. armed forces.	Japan surrendered.
1948	*Displaced Person Act*: 3,465 Chinese students, visitors, and seamen were granted permanent resident status.	Kuomintang–Communist Civil War (to 1949).
1949		People's Republic proclaimed. Chiang Kai-shek and Kuomintang to Taiwan. Many Chinese moved to Hong Kong, Taiwan, and overseas.

(continued)

TABLE 3.1 *(cont.)*

Year	Events in the United States	Events in China
1950		Land reform. China entered Korean War (to July 1953).
1952	*Immigration and Naturalization Act* Continued national origins quotas. Quota for skilled aliens whose services were urgently needed.	
1953	*Refugee Relief Act*: Allowed the entry of 2,777 refugees of the Chinese Revolution. It further granted a total of 2,000 visas to Chinese endorsed by the Chinese Nationalist Government.	
1957	*Act of Sept. 11, 1957*: Persons could not be deported if a spouse, parent, or child was a citizen of the United States or a permanent resident alien.	
1958		Great Leap Forward.
1959		Famine (to 1961).
1962	*Presidential Directive of May 25, 1962:* Permitted Hong Kong refugees to enter the United States immediately as "parolees."	
1965	*Immigration and Nationality Act Amendments* Repealed national origins quotas. Established 7-category preference system based on family unification and skills. Set 20,000-per-country limit for Eastern Hemisphere. Imposed ceiling on immigration from Western Hemisphere for first time.	
1966		Cultural Revolution started.
1972		President Nixon visited China.
1976	*Immigration and Nationality Act Amendments*: Extended 20,000-per-country limits to Western Hemisphere.	Zhou En-lai died; Mao Tse-tung died; Gang of Four arrested.
1980	*Refugee Act* Established first permanent and systematic procedure for admitting refugees. Removed refugees as a category from preference system. Defined refugee according to international rather than ideological standards. Established process of domestic resettlement. Codified asylum status.	Economic reform (1980–present).

TABLE 3.1 *(cont.)*

Year	Events in the United States	Events in China
1986	*Immigration Reform and Control Act* Instituted employer sanctions for knowingly hiring illegal aliens. Created legalization programs. Increased border enforcement.	
1989		Tiananmen Square incident.
1990	*Immigration Act* Increased legal immigration ceilings by 40%. Tripled employment-based immigration, emphasizing skills. Created diversity admissions category. Established temporary protected status for those in the United States jeopardized by armed conflict or natural disasters in their native country.	
1997	Immigration and welfare reform.	British Government returned Hong Kong to China on July 1.

only 5% were female (Wong, 1988). The married men became husbands or fathers of "mutilated" families (Sung, 1967), or split-household families (Glenn, 1983). They were physically separated from their wives and children in China. The economic function of the family was carried out by the Chinese male living in the United States, whereas other family functions such as taking care of the elderly parents and emotional nurturing the children were carried out by the wife and other relatives thousands of miles away in the villages in China. This type of "sojourner" family pattern had profound consequences on the personal and social development of family life of the early Chinese in the United States. One serious consequence was the delay for almost 70 to 80 years of the emergence and maturation of a substantial second-generation Chinese American population (Wong, 1988).

A limited number of Chinese women immigrated to the United States in the latter part of the 19th century. They were either prostitutes or wives of the small group of Chinese merchants. In the 1870 census, 61% of the 3,536 Chinese women in California listed their occupation as "prostitute" (Hirata, 1979). Hirata (1979) suggested that Chinese prostitution was an important element in the maintenance of split-household families by helping men avoid long-term relationships with women and ensuring that the bulk of their meager earnings would continue to support the family in China.

Although immigration law excluded the majority of Chinese from entering this country, it did allow entry of relatives of U.S. citizens of Chinese ancestry. When the 1906 San Francisco earthquake and fire destroyed most of the municipal records, this provided a loophole by which the Chinese could immigrate to the United States. American-born Chinese would visit China, report the birth of a son, and thereby create an entry slot which could be sold years later to someone wanting to immigrate. The purchaser, a "paper son," simply assumed the name and identity of the alleged son (Wong, 1988). The "paper family names" passed on from generation to generation.

The Second Wave: The Small Business Family (1920–1942)

The discriminatory Immigration Act of 1924 made it impossible for American citizens of Chinese ancestry to send for their wives and families. This law was changed in 1930 to allow wives of Chinese merchants and Chinese wives who were married to American citizens before 1924 to immigrate to the United States (Chinn, Lai, & Choy, 1969). As a result, sizable family units with second-generation American-born Chinese population were emerging in Chinatowns. At the same time, many first-wave laborers began to leave mining and railroads and used their savings to start their own small businesses, such as laundry shops or fishing, either alone or with partners. The small-producer families emerged during this period. This family type consisted of the immigrant and first-generation American-born family functioning as a productive unit (Wong, 1988). Although all family members participated in the family enterprise, there was a division of labor according to age and gender. There was also an emphasis on collectivity over the individual.

The Third Wave: The Reunited Family (1943–1964)

The liberalization and reforms of immigration policies during and after World War II were instrumental in partially rectifying past discrimination against the Chinese and slowly led to the development and normalization of family life among the Chinese in the United States. In 1943, the Chinese Exclusion Act of 1882 was repealed, making Chinese immigrants eligible for citizenship. In 1945, the War Brides Act was passed, allowing Chinese women to enter to this country as brides of men in the U.S. military. The Displaced Persons Act of 1948 gave permanent resident status to Chinese visitors, seamen, and students who were stranded here because of the Chinese civil war. The Refugee Relief Act of 1953 allowed a group of highly educated Chinese into the United States as refugees. During the period from 1943 to the repeal of the quota law in 1965, Chinese immigrants were largely female. After years or sometimes decades of separation from their husbands, many wives were reunited with their husbands for the first time. By the time they arrived in the United States, these women and their children had already established very powerful bonds which were far more intense than the marital tie. Reform in immigration policies also encouraged Chinese men to return to Hong Kong to find wives. These trans-Pacific marriages, with wives who were 10 to 20 years younger than their husbands, were usually arranged by matchmakers or relatives (Wong, 1988).

The Fourth Wave: The Chinatown and Dual-Worker Family (1965–1977)

Unlike the pre-1965 immigrants who came over as individuals, most of the Chinese immigrants who arrived under the Immigration Act of 1965 came as families. Many of them initially settled in or near Chinatowns in the major metropolitan areas. Approximately half of them were working class, employed as service workers or laborers. Most of husbands and wives sought employment in the labor-intensive, low-capital services such as garment sweatshops and restaurants. Unlike the small-business families, they tended to completely segregate work and family life, and family members had very little time to spend together. Economic survival was the primary goal for many families, especially the new immigrant families.

The Fifth Wave: The New Immigrant, Refugee, and "Astronaut" Family (1978–Present)

In the past two decades, there has been a tremendous influx of Chinese immigrants from China, Hong Kong, Taiwan, and Vietnam. Since 1979, after three decades of a closed-door policy, the United States started to admit immigrants from mainland China to join their relatives. The reestablishment of diplomatic relations between the United States and the People's Republic of China in 1978 also provided an opportunity for students and professionals from China to study in this country, and many elected to stay. The massacre at Tiananmen Square in June 1989 and its political aftermath increased the desire of many students to seek permanent residency in the United States. Another group of immigrants who came from Hong Kong worried about the 1997 transfer of British sovereignty to China. The recent political climate in Taiwan and the desire to seek higher education for their children also created an impetus for many Chinese to come to this country.

Many of the refugees from Vietnam, Laos, and Cambodia were ethnic Chinese. They constituted the second wave of Southeast Asian refugees. A significant number of them were survivors of hunger, rape, incarceration, forced migration, and torture. Although most of the original Southeast Asian refugees came under the sponsorship of churches and social services agencies, the new arrivals were often reunited families who were petitioned by family members.

Another recent phenomenon is the so-called astronaut families. These are the "frequent fliers" who set up two households, one for the children in the United States and one for the adults who work in their home country after they have received their green cards. The increased number of such families is a result of the economic boom of the Pacific Rim and the difficulty of finding suitable employment in the United States. In recent years, this phenomenon has applied not only to new immigrants but also to many Chinese American families who have lived in the United States for many years.

In summary, the influx of immigrants and refugees from many different parts of Asia and from many different socioeconomic and political backgrounds has contributed to the complexity of existing Chinese American communities.

DEMOGRAPHICS

According to the 1990 figures (U.S. Bureau of the Census, 1990), Chinese Americans, numbering more than 1.6 million, were the largest Asian Pacific American group, making up 22.6% of the Asian Pacific American population. Between 1980 and 1990, the Chinese American population doubled due to the new influx of immigrants. Currently, more than 63% of Chinese Americans are foreign-born, 23% do not speak English well, and 53% live in the Western parts of the United States. There are 542,121 Chinese Americans who reside in California, 147,250 in New York, and 55,916 in Hawaii. It is estimated that 13.3% of Chinese Americans live below the poverty level, 69.4% are high school graduates, and 72.5% speak a language other than English at home (Asian American Health Forum, 1990).

LANGUAGE

There is no single Chinese language. It is very important for clinicians to assess the primary dialect used by the client and to ask for an interpreter who is fluent in that dialect if he or she is not bilingual. There are many different dialects spoken by the different groups of Chinese Americans. Mandarin is the national dialect of China. However, many earlier immigrants who came from villages in the southern part of China still maintain their village dialects, such as Toishanese, Chiuchow, or Hakka. Chinese from cities such as Canton or Hong Kong use Cantonese as their primary dialect. Chinese who were born and raised in Shanghai speak the Shanghainese dialect, which is very different from the Mandarin Beijing dialect. Chinese from Taiwan mostly use Mandarin as their primary dialect, but some Taiwanese prefer the Taiwanese dialect. The Vietnamese Chinese are perhaps the most talented group of Chinese in regard to languages. Many can speak English, French, Vietnamese, and several Chinese dialects (e.g., Cantonese, Mandarin, Chiuchow, Fukien, and Hakka). Some American-born Chinese Americans who grew up with their monolingual parents and grandparents are capable of communicating with their elders in Chinese, but English is still their primary language. Acculturated immigrants are mostly bilingual and use both English and their native dialect, depending on the situation. It is important for the clinician to determine what dialect the family prefers to use in counseling sessions.

The written Chinese characters are less complicated than the variety of Chinese dialects. Generally speaking, there are two major styles: the "traditional" style practiced by the majority of Chinese from Hong Kong, Taiwan, and Southeast Asian countries and the "simplified" style of writing developed by the People's Republic of China.

COMMUNICATION STYLES

Eastern communication styles are very different from Western ones. In counseling sessions, Asian American clients often appear quiet, passive, polite, and formal and make a great deal of effort to avoid direct confrontation and offending others. Silence and lack of eye contact are also common forms of indirect communication. Among Asians, silence is a sign of respect and a desire to continue speaking after making a point during a conversation (Sue & Sue, 1990). Direct eye contact is considered a sign of lack of respect and attention, particularly to authority and older people.

THE TRADITIONAL CHINESE FAMILY

Traditional family in China had many unique characteristics. These characteristics were heavily influenced by Confucianism, with its emphasis on harmonious interpersonal relationships and interdependence. Family interactions were governed by prescribed roles defined by family hierarchy, obligation, and duties. Independent behavior or expressions of emotions that might disrupt familial harmony were discouraged. The family was patriarchal. Males, particularly the father and eldest son, had dominant roles. Marriages were commonly arranged, and it was socially acceptable for influential men to have mistresses. Husbands deal with the outside world and provide for the family. The spousal relationship was secondary to the parent–child relationship. Filial piety was highly cherished, and parents used respect and shame as a means of control. The father usually played the role of a stern disciplinarian whereas the mother was affectionate and caring. The eldest son was expected to carry on the family name and enjoyed special privileges; the eldest daughter was taught to assist the mother with household chores and to attend to younger siblings. The most elevated family dyad was the father–son dyad.

Throughout history, Chinese mothers have been portrayed as self-sacrificing, suffering, guilt inducing, and overinvolved with their children. Traditionally, in accordance with the custom of "thrice obeying," women were expected to comply with their fathers or elder brothers in youth, their husbands in marriage, and their sons after their husband's death. As wives, their value was judged by their ability to produce male heirs and to serve their in-laws. In many middle- and upper-class families, children were raised by wet nurses, who breast-fed the babies and took over the mothering roles. Grandparents and other extended family members also significantly influenced family life. Because of the strong bond and the intense sense of obligation, many sons never left their parents in their adult lives. Parents expected to be taken care of in their old age and never experienced the so-called empty nest period in their family life cycle.

CONTEMPORARY CHINESE AMERICAN FAMILIES

The patterns of family systems tend to be molded by economic, political, and sociocultural factors outside the family system rather than determined merely by emotional and psychological factors within the family (Tseng & Hsu, 1991). In the past generation, the traditional Chinese family has undergone tremendous transformation as a result of economic and political forces in the United States and Asia. As indicated previously, the structure and composition of Chinese American families are heavily influenced by U.S. immigration policy changes.

With the large number of Chinese immigrants from China, Hong Kong, and Taiwan, clinicians should recognize that economic and political changes in those countries have a dramatic impact on Chinese family system and values. Since the communist takeover of China in 1949, Confucian thought and religions were largely banned. A one-child family system has replaced the traditional extended family system. During the 10 years of the Cultural Revolution, many families suffered forced separation. Red Guard youths openly challenged their parents and teachers; filial piety and respect for the elderly no longer dominate life in China. In recent years, the economic boom in China has brought another wave of Western influences and urbanization.

After World War II, both Hong Kong and Taiwan underwent rapid growth in light industries and exports. The forces of industrialization, Westernization, urbanization, and economic affluence have brought a change in Chinese social and family structure. Although the older and middle-generational Chinese still embody some traditional beliefs, the younger generation has shown some evidence of their rejection of conservatism and traditionalism. Political history has also influenced traditional Chinese family values. In the case of Hong Kong, a British colonial past had a profound effect on the education, legal, and social systems. In Taiwan, a long period of Japanese occupation until the end of World War II has had a large impact on the society, especially among the older generation.

In summary, there are several distinct shifts in the contemporary Chinese American family: (1) The traditional Chinese extended family has gradually yielded to a more *nuclear family*, where functional relations apply instead of actual household structure; (2) the traditional patriarchal family has transformed in many cases to a *biarchal system*, where a mother shares decision making with the father; (3) the parent–child dyad has diminished in importance while the *husband–wife dyad* has increased; (4) favoritism of sons has slowly decreased because daughters now attain comparable education and careers and can be counted on to take care of aged parents; (5) the family life cycle has changed from arranged marriages and no empty nest period to one in which romantic love occurs before marriage and adult children leave the home; (6) successful childrearing is now measured mostly by the children's academic and career achievements; and (7) earning power is no longer solely the father's but is shared with other adult family members.

These observations are general ones. There is no one typical Chinese American family. There are many individual differences, and they represent a wide range of cultural values from very traditional (such as newly arrived family from a rural area in China or Vietnam) to very "Americanized" (such as a third-generation American-born professional family). The five types of Asian American families identified in Chapter 1 serve as a general guideline for understanding these differences.

COMMON PRESENTING MENTAL HEALTH PROBLEMS

Given the fact that no large-scale prevalence studies have been conducted on Chinese Americans, it is difficult to specify the rates of mental disorders within this population or to compare these rates with those for other ethnic minority groups. However, findings from the available research on prevalence and needs strongly imply that major mental health problems do exist among Chinese Americans, which is contrary to the widespread belief that Chinese Americans are a well-adjusted "model minority."

Somatization and Depression

Several research findings have reported the prevalence of somatization symptoms among the Chinese (Kleinman, 1982; Tseng, 1975; Marsella,

Kinzie, & Gordon, 1973). Many Chinese Americans who are treated for mental health problems complain of headaches, and back and chest pains. They have reported more somatic complaints than European Americans on the Minnesota Multiphasic Personality Inventory, even when Asian Americans and European Americans have mental disturbances of equal severity (Sue & Sue, 1974). Chinese American students seem to have a rather definite pattern of depression associated with somatic functioning (Marsella et al., 1973). Chang (1985) also found ethnic differences in the patterns of depressive symptomatology, and the Chinese were the most likely to exhibit somatic complaints.

There are many hypotheses on why Chinese tend to express their emotional problems in somatic symptoms. It may be a reflection of Chinese cultural values that emphasize avoiding shame and protecting the family's name from the negative stigma of mental problems. In addition, expression of physical complaints is more socially acceptable than expression of emotional complaints in Chinese culture. Somatization may be a socially acceptable means of suppressing direct depressive affect while allowing the individual to receive secondary gain. Many Chinese women, for example, may use the sick role to seek attention and emotional support from family members otherwise may not be available. In addition to the psychological and sociological explanations of somatization, clinicians need to understand the Chinese holistic view of health and illness based on traditional Chinese medicine. There is a strong belief in unity between the mind and the body, an organ-oriented conception of pathology that emphasizes close correspondences between human emotions and body organs. Somatic problems frequently are explained by traditional Chinese as resulting from weak kidneys, hot intestines, or *qi* energy imbalances.

Depression has been widely found among Chinese Americans, especially among the immigrants and refugees. This may, in part, be a result of social isolation, lowered status, grief (Lin, 1986), acculturation stress, war trauma, financial problems, and other social stressors. Many experience symptoms of exhaustion, weakness, dizziness, diffuse bodily complaints, and difficulty with sleep and appetite, as well as a sense of hopelessness. They may meet the official diagnostic criteria for a major depressive disorder. However, from the traditional Chinese patient's perspective, the chief problem is not depression but "neurasthenia," an official diagnosis in China and a diagnosis widely offered by traditional herbalists in Chinatown.

Suicide

In an earlier study in San Francisco's Chinatown, Bourne (1973) reported a high suicide rate among the Chinese. From 1952 to 1968, the suicide rate among Chinese was 27.9 per 100,000 population per annum, which was three times higher than the reported rate for the national average. The study also found that the frequency of Chinese men committing suicide was four to five times more than that of Chinese women. Barbiturate ingestion was noted to be the most common method of suicide of Chinese men. Lonely elderly men who came to the United States as sojourners, and who were despondent over physical illness, constituted a very high-risk group. Suicide attempts for Chinese women were usually precipitated by such interpersonal conflicts as chronic family strife, desertion by husband, or parental scolding. Yap (1958) borrowed Lindemann's concept of hypereridism to explain the high frequency of interpersonal stresses as a precipitating factor for female suicide. In traditional Chinese culture, women were denied opportunities for self-expression and assertion. Interpersonal conflicts may produce a hyperidic state, which exerts an impersonal pressure that slowly leads to despair and cannot be alleviated by threats or appeals. Under such circumstances, an acute quarrel or even a minor reprimand can set off an impulsive, poorly planned suicide attempt. For Chinese women, the most frequent method for suicide was hanging. A popular traditional belief held that the ghosts of those who died by hanging could return to torment the living as a means to achieve final and lasting vengeance.

In a more recent study of the percentage of all deaths of 15- to 24-year-olds attributed to suicide, Chinese Americans have a higher rate in comparison with European Americans in that age range. The rate for female Chinese is 20.8% versus 8.8 for European American females. Foreign-born Chinese Americans have higher suicide rates than do American-born Chinese Americans (Yu, Chang, Liu, & Fernandez, 1989).

Schizophrenia

There is an absence of epidemiological data in the United States on schizophrenia prevalence for Chinese Americans. The prevalence data indicate a band of prevalence rate ranging from roughly 2 to 10 cases per 1,000 population across a range of populations (Sartorius & Jablensky, 1976). The prevalence of schizophrenia in China ranged from 0.77% to 4.80% (Lin & Kleinman, 1981). In Chinese culture, mental illness is stigmatized and a mentally ill member usually brings shame upon the entire family.

Other Psychological Problems

Other common manifestations of psychological problems among Chinese Americans include anxiety disorder; dissociative disorder; posttraumatic stress disorder; paranoia; hypersensitivity; identity confusion; low self-

esteem; conduct disorder; drug, alcoholism, and gambling (a serious problem in the Chinese community which has not been properly studied)
addictions; family problems (intergenerational conflicts, marital disharmony, in-law problems, domestic violence, child abuse, and neglect); difficulties at work, in school, and in dating; and impaired interpersonal skills.

CLINICAL CONSIDERATIONS

Conceptualization of Mental Illness and Emotional Difficulties

Western-trained clinicians have paid a great deal of attention to either the
intrapsychic influences or the biological explanation of the cause of
mental illness. The views of many traditional Chinese are still highly
influenced by their religious and spiritual beliefs and, most important, the
concepts of health and disease in traditional Chinese medicine. Generally
speaking, several common popular explanations of factors may contribute
to the development of mental illness (Lee, 1982).

1. *Imbalance of* yin *and* yang *and disharmony in the flow of* qi. In
traditional Chinese medicine, humankind is viewed as a microcosm within
a macrocosm. The energy in each human being interrelates with the
energy of the universe. *Qi* (energy) and *jing* (sexual energy) are both
considered vital life energies which are kept in balance by the dual
polarities of *yin* and *yang*. If there is an imbalance of the *yin* and *yang*,
the immunity of the body is disturbed and the body is susceptible to
illness. Another important concept is that the universe and the human
are subjected to the laws of the five elements: fire, earth, metal, water,
and wood. The five elements correspond to the five visceral organs and
five emotions: joy from the heart, sorrow from the lungs, anger from the
liver, fear from the kidneys, and compassion from the spleen (Table 3.2).
There is a strong belief in unity between the body and the mind. For
example, the literal Chinese meaning of the written character "joyless" is
"the heart locked inside the door." The character "happiness" is "the heart
opened inside the door." The presence of emotional problems is thought
to result from an imbalance of *yin* and *yang* or the excessive decrease or
accumulation of *qi*. Emotional disturbances are often reflected in somatic
symptoms.

2. *Supernatural intervention.* Mental illness is seen as some form of
spiritual unrest meted out to the individual through the agency of a ghost
or vengeful spirit. It is a sign of punishment caused by the transgression
of family rituals in ancestor worship (Lin & Lin, 1981).

3. *Religious beliefs.* Mental illness is viewed as *karma,* caused by deeds
from past lives or punishment from God.

4. *Genetic vulnerability or hereditary defects.*

TABLE 3.2. Key Concepts of Five Elements

Five phases	Direction	Season	Organs	Orifices	Emotions	Color
1. Wood	East	Spring	Liver	Eyes	Anger	Green
2. Fire	South	Late summer	Heart	Ears	Joy	Red
3. Earth	Middle	Summer	Spleen	Nose	Compassion	Yellow
4. Metal	West	Autumn	Lungs	Mouth	Sorrow	White
5. Water	North	Winter	Kidney	Genitals	Fear	Black

5. *Physical and emotional strain and exhaustion* caused by external stresses such as failing in a business venture, ending a love affair, or the death of a family member.

6. *Organic disorders.* Mental illness is conceptualized as a manifestation of physical disease, especially brain disorders, diseases of the liver, hormonal imbalance, and so forth.

7. *Character weakness.* Mental health is achieved through self-discipline, exercise of will power, and the avoidance of morbid thoughts. Persons who are born with a weak character will not be able to achieve mental health and are more vulnerable to emotional problems.

Indigenous Healing Practices in the Chinese Community

Despite the existence of an advanced, highly institutionalized U.S. medical system and the availability of mental health professionals, it is evident that Chinese clients still utilize many types of traditional healing methods for physical health or emotional problems. Various indigenous healing practices are available in major Chinatowns and refugee communities. The most popular ones are herbal medicine, acupuncture, and therapeutic massage. Religious faith healing is also perceived to be helpful. The sick person believes that there is a supernatural power and sickness can be cured through the very power of his or her faith. Religious faith-healing ritual treatments are usually conducted by Buddhist monks or priests. Many go to temples to chant and receive counseling from their spiritual leaders. Other practices such as geomancy and fortune telling are also being used to prevent or to remove "bad spirit."

Nutrition is another popular means to restore health. According to Chinese traditional medicine, foods are categorized in five groups: hot, cold, allergic, moderate, and nutrient. Chinese are usually very conscious of good nutrition. Therapeutic cuisine that gives "good *qi*" is very popular in treating health and emotional problems. In addition, many Chinese practice health exercises such as *tai chi chuan* and *qi-gong* to bring harmony to their body and mind.

There are a number of similarities between the indigenous healers and Western health practitioners. Both have diagnostic tools that help them identify the nature of the problems; both are able to provide interpretations to their respective patients; and both have treatment methods to treat the problems presented to them. Beyond these similarities, there are important areas of difference. One of the most prominent is found in their methods of categorizing health problems. The primary distinctions that traditional healers are likely to make in the diagnosis and treatment of illnesses are in terms of their basic cause: Illnesses are regarded as either natural or supernatural in origin. Western health professionals are more biopsychologically oriented. Whereas indigenous systems of healing tend to treat illness, modern professional health care workers tend to treat disease. They usually treat a single individual patient, out of the context of his or her family, social network, and community. The holistic nature of Eastern healing systems recognizes that illness is a psychosocial process.

Dealing with Psychological Problems

Most Chinese Americans try to deal with their psychological problems without seeking professional mental health counseling. Traditional families usually seek help from family members first because it is considered the collective responsibility of the family to take care of the disturbed member as long as possible. Such problems are kept from outsiders for fear of the shame, guilt, and stigma that this knowledge might bring upon the family. The family often tries to deal with the problem by denying the seriousness of the illness, or by extorting or reasoning with the patient to "correct" his or her behaviors (Lin & Lin, 1981). Each family member may contribute his or her own proposal for treatment. When the family and the troubled person are not able to resolve the problem, they often turn to certain trusted outsiders and helpers within the ethnic community, such as community elders, spiritual leaders, indigenous healers, and physicians (Sue & Morishima, 1982). When these efforts fail, assistance from other agencies and providers, including psychiatrists and other mental health professionals, is sought while the troubled family member is still kept at home. Family members usually resist hospitalization until all other efforts have failed. The introduction of the label of mental illness seems to hasten the transition from intrafamilial coping to hospitalization of the troubled member, who ultimately is rejected, scapegoated, and blamed for things that went wrong within the family (Lin & Lin, 1981; Gaw, 1993). Providers thus need to be keenly aware of the help-seeking behavior and the family dynamic involved in coping with mental illness in Chinese families.

Treatment Expectations

For many clinicians, the success of a case is measured by the emotional growth of the client or the psychological understanding of the problem.

Although some of the acculturated Chinese may expect "insight" therapy, the majority of Chinese immigrants and refugees expect more concrete help to produce physical and behavioral changes and the immediate alleviation of such symptoms as the inability to work, eat, sleep, and assume allocated family roles. Many come in with physical complaints, expecting medication from the doctor.

Process of Healing

A traditional Western treatment model usually goes through a rather complicated and lengthy sequence of steps with each client: initial assessment, psychosocial evaluation, formulation of diagnosis, development of treatment goals, actions to achieve these goals, and, finally, termination. The major activity in the treatment process is verbal communication, or "talk therapy," between the clinician and the client. Chinese clients will probably have difficulty understanding such a therapeutic process. They seek help from mental health agencies only as the last resort after they have exhausted all other resources, and they usually come in for help in a state of crisis with expectation of an immediate "cure." They are used to traditional Chinese healing practices, which usually include a brief physical observation, diagnosis, and prescription writing—all in one session. They expect a rapid diagnosis and do not understand the purpose of lengthy evaluation and the apparent lack of treatment in the initial process. They may also get upset with initial interviews that probe into their family and personal backgrounds, which they perceive as having nothing to do with the presenting problem. For immigrants and refugees who have suffered many losses and separations, this process can be extremely stressful. To reveal family secrets to an outsider also evokes a sense of guilt. Consequently, many Chinese clients drop out of treatment (Lee, 1982).

Perception of Mental Health Professional Roles

Many mental health disciplines (e.g., psychiatry, psychology, social work, marriage counseling, and family therapy are not widely recognized in some Asian countries. Many Chinese do not have the sophistication to understand the roles of the clinicians or their special professional orientations. Because the role of a physician is more clearly understood and respected, Chinese patients may expect clinicians to conduct themselves in the traditional role of physicians who prescribe medication. Therefore, especially in the initial stage of the therapeutic relationship, it is very important for clinicians to explore their clients' exposure to mental health professionals in the past and their experiences. Mental health disciplines function quite differently in different Asian countries. It is also very helpful for the clinician to explain his or her role to the client and at the same time to explore the client's expectations with regard to the clinician's role.

ASSESSMENT AND TREATMENT OF CHINESE AMERICAN FAMILIES

For many Chinese immigrants and refugees with language limitations and cultural differences, family and community networks often provide the sole means of support, validation, and stabilization. To treat Chinese American families effectively in therapy, the clinician must be able to both conceptualize and intervene at multiple levels and in multiple systems. This approach is built on the structural family systems model (Minuchin, 1974), an ecostructural approach (Aponte, 1976), and the multisystems model (Boyd-Franklin, 1989). In addition, the clinician also needs to incorporate the Eastern holistic way of thinking into clinical practice. Based on these perspectives, a model that takes into the account not only the psychological and biological influences but also the cultural, social, political, and spiritual forces and their impact on the individual, the family, and the community (Lee, 1989, 1990). The multisystems model provides an overall framework that allows a clinician to provide treatment successfully at whatever level or levels are relevant to the family situation. This model proposes intervention at the following levels:

1. Individual family member.
2. Family subsystems (husband–wife; parent–child; siblings).
3. Family as a unit.
4. Extended family members.
5. Work group, nonblood kin, friends, neighbors.
6. Chinese community.
7. American mainstream systems.

The multisystems model allows the clinician to organize complex data and to plan and prioritize intervention. It does not require that the clinician intervene at all levels (Boyd-Franklin, 1989). Different families may require different levels of involvement. For some Chinese families who enter treatment, the clinician may make the decision that one or more family members needs individual work for a variety of reasons. For example, many Chinese young adults struggle with the dilemma of how to be differentiated and individuated within a close extended family and yet not become either too enmeshed or totally cut off. They may need individual counseling to find a balance between cultural and familial expectations and their own needs. Or, when communication has totally broken down between the teenagers and parents, both subsystems may need to be "coached" before they can meet together for family therapy. Some families may enter treatment with an overwhelming number of survival issues instead of problems related to family structure or dynamics. The primary intervention should be at the community resources level. The clinician assumes the role as the system guide or facilitator, helping the family to navigate effectively within the service systems. The flexibility with which the clinician approaches this model is the key to its effectiveness.

To work with Chinese families more effectively, the clinician may need to postpone extensive evaluation until trust is established. The basic components of the therapeutic process consists of the following six steps:

1. Joining and engaging (building social and cultural connection and trust).
2. Initial assessment (focusing on presenting problem and observation of family dynamic).
3. Problem solving (helping to solve the presenting problem and establishing credibility).
4. In-depth information gathering and evaluation (focusing on family history, family dynamic, and other sociocultural factors).
5. Intervention (restoring healthy functions of family members and restructuring the family and the multisystems).
6. Termination (summarizing the accomplishments and future planning).

Joining and Engaging Chinese American Families

Because of the reluctance with which many Chinese American families come to treatment, the joining process is the most difficult and challenging.

1. It is important for the clinician to make the first appointment with the "decision maker" (e.g., the parents) and not simply to send messages through the English-speaking children. Joining frequently involves outreach to key family or extended family members (e.g., a resistant father or an overprotective grandmother) who may object to or sabotage certain aspects of the treatment. Therefore, it is important for the clinician to reach out by means of letters, phone calls, and home visits to engage these crucial family members. The clinician must be sure to set an appointment time that is convenient to the working parents because they may value work more than therapy. Detailed explanations about the reasons for such an appointment and the location of the agency may be necessary.

2. Many immigrants do not understand the role of mental health professionals and may confuse him or her with a physician. A brief explanation of the health professional's role and training background may be helpful.

3. During the first session, the clinician should address the family in

a polite and formal manner. In addition, he or she needs to pay attention to "interpersonal grace" and show warm expressions of acceptance, both verbally and nonverbally. Greeting the family with a smile, hanging up his or her coat, offering a cup of tea, and providing comfortable chairs to the older family members are pragmatic ways to convey genuine concern and can go a long way toward creating a positive relationship (Ho, 1987).

4. Many Chinese are used to receiving "counseling" from their friends or village elders whom they know personally. They may ask the clinician many personal questions (e.g., his or her country of origin, marital status, and number of children). The clinician needs to feel comfortable in answering such questions. Appropriate self-disclosure may facilitate a positive cultural alliance and a level of trust and confidence.

5. Forming a social and cultural connection with the family during the first session is very important. When the clinician has lived in the same Asian country or has extensive experiences in working with Chinese, it is beneficial to disclose familiarity of that culture to make the cultural connection. When the clinician is not very familiar with the client's culture, it is important to show his or her interest and appreciation of the client's cultural background. Pictures of Asian countries and culture on the office wall can also convey the clinician's interest.

6. Because many Chinese family members are not used to verbal communications in therapy, asking nonthreatening personal questions can put the family at ease. Engaging the clients in small talk may help. Before rapport has been established, it is important to avoid direct confrontation, not to demand greater emotional disclosure, or to avoid culturally taboo subjects such as sex or death.

7. For many Chinese, public admission of mental health problems can bring intense shame and humiliation. The clinician may counter those emotions by empathizing with clients and encouraging them to verbalize this feeling. It is important to assure family members of confidentiality and anonymity. One helpful technique is to reframe the client's courage in seeking help as love and concern for family members. If appropriate, mobilizing the family's sense of obligation to get help to achieve family harmony or for the sake of the children can be very effective.

8. Many Chinese clients come to their first session believing that the clinician is an authority who can tell them what is wrong and how to "fix" their problems. It is helpful for the clinician to establish credibility right away. Professional mannerism and an air of confidence are important ingredients.

9. Many Asian Americans do not comprehend the significance of sometimes lengthy procedures of evaluation. They are either not used to detailed history taking or do not understand the relationship between the questions and the presenting problems. Some may even suspect that such information will be put to political use, thus jeopardizing their immigra-

tion status. The clinician needs to help the client understand the reasons behind such questions.

10. Most of the families come to the first interview during a family crisis. The clinician should plan to allow more time than the usual 1-hour session, especially when an interpreter is used.

Initial Assessment

There are two major tasks for the clinician in this phase: (1) to observe the family and to begin the formation of initial hypotheses about the family structure and (2) to assess the presenting problem(s) and family members' readiness for therapy. Questions that the clinician might consider are:

1. Who referred the family? (Many Chinese families are not self-referred.)
2. What are the problems as perceived by each family member (as distinct from the goals of the referral agency or the clinician)?
3. What are their expectations? (Many do not have any working experience with Western-trained mental health professionals.)
4. How does the family feel about the counseling? (Many Chinese feel that mental health treatment is for "crazy people.")
5. Who came to the session, who is missing, and why?
6. Who is the family's spokesperson?
7. What is the communication pattern among the family members?
8. What is the primary dialect of each member? What dialect is commonly used by all family members? (The dialects may be different among the children, parents, and grandparents.)
9. What are the boundaries in this family?
10. Who has the power in the family?
11. How is the family responding to the clinician? Are key members beginning to trust the clinician?
12. Do the family members have a sense of hope that the clinician can help them to solve the problems?

Problem Solving

A problem-focused family therapy approach with Chinese American families appears to be very effective. From a multisystems perspective, problem solving is a cyclical process. It does not occur one time but throughout treatment. In the initial stage of treatment, it is important to respect the family's priority for which problem(s) require immediate attention. Many immigrant and refugees families are "multiproblem families" whose members feel overwhelmed by a vast number of problems.

The clinician should spend early sessions helping the family to identify the most urgent problems and then to remain focused on these problems. It is important to start with a problem that can be addressed and solved quickly to establish credibility and to gain the trust. However, it is very important for the clinician not to offer an inappropriate "instant quick fix" just because the family members are pushing for solutions.

In-Depth Information Gathering

Information gathering with Chinese American families often occurs at a point later in the treatment process. Many Chinese will not share important family background information or "family secrets" until they feel that the clinician is no longer an outsider and is part of the family. In working with clients who have suffered from psychological and physical trauma (e.g., the "boat people" from Vietnam and Chinese who were tortured during the Cultural Revolution), it is extremely important not to force the clients to deal with their psychological traumas prematurely. Skillful assessment of the family's readiness to share their trauma stories is very important.

Based on the multisystems/holistic model, the clinician should gather information not only on the internal family system but also on the external factors, which include many environmental stressors. In providing culturally competent services to Chinese families, the clinician needs to understand the social, psychological, physical, cultural, and political impacts on the client, his or her family, and the community in which they live. Effective assessment must take into consideration the Chinese holistic view of health and illness and their culturally specific ways of coping with emotional difficulties. The assessment must include information beyond traditional intake data. Relevant personal, familial, and community information and cultural mapping are extremely helpful in the assessment of Chinese families who have undergone rapid social change and cultural transition (Ho, 1987). Effective techniques include the use of family genograms (McGoldrick, 1985), family albums, stories, and so on.

Information gathered on each family should include (1) demographic information (years in the United States, country of origin, immigration status); (2) personal data (language and dialect spoken, physical health and medical history, educational level, occupation, income, marital status); (3) family data (family composition, birth order, roles, communication style, decision making, extended family network, parent–child relationship); (4) social and cultural data (individual's migration and relocation history, community work and organization membership, religious affiliation, help-seeking pattern); and (5) psychological data (role and process of adaptation and acculturation of family member, member's perceptions of problems and solutions, extent and kind of interruptions to the family life cycle). Based on the assessment model discussed in Chapter 1, Table 3.3 provides a summary of the kind of information needed in each key area.

Special Intervention Strategies

The treatment approaches I suggested in Chapter 1 are mostly applicable to Chinese American families. Effective strategies include forming a social and cultural connection with the family during the initial stage, acknowledging the family's sense of shame, establishing expertise and credibility, building alliance with members with power; restructuring social support networks, and mobilizing the family's cultural strength, holistic approaches to health, and religious belief. In addition to the need to be flexible in providing services to family members at the individual, family, or community level, clinicians also need to assume flexible roles. In addition to being the therapist, he or she may play the roles of teacher, advocate, interpreter, facilitator, mediator, and so on. As many Chinese families often do not see the connections between talking about their problems and actual changes, the use of educational approaches such as psychoeducation, role play, and assignment of tasks at home can be very effective. The clinician also needs to understand the family's communication style and be skillful in overcoming language barriers, especially when an interpreter is used.

To summarize the key recommendations, the following seven (CHINESE) strategies are found to be effective in working with Chinese American families:

C = Credibility. Improve credibility by displaying academic and professional expertise, demonstrating an air of confidence and maturity, showing familiarity with a family's cultural background and community resources, and providing effective solutions to deal with presenting problems.

H = Healing. Give positive healing energy to the family at a time of vulnerability and respect the Eastern holistic view of health and illness.

I = Inquiry. Ask the right question at the right time. Be tactful in the art of elicitation. Do not force clients to reveal family secrets and unresolved pain prematurely.

N = Negotiation. Negotiate cultural and value differences between the clinician and the clients and among family members.

E = Education. Educate the family members about the illness, the cause, problem-solving strategies, and community resources.

S = Strengths. Respect and utilize available strengths of the individ-

TABLE 3.3. Assessment Guidelines for Chinese American Immigrant and Refugee Families

Area of assessment	Assessment content
1. Family's ethnocultural heritage	Country of origin: paternal and maternal ancestry Province/city/village of origin Generations in United States Cultural identity of each family member
2. Family migration stress and relocation history	Premigration experience (life before migration) Type of community where the family lived Socioeconomic status Significant political events Family composition Educational, health and mental health systems in the home county Traumatic events encountered Migration experience (the escape/relocation process) Decision to leave: why, when and who Degree and type of hardships during escape Stress induced by legal immigration process: uncertainty of sponsorship, duration of waiting
3. Degree of loss and traumatic experience	Postmigration (life immediately after the arrival in United States) School adjustment Job and financial worries Changes in living environment and neighborhood Significant changes in family composition and relationship Learning and adjusting to Western values Problems with housing, transportation, child care, legal issues Racism and minority status
4. Postmigration experience and cultural shock	Separation and losses of family members, relatives, and friends Financial and material losses Loss of spiritual and cultural communities Physical trauma Psychological trauma
5. Acculturation level of each family member	Individual family member acculturation rate depends on: Years in host country Age at time of migration Exposure to Western culture Professional affiliation Contacts with American peers English-speaking ability Work or school environment

TABLE 3.3 *(cont.)*

Area of assessment	Assessment content
6. Work and financial stresses	Unemployment Underemployment/downward mobility Long working hours Language difficulty Racism at workplace "Glass ceiling" issue
7. Family's place of residence and community support	Type of neighborhood Availability of support system Help available from community-based service agencies Community stigma
8. Family dynamic	Family membership/composition Leadership Decision making Role assignments Communication patterns
9. Family problems	Intergenerational conflicts In-law conflict Marital difficulty Role reversal Addiction, substance abuse, gambling
10. Family strengths	Functional coping strategies Strong family bond Support from the ethnic community and networks
11. Physical health and medication history	Medical history of client and family members Exposure to Western and herbal medicines Consultation with physician and indigenous healers
12. Family's concept of presenting problem, help-seeking behavior, and treatment expectations	Symptoms and problems as perceived by family Causes of the problems as perceived by family Relationship with traumatic events Family help-seeking behavior Treatment expectations

ual, the family, and the Chinese American community. In addition to the rich and long history of Chinese culture, the most important strength the Chinese family possesses is its survival spirit.

E = Empathy. Show understanding and compassion to help build trust and rapport. Effective listening skills, caring, and acknowledging a family's pain and problems can be very therapeutic.

Termination

The process of termination should take into consideration the Chinese client's concept of time and space in a relationship. The client and family members may regard the clinician as a family member and may want to maintain contact with the clinician even after they have successfully achieved their treatment goals. For many Chinese clients, especially those who experienced many losses and separations, a good relationship is a permanent one that is to be maintained and treasured. They may like to contact the clinician on special occasions, perhaps bringing food to the office during Chinese New Year or reporting special family events such as the birth of a grandchild or a death in the family. The traditional psychodynamic therapeutic concept of separation anxiety during the termination phase may not apply when working with Chinese clients.

CASE EXAMPLE: A CHINESE WOMAN DEALING WITH LOSSES

Presenting Problem

Mrs. L, age 52, was referred to an outpatient mental health clinic in Chinatown from the emergency room of a public hospital. She went to the hospital with complaints of shortness of breath, dizziness, insomnia, and fear of "ghosts." She suffered from acute anxiety attacks and talked in a whisper.

During the first interview, she related one particular precipitating event—the death of an old Chinese man who was a tenant in her attic. He had died and had lain undiscovered for a long time. She found the body and was highly traumatized.

Evaluation and Assessment

Because of Mrs. L's life experiences as a Chinese immigrant and her unique cultural background, the evaluation and assessment of her case must include information beyond traditional intake data. Based on the suggested assessment guidelines in this chapter, the following vital information on the patient and her family was obtained.

Major Stressors: Migration Stress Caused by War and Relocation

Mrs. L was born in a rural farming village in Kwantung, China, the oldest daughter of three children in a Chinese, Toisanese-speaking family. Her father worked as a farmer while her mother took care of the household responsibilities. She spent most of her childhood helping in the farm and taking care of her younger brother. She experienced many losses, separations, and deaths in her lifetime.

- Age 8. Mother died of starvation in a Chinese village during the war with Japan.
- Age 9. Younger brother died of high fever and lack of medical care.
- Age 10. Father remarried and stepmother physically abused her.
- Age 13. Stepbrother was born and Mrs. L acted as the caretaker of her stepbrother.
- Age 15. Communists overran the village. Many family members, including her father, were tortured due to landlord status.
- Age 17. Entered arranged marriage to her husband, whom she had never met. Moved to another village and lived with her in-laws.
- Age 18. Husband left the village to go to work in Guangzhou. He came home for an occasional visit.
- Age 19. Birth of her oldest daughter.
- Age 21. Birth of her son, who died 3 years later of a fever. Upon the advice of others, Mrs. L fed the child "holy ashes" and could not forgive herself for his death.
- Age 22. Adopted a son, who is her brother's son.
- Age 24. Husband came to the United States to join his father, who had immigrated many years before. Mrs. L continued to live with her mother-in-law.
- Age 27. Mother-in-law was found to be guilty of adultery, and was beheaded in public, then her body was thrown into a deep well. Mrs. L witnessed this incident and was unable to talk about it for a long time.
- Age 30. Mrs. L left everything behind, moved to Hong Kong by herself, and waited there for her immigrant visa to the United States.
- Age 34. She was reunited with her husband in the United States.
- Age 36. She gave birth to another daughter. Husband demanded a son and insisted that she try fertility drugs and operations to give him a son.
- Age 40. Eldest daughter came to the United States; she later married and moved to a suburb. Mrs. L tried in vain to bring her adopted son to the United States.

- Age 40–52. Bought an old house and lived there with husband and younger daughter. Her husband took a job as a chef in a suburban restaurant, and came home only once a week. Her younger daughter dated an Irish young man and threatened to leave home once she graduated from high school.

Family Stress Caused by Intergenerational Conflict

Mrs. L gave birth to a daughter 2 years after she came to the United States. Her husband was very disappointed. Like most traditional Chinese parents, they raised their daughter the "Chinese way," expecting their daughter to be hardworking, obedient, dependent, and polite and to take care of them in their old age and bring honor to the family. However, like many acculturated adolescents, their daughter identified with American values, with their strong emphasis on independence, self-reliance, and assertiveness. As an American-born Chinese American, Mrs. L's daughter spoke very little Chinese and was not able to communicate with her parents. She also resented her monolingual parents' dependency on her as the cultural broker and interpreter in negotiations with the outside world. She spent most of her time dating non-Chinese boyfriends and threatened to leave home as soon as she finished high school.

Work and Financial Stresses

Mrs. L worked in a sewing factory with low pay and long hours. As a result of her "poor health" (e.g., dizziness and headaches), she was not as productive as other workers and was fired several times. Mr. L worked in a Chinese restaurant located 3 hours from the city and came home once a week on Mondays. Mrs. L felt very lonely as her husband and daughter were gone most of the time.

Other Stressors

Other stressors included legal problems (Mrs. L wanted to apply for her son to come from China), health problems (Mrs. L suffered from severe headaches, dizziness, and anxiety attacks and Mr. L had a heart condition and had been recently hospitalized), and stress caused by the living environment (the family lived in a high-crime neighborhood, and Mrs. L had been robbed three times on the streets).

Assessment of Strengths

In spite of the trauma of war, relocation, and years of separation, the family members demonstrated a great deal of love and caring with each other and a strong sense of commitment and obligation to take care of each other. Mrs. L's daughter and her husband visited every week and provided Mrs. L a great deal of support. A lovely granddaughter brought much joy to the family.

Assessment of Culturally Specific Responses to Mental Health Problems

At the beginning of the evaluation, all family members denied that the somatic complaints were related to mental health problems. They attributed all symptoms to physiological causes. Mrs. L declared that she was "not crazy" and did not understand why she was referred to a mental health clinic.

The family's belief in the physical cause of the patient's problems was not openly challenged by the therapist. Instead, family members were encouraged to talk about traditional Chinese medicine and cultural beliefs. After several interviews, Mrs. L revealed her belief that her dizziness was caused by too much "wind" in her body because she went back to work in the farm soon after the delivery of her baby. She was convinced that her poor health was highly related to having sexual intercourse during her "period." She also believed that she might be possessed by a male ghost (the old man who died in the attic), who made her lose her ability to speak. She consulted with a local fortune teller in the community to find out whether the apartment was haunted. The patient also sought help from several herbalists and several Western-trained Chinese physicians located in Chinatown. Getting help from mental health professionals was considered the last resort, and the family entered treatment with extreme anger, resentment, and a sense of hopelessness.

Treatment

It is beyond the scope of this chapter to discuss the treatment approaches of this case in detail. The patient came in for weekly therapy for 9 months and had a successful treatment outcome. Mrs. L's anxiety attacks disappeared after a few sessions, and her somatic symptoms decreased gradually over the course of treatment. In addition to individual therapy, Mr. L and the two daughters were also involved in family therapy. Several important treatment strategies contributed to success in this case:

1. Forming a social and cultural relationship with the patient and her family members during the initial phrase of treatment. The clinician acknowledged with understanding their anger, denial of mental health problems, and feelings of shame.

2. Encouraging the patient and other family members to openly discuss their cultural viewpoints on the causes of the problem, their past efforts in coping with the problems, and their treatment expectations.

3. Educating the family about the Western concept of psychosomatic complaints and depression, including their diagnostic procedures and treatment process. In this case, it is important to work closely with the physician to rule out organic causes.

4. Demonstrating care by assuming multiple helping roles. The clinician helped the client with legal and immigration problems in applying for her adopted son to come to the United States and to find a low-pressure job.

5. Creating a supportive environment for the client. Mrs. L was referred to the women's support group in the clinic. She was able to form new social relationships and enjoy outings and other recreational activities.

6. Establishing credibility and authority by being the problem solver for the family. Mrs. L and her family members received concrete advice on how to deal with conflicts within the family, such as the intergenerational conflict with the daughter.

7. Providing a safe environment for the client to work through losses in the past. Mrs. L was able to discuss her feelings regarding the death of her mother and her brother, the violent death of her mother-in-law, and the loss of her young son.

8. Mobilizing the client's family strengths. These strengths included a strong desire to return to work and family obligations toward each other. In addition, the community resources available in Chinatown were also utilized.

CONCLUSIONS

This chapter provided a brief overall description of Chinese American families and the demography, migration, language, and unique family characteristics of traditional and contemporary Chinese families. Special clinical considerations in treating Chinese American families were discussed. In providing culturally competent services to this population, clinicians need to understand the cultural meanings of the Chinese concept of mental health problems, health-seeking pattern, the process of healing, ways to deal with psychological problems, and treatment expectations. A practical guideline in assessing and treating Chinese American families based on a *multisystems/holistic* model is also offered. Clinicians can try to incorporate this model into their clinical intervention, with the goals of establishing trust and credibility, improving communication, overcoming cultural barriers, and obtaining more effective treatment outcomes. The most challenging task in working with Chinese Americans is to integrate the very rich cultural strengths of the East with the best modern Western medicine and psychology can offer. I believe that such an integrated model will not only benefit the treatment of Chinese Americans but can also benefit clients from many different cultures.

Chinese American families are in transition. From the pioneer family to the newly arrived immigrant family, Chinese American families have undergone numerous changes and are continuing to evolve. With the present political and economic trends in the United States and Asia, Chinese American families may undergo more rapid changes. We need to stay in tune with these changes and be flexible in designing culturally competent clinical service for this underserved population.

REFERENCES

Aponte, H. (1976). The family–school interview: An ecostructural approach. *Family Process, 15*(3), 303–311.

Asian American Health Forum. (1990). Asian and Pacific Islander American population statistics (Monograph Series No. 1). San Francisco: Asian American Health Forum.

Bourne, P. (1973). Suicide among Chinese in San Francisco. *American Journal of Public Health, 63*(8), 744–750.

Boyd-Franklin, N. (1989). *Black families in therapy: A multisystems approach.* New York: Guilford Press.

Bunge, F. M., & Shinn, R. S. (1981). *China, a country study.* Washington, DC: U.S. Government Printing Office.

Chang, W. (1985). A cross-cultural study of depressive symptomatology. *Culture, Medicine, and Psychiatry, 9,* 295–317.

Chinn, T. H., Lai, M., & Choy, P. (1969). *A history of the Chinese in California: A syllabus.* San Francisco: Chinese Historical Society of America.

Gaw, A. (1993). Psychiatric care of Chinese Americans. In A. Gaw (Ed.), *Culture, ethnicity, and mental illness* (pp. 245–280). Washington, DC: American Psychiatric Press.

Glenn, E. N. (1983). Split household, small producer and dual wage earner: An analysis of Chinese-American family strategies. *Journal of Marriage and Family, 45*(1), 35–46.

Hirata, L. C. (1979). *Free, indentured, enslaved: Chinese prostitutes in nineteenth century America.* Boston: Houghton-Mifflin.

Ho, M. K. (1987). *Family therapy with ethnic minorities.* Newbury Park, CA: Sage.

Kleinman, A. M. (1982). Neurasthenia and depression: A study of somatization and culture in China. *Culture, Medicine, and Psychiatry, 6,* 117–189.

Lee, E. (1982). A social systems approach to assessment and treatment for Chinese American families. In M. McGoldrick, J. K. Pearce, & J. Giordano (Eds.), *Ethnicity and family therapy* (pp. 527–551). New York: Guilford Press.

Lee, E. (1989). Assessment and treatment of Chinese-American immigrant families. *Journal of Psychotherapy and the Family, 6*(1/2), 99–122.

Lee, E. (1990). Family therapy with Southeast Asian refugees. In M. P. Mirkin (Ed.),

The social and political contexts of family therapy (pp. 331–354). Needham Heights, MA: Allyn & Bacon.

Lin, K. M. (1986). Psychopathology and social disruption in refugees. In C. William & J. Westermeyer (Eds.), *Refugee mental health in resettlement countries* (pp. 61–73). Washington, DC: Hemisphere.

Lin, K. M., & Kleinman, A. (1981). Recent development of psychiatric epidemiology in China. *Culture, Medicine, and Psychiatry, 5,* 135–143.

Lin, T., & Lin, M. (1981). Love, denial and rejection: Responses of Chinese families to mental illness. In A. Kleinman & T. Lin (Eds.), *Normal and abnormal behavior in Chinese culture* (pp. 387–401). Dordrecht, The Netherlands: D. Reidel.

Marsella, A., Kinzie, D., & Gordon, P. (1973). Ethnic variations in the expression of depression. *Journal of Cross-Cultural Psychology, 4,* 435–458.

McGoldrick, M. (1988). *Genograms in family assessment.* New York: Norton.

Minuchin, S. (1974). *Families and family therapy.* Cambridge, MA: Harvard University Press.

Sue, D. W., & Sue, D. (1990). *Counseling the culturally different: Theory and practice* (2nd ed). New York: Wiley.

Sue, S., & Morishima, J. (1982). *The mental health of Asian Americans.* San Francisco: Jossey-Bass.

Sue, S., & Sue, D. W. (1974). MMPI comparisons between Asian American and non-Asian students utilizing a student health psychiatric clinic. *Journal of Counseling Psychology, 21,* 423–427.

Sung, B. L. (1967). *Mountains of gold.* New York: Macmillan.

Tseng, W. (1975). The nature of somatic complaints among psychiatric patients: The Chinese case. *Comparative Psychiatry, 16,* 237–245.

U.S. Bureau of the Census. (1990). *1990 census of population.* Washington, DC: U.S. Government Printing Office.

Wong, M. G. (1988). The Chinese American family. In C. H. Mandel, R. W. Habenstein, & R. Wright (Eds.), *Ethnic families in America* (3rd ed). New York: Elsevier Science.

Yap, P. M. (1958). Hypereridism and attempted suicide in Chinese. *Journal of Nervous and Mental Disease, 127,* 34–41.

Yu, E., Chang, C. F., Liu, W., & Fernandez, M. (1989). Suicide among Asian American youth. In M. Feinleib (Ed.), *Report of the Secretary's task force on youth suicide* (pp. 157–176). Washington, DC: U.S. Dept. of Health and Human Services.

4

East Indian American Families

SUDHA PRATHIKANTI

HISTORICAL BACKGROUND

The civilization of India dates back to 6500 B.C., with ancient and sophisticated traditions in medicine, astronomy, and the physical sciences, as well as in religion, philosophy, and the arts. The ancient people of India encoded and preserved their collective knowledge in a vast body of Sanskrit verses called the Vedas. In several regions throughout India, the study and practice of the original Vedic disciplines continue with remarkable integrity to this day. European colonials propagated the theory that the elaborate Vedic culture of India was a somewhat late historical development, brought to natives of the subcontinent by Aryan invaders from the north. However, scholars have now refuted the Aryan invasion theory as spurious, demonstrating both the antiquity and the indigenous origins of India's Vedic heritage (Talageri, 1993; Frawley, 1994; Rajaram, 1993; Misra, 1992).

For several millenia, the formidable Himalaya mountain range afforded little contact between the native people of India and other ethnic groups. However, by 2500 B.C., a flourishing sea trade had developed between India and the people of Persia and Mesopotamia (Thapar, 1966). The various kingdom-states of India became well-known for silk and spices, and many of India's technical advances in areas such as mathematics and medicine began to spread westward to Europe via Persia. India's enticing material and cultural wealth set the stage for a series of foreign conquests and colonizations of the subcontinent, beginning with Alexander of Macedon in 327 B.C. and later including invasions by the Mongols, the Muslims, the French, the Portugese, and the British (Basham, 1996). After centuries of colonization, India finally won its independence from Britain in 1947 and established itself as the world's largest democracy.

With historical influences from so many ethnic groups, the 800 million people of India today form a complex mosaic of cultures. Descendants of the original Vedic people came to be called Hindus, and they comprise the single largest religious–cultural group. However, India is also the birthplace of Buddhism, Jainism, and Sikhism, and over the centuries, it has been home to followers of Islam, Christianity, and Judaism. Tolerance for religious diversity has been the norm among the Hindu majority for centuries, although communal strife between religious groups has increased since independence. Hindi is the national language, but English and 14 major Indian languages are also spoken, along with hundreds of regional dialects. About 70% of India's people live in rural areas, while the rest of the population is concentrated in large urban centers. Centuries of British occupation with rampant exploitation of India's wealth exerted a devastating economic impact, and India's recovery in the post-independence era has been complicated by a burgeoning population. Modernization has been intense but unevenly distributed; for example, the Indian city of Bangalore has become a leading global producer of computer software, but many rural areas throughout India remain without adequate telephone access. As India approaches the 21st century, the challenges in addressing the needs of her large and diverse constituency are readily apparent.

MIGRATION TO THE UNITED STATES

People of East Indian origin first arrived in the United States in the middle to late 1800s and were mainly farmers settling in California (Chandrasekhar, 1982). However, these immigrants were greeted with open hostility by local American communities; antimiscegenation laws were quickly enacted against Indians, and they were not allowed to buy or own real estate or to become U.S. citizens (Takaki, 1989). In the face of such intense discrimination, most of the early Indian immigrants returned to India by the turn of the century, although a few stayed on in the United States and intermarried with local people of Mexican origin.

Between 1917 and 1965, federal immigration laws aimed against people of Asian origin made it either impossible or very difficult for Indians to settle in the United States (Arnold, Minocha, & Fawcett, 1987). The Immigration and Naturalization Act of 1965 finally ended racial discrimination in immigration policy; entry into the United States was to be determined not by race but by the skills the potential immigrant could offer. During the 1960s, the United States was involved in the Vietnam War and needed physicians, engineers, and other technical specialists. Thus, the second wave of Indians who entered the United States in the late 1960s and early 1970s was largely composed of young, well-educated, English-speaking physicians, scientists, and engineers (Chandrasekhar, 1982). These Indian professionals generally achieved financial success and most obtained U.S. citizenship.

Between 1980 and 1990, the number of Indians settling in the United States increased from 362,000 to 815,000 (U.S. Bureau of the Census, 1980; U.S. Bureau of the Census, 1990). Although many of the new arrivals continued to be highly educated in technical fields, there was an overall shift in demographics towards a less educationally elite Indian immigrant group. This demographic shift occurred during the 1980s as a large number of professionals from the second wave sponsored entry of their Indian relatives into the United States through the Family Reunification Act. The sponsored family members—the "third wave" of Indian immigrants—were generally not as well educated or technically oriented as their immediate predecessors (Passano, 1995). These newer immigrants tended to open small businesses or to enter vocational trades and do not have as much familiarity with the English language or with Western cultural practices. A cultural "chasm" may be developing between Indian immigrants of the second and third waves.

TRADITIONAL FAMILY ORGANIZATION AND VALUES

Despite the wide range of cultures present in India, Hindu values are pervasive and tend to inform many of the traditional structures of family and community life (Almeida, 1990; Bassa, 1978). In the Indian context, the concept of family does not usually connote a dyad of parents with their biological offspring, or even a multigenerational household. Instead, as noted by Das and Kemp (1997), family generally refers to a large, flexible, and fluid entity encompassing several households—households that may be scattered over different geographical regions but composed of members who think of themselves as one. A household may range in size from a single parent and child to a "joint family" with more than 20 people; yet, members of any given household tend to see themselves as part of a much larger kinship network that will assist with key educational, financial, or interpersonal decisions throughout the lifespan of the various members. For example, it is common for children to move between households to complete their schooling in a city remote from their parents' home. A young woman may move in with her aunt and uncle so that they can help her find a suitable marriage partner. An elderly widow in poor health may come to live in her great-nephew's household because of convenient access to a hospital. Das and Kemp (1997) note that "this fluidity and flexibility enable many families to be resilient in times of difficulty" (p. 25).

Although the extended Indian family may be relatively fluid in supporting and accommodating individuals from multiple households, clear-cut roles and norms govern interactions among its various members. Hindu culture emphasizes the sacredness of dharma, which is the living of life according to well-defined rules of right conduct (Basham, 1996). The traditional Hindu family is pervaded by an elaborate order and hierarchy in which variables such as age, gender, birth order, and marital status have tremendous salience in how individuals locate their psychic and behavioral "place" in family and community life (Kakar, 1978; Brown & Coelho, 1986). The dharma for each family member is defined explicitly by kinship ties as well as developmental stage in the life cycle. Traditionally, caste was also a significant factor in determining the vocation and community dharma adopted by an individual, but in modern-day India, education and economic class have generally replaced caste in influencing occupational and social roles (Krishnamurthy, 1989; Liddle & Joshi, 1986; Nandy, 1980)

In living a dharmic life, an individual ideally contributes to the smooth functioning of family and community; each person carries out a valued role and is interdependent on others to maintain the integrity of the societal unit as a whole. Sacrifice of individual wishes and desires is expected when these conflict with one's dharma within the family. Failure to make the appropriate sacrifice is viewed as bringing significant hardship—as well as shame and possible social ostracization—to the entire family. Family members collectively use guilt, shame, and a sense of moral obligation to bring the truant individual back to the dharma he or she may transiently abandon (Derne, 1995; Sodowsky, Kwan, & Pannu, 1995; Sue, 1981).

Exquisite attention is paid to fulfilling the dharma appropriate for a given time and place in one's life cycle. In the original Vedic tradition, the first quarter of one's life should be dedicated to study and moral development; in the second quarter, one should work, marry, and experience the joys and struggles of family life; in the third quarter, one begins to turn over family and vocational responsibilities to the next generation; the last quarter is dedicated to spiritual inquiry and contemplation (Basham, 1996). Within this developmental framework, the goal of the first three stages is to achieve a stable and emotionally mature ego; in the final stage, one moves beyond identification with the individual ego and seeks union with the *atma,* or universal self. In practice, older people may often have difficulty with the task of relinquishing control to the next generation (Das & Kemp, 1997) and may not feel ready to focus primarily on spiritual pursuits. Nevertheless, elders often seek to integrate the spiritual with the material in their life activities, and to set an example of this balance for the younger generation. The Vedas do not exclude women from this four-stage developmental process, but historically, these stages were applied primarily to men. Women's developmental process was often seen as an evolution from daughter to wife to mother (Madan, 1987; Pandey, 1991). Throughout India's history, however, there are many notable examples of women who chose to renounce their family relationships and become spiritual seekers in the original Vedic tradition (Ramanujan, 1982; Ramakrishna Vedanta Centre, 1972).

Complex and well-defined rituals mark the various milestones of one's life, from the moment of birth into marriage, parenthood, loss of loved ones, and impending death (Basham, 1996; Madan, 1987). These rituals reinforce the notion of an orderly progression through life, with family and community members actively involved in helping the individual make important transitions to a new developmental phase.

Among Indian families, marriage is seen as the permanent alliance of two families, not merely the union of two individuals. For this reason, the choice of marriage partner is largely left to elders in the family, and most marriages are arranged (Bumiller, 1990; Liddle & Joshi, 1986). Although young people today have the opportunity to meet their future partner on a few occasions prior to the marriage, these meetings often take place in the company of other family members. Dating and courtship in the Western style are not permitted, and premarital sexual activity is strongly prohibited, particularly for young women (Saran, 1985). Even after marriage, public displays of affection between husband and wife are infrequent, and it is much more common to observe men and women in affectionate physical contact with friends and family of their own gender (Jayakar, 1994). Divorce tends to be rare in India, although this is changing slowly with increasing urbanization and more options for women's economic independence outside marriage.

In most regions of India, people traditionally follow a patrilocal pattern of family residence (Das & Kemp, 1997). When a woman marries, she leaves her natal family and moves into her husband's household; this household may include the husband's parents, any unmarried sisters, and his brothers and their spouses. In addition, it is common to find in the household an elderly relative or two: perhaps a grandparent or a widowed great-aunt. Within the family hierarchy, the eldest male is generally invested with the authority to make final decisions affecting the educational, financial, or interpersonal lives of the various household members (Derne, 1995; Ananth & Ananth, 1996). For example, he may decide on the future career for his daughter, the timing of his son's marriage, or the amount to spend on building a new home. His wife often carries the most weight in making decisions that involve the day-to-day operations of the household and the duties assigned to each member, particularly to any daughters or daughters-in-law. If the family patriarch dies, his eldest son technically assumes his responsibilities; in practice, however, the surviving widow often becomes invested with considerable power, consulting on and approving any major decisions facing the family.

In day-to-day family life, open expression of conflict is not the norm between household members (Ananth & Ananth, 1996). A direct display of anger may be equated with a shameful lack of patience and self-control. More often, disagreement and unhappiness are communicated by an individual's subdued behavior and demeanor. Elders in the family then mediate between the two people in conflict, encouraging each person to adjust and accommodate to the other's differences rather than trying to effect a major change in the situation. Most household members are quite reticent to discuss their family conflicts with "outsiders," but among the members of a given household, there are few secrets or strictly private conversations (Das & Kemp, 1997). Possessions are frequently shared by multiple members, and it is unusual for children to have their own rooms. Unannounced visits between family members living in different households constitute the norm and can occur at any hour of the day. In many Indian families, the attitude towards privacy and personal space is exemplified by the following custom: The main door to the household is generally closed from the outside world, but doors within the family home are almost always kept open.

In a multigenerational household, it is common for grandparents or aunts and uncles to have as much input in childrearing as the parents. Young children within a joint family typically enjoy great freedom and are much indulged by their elders. They are rarely punished for pranks and misbehavior, and they are fed, comforted, and played with on demand (Das & Kemp, 1997). They are generally taught by example rather than by explicit instruction, and the emphasis is on making the child aware of social roles rather than to master sensorimotor tasks or to discover unique talents and personality traits (Ananth & Ananth, 1996). By school age, children are expected to show a considerable degree of focus and self-discipline, and the willfulness of their early years is no longer tolerated (Roland, 1989). The dharma of a child is to respect, learn from, and defer to authority figures such as parents and teachers. Children's love for family members often becomes measured by their obedience to elders. Disobedience is perceived as a rejection of both dharma and familial affection, resulting in considerable shame, hurt, and perhaps bewilderment on the part of parents and other elders.

Male children tend to enjoy more attention and privilege than their sisters, particularly as they grow older (Bumiller, 1990; Mitter, 1991). Within the patrilineal tradition of most Indian families, it is male children who ensure continuity of the family name and blood line. Male children are also expected to provide for their aging parents and to perform important religious rituals on the family's behalf, including the symbolically significant last funeral rites for their parents. In addition, when a son marries, the bride's dowry comes to his family, thereby increasing the family's resources. Clearly, this patriarchal social structure creates a bias toward sons, and female child neglect, selective abortion of female fetuses, and even female infanticide have been reported. (Skultans, 1991; Kristof, 1991; Singh, 1990; Bumiller, 1990; Krishnaswamy, 1988; Patel, 1988).

Nevertheless, daughters in the majority of Indian families are well loved and well cared for, frequently enjoying very close relationships with their natal families even after marriage. However, girls often contend with more household responsibilities and more discipline for misbehavior than do their brothers (Das & Kemp, 1997; Mitter, 1991). A girl's future "marketability" as a wife and daughter-in-law will be strongly linked to her decorum and her capacity for caretaking activities in her husband's household, even though she may be well educated with a professional career. In most households, a young wife tends to gain more status once she becomes a mother—particularly if her child is a son; she may not have access to the same power as male members of the family, but she is honored in her role as a mother (Ibrahim, Ohnishi, & Sandhu, 1997). The freedom and authority accorded to women in a given household vary considerably according to the education and socioeconomic class of the family, as well as the regional customs. In more urbanized and educated families, as well as in a few matrilocal and matrilineal families in South India, decision-making power may be shared between the genders in a relatively egalitarian manner.

Whereas Indian women may be circumscribed to relatively narrow roles within the domestic sphere, a significant number have enjoyed a remarkable degree of power and equality in other arenas of life. Since 1947, the number of women physicians in India has been virtually equal to the number of men in most medical specialties (Jayakar, 1994); this occurred long before the class action lawsuits of the 1970s resulted in a gradual increase in women medical students in the United States. Women lawyers in India have long argued cases in both civil and criminal courts, and there is an illustrious legacy of female social activism over the last two centuries of Indian history (Kumar, 1993). In India, a strong and capable woman was the head of government well before England could make a similar claim, and even today, the number of prominent women political leaders in India outnumber their counterparts in the United States. In addition, Hindu conceptualization of the divine feminine and the widespread worship of female deities— particularly the awesome figure of Durgakali—have a profound influence on the Indian psyche. As noted by Kakar (1978), the impact of religious myth in India "cannot be underestimated," and there are striking examples of how female deities such as Durgakali have been used to effect enormous social change in the Indian political landscape (Kumar, 1993).

It is important to note that many of the traditional patterns of family life described earlier are changing dramatically with increasing urbanization in India and the development of an affluent middle class (Anant, Rao, & Kapoor, 1986; Bassa, 1978). Although rural families often continue to function in the traditional manner, many urban dwellers are in transition to other models of family life. For example, urbanites may retain traditional family values of self-sacrifice and respect for elders but may choose more flexible gender roles and a more Western-style nuclear household. Historically, the Indian people have demonstrated a remarkable capacity to absorb large-scale demographic and sociopolitical changes while retaining a core set of ideological constructs.

EFFECTS OF CULTURAL TRANSITION ON THE FAMILY SYSTEM

Indian families coming to the United States respond variably to the challenges of acculturation, influenced by such factors as preimmigration socioeconomic and educational status, motivations for leaving their native country, marketable skills, degree of support from extended family in the United States, and the degree of hostility or acceptance they encounter in the new environment (Brody, 1973). As noted earlier, most of the second wave of Indian immigrants came from relatively elite professional backgrounds, having a preexisting familiarity with English and some exposure to Western cultural practices. These individuals emigrated to the United States to maximize their educational and economic opportunities, and they have tended to adopt selectively sociocultural norms of the U.S. culture that facilitate the attainment of their goals.

For example, Ibrahim et al. (1997) note that South Asian culture traditionally values a modest, self-effacing personality; the more accomplished one is, the more humbly one is expected to behave. Public recitation of one's own merits is considered shameful, so one depends on others in the community to attest to his or her virtues. Unfortunately, U.S. employers and supervisors can misperceive this humble attitude as a reflection of mediocrity or low self-worth, and a highly accomplished Indian immigrant may be denied promotion or may be seen as an ineffective worker. Thus, most Indian professionals have learned to adopt the dress, etiquette, and confident, extroverted manner of their colleagues in the workplace so that appropriate advancement will follow. Yet, they tend to retain the food preferences, family values, and religious ideology of their native culture (Sodowsky & Carey, 1988). Indian women professionals seem especially adept at changing their dress, behavior, and demeanor to adjust to the environment of the workplace versus the family home (Saran, 1985; Sethi & Allen, 1984). Although this sort of "cultural switching" might be adaptive up to a certain point (Chin, 1994), it may also pose a major psychological strain for some Indian American women (Ramu, 1988; Mandelbaum, 1986).

In addition to the selective adoption of new cultural behaviors in the workplace, immigrant Indians may also exhibit considerable change in certain traditional behaviors within the household. Indian families living in North America may show an increase in mutual decision making between husbands and wives, and children may be allowed more input regarding their career decisions (Siddique, 1977; Lessinger, 1995). Sodowsky et al. (1995) note a reduction in certain gender-specific cultural behaviors among Indian American families; for example, wives may be much more involved in banking and other extrahousehold financial matters that were traditionally left to their husbands. Some of these external behaviors may be amenable to change because of pragmatic realities, such as the time restrictions of a husband's job or a child's increased knowledge about the U.S. educational system. However, core values in areas such as religious ideology or sexuality may be much more resistant to change (Wakil, Siddique, & Wakil, 1981; Sodowsky et al., 1995).

In general, families from the second wave have experienced relative success in the United States vis-à-vis economic and occupational measures. Yet, these immigrant families may often remain vigilant to the actual and potential discrimination against them as a visible ethnic minority (Hutnik, 1986; Jiobu, 1988). Social ease in a dominant white culture may be difficult to achieve due to their recollection of being a colonized people in British-ruled India as well as being a marginalized and oppressed immigrant group in other countries of the former British Commonwealth. In the past decade, several incidents of racially motivated assaults and vandalism against East Indians have been documented in the United States (U.S. Commission on Civil Rights, 1992; Lee, 1991). In facing external adversity such as racism, the powerful bonds of affection and loyalty found in the traditional Indian family can be a source of great emotional strength and support to its members. In addition, religious concepts such as karma and destiny can sometimes be very helpful in dealing with external adversity; within this framework, "certain challenges are simply preordained and must be handled appropriately" (Ibrahim et al., 1997, p. 45), and individuals are unlikely to internalize blame for a situation such as a racist attack. However, this same asset can become a liability if appropriate actions to safeguard the vulnerable family member do not ensue.

The more recent third wave of Indian immigrants came to this country primarily to be reunified with extended family members. These newer immigrants may not be as well educated as their predecessors

(Passano, 1995) and may be less likely to speak fluent English, to pursue ambitious technical careers, or to socialize with members of the dominant white culture. Clearly, the acculturation issues and adaptation process confronting an immigrant of the third wave would be significantly different from those a second-wave immigrant might experience. On the one hand, the presence of a preexisting kinship network in the new country may lessen the emotional distress associated with migration. On the other hand, less familiarity with English and Western cultural norms may lead to increasing insulation from the mainstream environment and an over-reliance on more acculturated family members for negotiating even the most basic tasks in the outside world. Ananth and Ananth (1996) point out the special vulnerability of elderly individuals in this immigrant group: To join their children in the United States, older adults may give up a familiar and cherished place in their native communities only to feel overwhelmed by the lack of useful roles or dignity for elders in the new culture.

Within a given Indian American family, emotional difficulties can arise because of the discrepant acculturation of its various members (Sodowsky et al., 1996). For example, first-generation Indian parents who came to the United States in the 1960s may strongly endorse high academic achievement for their children and the pursuit of a professional career; in their experience, this will provide the most financial security and serve as a buffer against some of the more extreme forms of discrimination experienced by people of color in a dominant white culture. In addition, these parents may want their adolescent children to refrain from dating because they fear that dating will lead to premarital sexual activity or to loss of cultural identity through interethnic marriage. In contrast, their second-generation daughter may feel more secure than the parents about her place in the dominant culture; therefore, she may resent the constant push toward medical school because she wants to explore her potential as a musician. She may not understand her parents' fears about adolescent sexuality or interethnic romantic relationships and feels aggrieved when she cannot date or go to dances like other girls in her high school.

Table 4.1 illustrates several attitudes about family life that may become the focus for conflict in an Indian American household because of differences in acculturation between older and younger members.

Members of the household may attribute their conflict to a "generation gap," although the discord might be more representative of an "acculturation gap." In the context of intrafamilial cultural conflict, some Indian American parents may adopt a more rigid and conservative stance in enforcing the values of the native culture (Jayakar, 1994); their children may respond with an increase in provocative acting-out behaviors. Sodowsky et al. (1996) suggest that parents who apply excessive pressure and

TABLE 4.1. Values Orientation in the Indian American Family

First generation	Second generation
1. Expectation of self-sacrifice for good of the family	1. Expectation of family assisting in self-actualization
2. Authoritarian and hierarchical decision making	2. Endorse democratic decision making
3. Elders accorded more respect than their juniors	3. Idealization of youth/subtle devaluation of old age
4. Males accorded more overt authority than females	4. Endorse little difference in authority based on gender
5. Expectation of filial piety and obedience	5. Expectation of separation and autonomy from parents
6. Indirect expression of anger as the norm	6. Direct expression of anger as the norm
7. Accommodation and tolerance in face of conflict	7. Confrontation and negotiation in face of conflict
8. Emphasis on academic achievement/professional career	8. Exploration of career options based on interests/talents
9. Little emphasis on sports/extracurricular activities	9. Emphasis on becoming well-rounded person
10. Modesty in dress with limited exposure of body parts	10. Comfortable with displaying body in public
11. Few open displays of heterosexual affection	11. Comfortable with open displays of heterosexual affection
12. Discouragement of dating/adolescent sexual expression	12. Acceptance of dating/adolescent sexual expression
13. Expectation of arranged marriage within same ethnic group	13. Selection of own mate/acceptance of interethnic marriage
14. Importance of preserving religious/ethnic identity	14. Importance of creating multicultural identity

Note. Adapted from Juthani (1990).

restrictions on children in the hope of strengthening Indian identity may actually drive the children away from their native culture. The few studies examining family environment and ethnic identity seem to indicate that feelings of ethnic pride are more likely to emerge in families marked by warmth and independence (Rosenthal & Feldman, 1992), and that supportive family relations may be an important prerequisite for minority youth to explore their cultures of origin (Phinney & Chivera, 1992).

Some Indian parents first emigrating to the United States in the 1960s and 1970s may have been overly anxious to have their children assimilate into the new culture. They may have believed that rapid assimilation would result in less discrimination and rejection of their children in school and the mainstream environment. As a result, their children may have grown up with little knowledge of the history, language, religious customs, or kinship traditions of their native culture. A few families may even refuse to identify Indians as people of color, and their children may claim that they are white. Yet, by the time their children reach college age, some of these parents may start regretting the loss of ethnic identity. As the parents contemplate the impending marriages of their children to non-Indians or the notion of growing old in America without the traditional family support structure, they may begin a zealous campaign to reclaim the family's Indian identity. Unfortunately, this often results in confusing and internally dissonant experiences for their sons and daughters. Young adult children may suddenly be asked to attend religious functions at the temple or to begin dating only Indians. In some extreme cases, parents may even insist that the children return to India for a time so that they can "become Indian again" and perhaps come back with an Indian spouse. Adolescent girls and young women seem particularly vulnerable to coercive tactics on the part of their families, perhaps because Indian females are seen as the primary transmitters of culture from one generation to the next.

First- and second-generation Indian American women increasingly report domestic violence within their marriages to men of the same ethnicity (Maitri, 1997; Passano, 1995; Manavi, 1992). It is not yet clear whether the rate of domestic violence occuring in the Indian American community is similar to the 7% overall prevalence rate of domestic violence in the United States (Violence against Women Act, 1990). It is common practice for Indian American men to have arranged marriages in India and then return to the United States with their new brides (Gupta, 1991; Luthra, 1989; Saran, 1985). The perception is that an Indian-born and -raised woman is more likely to adapt and make compromises in the husband's family. For the subgroup of these Indian immigrant brides who encounter domestic violence within their new households, loss of access to the natal family in India appears to exacerbate the mistreatment and emotional difficulties they endure. It is common for multiple family members in the husband's household to be involved in the emotional and physical abuse of these young women. The husband and in-laws in the United States might threaten a woman with the shame of divorce or deportation to make her comply with their demands. Despite the fact that divorce is commonplace in the dominant U.S. culture, it still carries a heavy stigma for women in Indian American communities.

Patel and Gaw (1996) reviewed the literature on suicide among immigrants from the Indian subcontinent. They did not find any studies originating in the United States; most of the studies were conducted with Indian immigrants in Great Britain, South Africa, Fiji, Singapore, and Malaysia. The authors found that suicide rates of young women immigrants were consistently higher than those of their male counterparts; moreover, the suicide rates of these immigrant women were higher than those of their female counterparts on the Indian subcontinent. Family conflict with the in-laws appeared to be a major predisposing factor in many suicides, and the authors cite domestic violence, depression, and anxiety as probable contributors to the high rates of suicide in this population. It is unclear whether these results can be extrapolated to the Indian immigrant population in the United States; however, they suggest that investigation of psychological difficulties in young Indian American women may be especially warranted.

CLINICAL CONSIDERATIONS AND TREATMENT STRATEGIES

Within Ayurvedic medicine and other indigenous healing traditions of India, the psyche does not appear as a discrete entity whose health or injury results in the individual's emotional well-being or distress. In the Ayurvedic framework, a person simultaneously exists as a physical body, a reincarnating soul, and a social being invested with a particular dharma; the sense of emotional distress is viewed as a manifestation of disturbance within *any* of these three realms (Kakar, 1982). Moreover, disturbance in one realm of being simultaneously affects functioning within the other two realms. The person is always a whole, an integrated being whose overall balance of humors is adversely affected by disruption in any one realm. Thus, psychological distress or mental illness is primarily a reflection of the overall imbalance in humors.

In the Ayurvedic tradition, there have never been treatments designed to address mental illness as a phenomenon distinct from the underlying three aspects of being. Mental illness is largely a signal of humoral imbalance stemming from physical illness, social disruptions, or karmic tendencies of the reincarnating soul. The remedies for humoral imbalance involve prayers, purification rituals, soothing ointments, dietary instructions, and behavioral changes; the remedies are designed to mitigate karmic influences and restore harmony to the suffering person's physical body and relational matrix (Kakar, 1982). Because of the interrelated nature of body, soul, and social being, treatment within any one realm can have restorative effects on the other two, regardless of the realm in which the primary disruption occurred. As humors are brought back to balance, the person's overall functioning and emotional well-being are restored.

Ayurvedic concepts have subtly but profoundly influenced the ways in which many people in India tend to present psychological problems (Obeyesekere, 1977). For example, it is easier to comprehend why so many patients seem to "displace" their emotional pain into somatic complaints or into complaints about extrapsychic structures such as destiny or family dharma. After all, Ayurveda views psychological difficulties as a manifestation of disruption in the body, the transmigrating soul, or the fulfillment of social duties. Within this framework, the exploration of one's intrapsychic conflicts or the reconstruction of distant childhood memories may appear irrelevant or decidedly odd. In addition, descriptions of the family system that appear to assign personal blame to family elders may be quite ego-dystonic. Instead, distressed individuals may find it more ego-syntonic to frame family conflicts as failures to perform expected duties or obligations.

In addition to Ayurvedic physicians, numerous other indigenous healers are available to people in India experiencing psychological problems (Kakar, 1982). Various gurus and mystics specialize in restoring moral and spiritual well-being to the suffering individual. Also, the therapeutic efforts of innumerable palmists, herbalists, and diviners combine elements from classical Indian astrology with folk beliefs and magic; many of these practitioners may attempt to address the karmic influences impacting on the person in distress. As Kakar (1982) points out, the role of the sacred is prominent in all the healing traditions of India; it is the sacred that links Ayurveda's concern with the wholeness of the person and the guru's concern with the abandonment of dharma and the palmist's concern with the machinations of karma. The disappearance of the sacred from Western healing sciences, including psychiatry and psychotherapy, might contribute to the attitudes of distrust and alienation with which many Indian people (especially rural dwellers) react to these disciplines.

When experiencing psychological distress, the help-seeking behavior of people in India varies considerably with degree of education and urbanization. In a rural or less-educated population, the distressed person or family may turn to local shamans, priests, or elders in the community. In a more educated or urbanized population, distressed individuals may turn primarily to physicians or to extended family members for support. In more recent years, it is gradually becoming more acceptable for urbanites to seek help from Western-trained mental health professionals.

Among Indian Americans in the United States, large numbers of medical professionals have information about—and access to—mental health services. Yet, as a group, Indian Americans tend to underutilize mental health services. The following factors may keep Indian American families from seeking psychotherapy or counseling (Das & Kemp, 1997; Jayakar, 1994):

1. There are strong cultural prohibitions against revealing interpersonal conflicts to anyone outside the family. Disclosures about mental illness or emotional "instability" are seen as bringing particular shame and stigma to the entire family.
2. The family may not wish to undermine the myth of the "model minority," which many members of the dominant culture apply to Indian Americans. In general, Indian American families may

fear that the entire ethnic group will suffer if their problems come to light.

3. There may be dissonance with standard psychotherapeutic goals of separation and individuation from primary attachment figures. Family members may be reluctant to sacrifice group obligations and loyalty to further individual interests.

When members of Indian American families do seek help for their emotional distress, their clinical presentations may include some of the following features (Ananth & Ananth, 1996; Jayakar, 1994; Guzder & Krishna, 1991; Dasgupta, 1986):

1. Multiple somatic complaints, which may lead them to medical doctors rather than a psychotherapist. Conversion disorders are not uncommon but are not as prevalent as in the population in India.

2. Attribution of illness to multiple external factors, which can range from economic difficulties to supernatural/karmic forces. Family members may believe that the solution to mental illness lies in changing jobs, moving to another city, or even getting married.

3. Severe depressions and psychotic states, which may result from individuals being sheltered in the family home until the most extreme decompensations have occurred.

4. Controlled emotional expression, which may be mistaken for anhedonia or the emotional blunting of schizophrenia.

5. Difficulty in elaborating on incidents from childhood. Phrases such as "good mother" or "normal childhood" might be the only descriptions given. There may be a great deal of skepticism about the relevance of childhood issues to current dilemmas and a reluctance to assign blame to elders.

6. Extreme reticence in addressing any sexual concerns, including sexual orientation, knowledge of sexual facts, acknowledgment of erotic feelings, or history of sexual abuse. The taboo against discussing sexual matters is especially strong for women, who may be labeled as "loose" because of such dialogues.

7. Marital difficulties due to enmeshed relationships between mothers and their adult sons. Close bonds between a husband and his mother/family of origin often take precedence over the bond between a husband and wife. A wife's intimacy needs are expected to be fulfilled though her own children, especially her son, rather than her husband.

8. Vulnerability of a wife to mistreatment from her mother-in-law. In the traditional household, the mother-in-law is culturally

sanctioned to have enormous control over the daughter-in-law's duties and behavior.

9. Ambivalence and depression/anxiety among Indian American women regarding retention of traditional gender roles and behaviors within the family.

10. Struggles between parents who want to prevent their children from becoming too "Americanized" and children who respond with acting-out behaviors or depression and social withdrawal.

11. Extreme feelings of failure and anxiety when faced with academic disappointments or inability to establish a certain kind of career. The dejection of the unsuccessful family member may become magnified to an intolerable level if the family experiences the situation as a catastrophic injury to the group as a whole.

12. Social isolation and extreme helplessness in functioning in the mainstream environment. This tends to occur with elderly parents who are reunified with adult children in the United States as well as with young brides from India who have recently married Indian American men. These immigrants are especially vulnerable to neglect and abuse in their new households.

13. Fear, frustration, or helplessness in the face of personal or institutional racism. Young school-age children and traditionally attired immigrants are particularly vulnerable targets for racially motivated personal assaults, whereas middle-class professionals may be confronted with more subtle institutional racism.

Many Indian Americans express a preference for a mental health professional of the same ethnicity (Ananth & Ananth, 1996; Jayakar, 1994). They may feel that a clinician of Indian origin will better understand the importance of their family and cultural values. However, a few Indian Americans may deliberately avoid a clinician of the same ethnicity out of a fear that the larger Indian community may learn of their family's problems. Family members' expectations for treatment vary considerably according to the education, age, and acculturation level of the individual. Members of the younger generation may feel quite comfortable with an open-ended, collaborative approach on the clinician's part. However, older members of the family may view such a therapeutic approach as a reflection of incompetence because they may expect a more directive style in which specific instructions are given and a clear-cut end point to the therapy is apparent. Problems may arise if a therapist wishes to speak with individual members in private; family cohesion may feel threatened and occasionally members may insist that individual sessions are "unnecessary" because there are no "secrets" between them. Awkwardness may be created if the therapist emphasizes that every member's point of view is to be equally weighted in understanding the conflict the family is having;

this may fly in the face of the older generation's belief that the opinion of elders should count for more. In addition, the age and gender of the mental health provider may have a significant impact on the progress of therapy: Some of the older men may have a difficult time accepting suggestions from a younger woman clinician. Once the treatment alliance is established, however, many older individuals may show exceptional adherence to the clinician's recommendations, particularly with respect to any medications and somatic treatments.

When working with Indian American families, the clinician may find the following suggestions useful (Ibrahim et al., 1997; Ananth & Ananth, 1996; Jayakar, 1994):

1. Communicate respect for the family and for the culture, taking the initiative to learn something of the migration history and socioeconomic variables affecting the family's specific ethnic subgroup in the Indian American community. This knowledge can be gained by consulting with South Asian colleagues and by independent reading, as well as by direct and respectful questions during therapy sessions with the family.

2. Have a clear understanding of the different levels of acculturation present among the various family members before planning any interventions. Outward signs of acculturation (adoption of Western dress, manners, speech patterns) may coexist with significant retention of traditional values and behaviors within the family system.

3. Recognize the importance of age, gender, and life stage in evaluating each family member's expectations of himself or herself within the family system. As the counselor becomes aware of these expectations, he or she should verbalize that awareness to family members, helping them to feel that their cultural norms are being understood. This may be particularly helpful for adolescents and young adults negotiating conflict between the developmental tasks of their peer group in the mainstream culture and the traditional roles they may be expected to play within their families.

4. Clarify the spiritual identity of different family members before deciding on the goals and outcome of therapy. For many Indian Americans, a major source of anxiety involves keeping a balance between spiritual/religious ideals and certain interpersonal or occupational choices important for individual ego development. However, this anxiety may often be unconscious, in which case the clinician should make direct explanations to the family about how their behaviors and verbalized thoughts appear to indicate a dilemma.

5. Respect the individualism *and* communal identity of each family member, recognizing that family members are simultaneously concerned with personal development as well as relational ties.

6. Intrafamilial conflict around the traditional distribution of power and the traditional patterns of alliance may require diplomatic and carefully executed shifts in family structure for the tension to resolve. The marital dyad often needs to be strengthened while paradoxically acknowledging the importance of the mother-in-law; the mother's authority may need to be increased while allowing the father to feel indispensable in decision making; parental empathy and pride toward a daughter may need to be encouraged while praising the son.

7. Recognize the role of humility in the cultural identity of various family members. Do not confuse poor self-esteem with the culturally normative attitude of downplaying one's accomplishments in a group setting.

8. Pay close attention to nonverbal attitudes which may be communicated to the family in subtle nuances of gesture, posture, and demeanor. In South Asian cultures, nonverbal messages are often given more credence than verbal ones.

9. Use a relational, interactive style with the family in exploring their bicultural experiences and value systems. An impassive, silent demeanor on the therapist's part will not be effective in having family members reveal their conflicts and anxieties, and may even be mistaken for incompetence.

10. Multidimensional interventions may be more helpful than psychodynamic psychotherapy alone. For example, consider role-playing or guided imagery to bring up repressed feelings, and consider cognitive-behavioral techniques for coping with painful affects. Consider integrating traditional cultural practices such as meditation into the "homework" assigned to the family between sessions.

SUMMARY

"Being in their place is what makes [things] sacred," said anthropologist Claude Lévi-Strauss (1966, p. 10), and in India, secular existence becomes sacred when one is acting in harmony with one's dharmic place in the social order. Family life is permeated with attention to well-defined kinship roles and hierarchical structures, allowing for maximum stability and cohesion of the family unit from generation to generation. For Indian Americans, the traditional family structure can be a source of both strength and conflict as family members adapt to the environment of the dominant U.S. culture. Women and adolescents may be especially vulnerable to intrapsychic and intrafamilial tensions stemming from bicultural adaptations. Western mental health disciplines tend to emphasize a need for family members to separate and individuate from primary attachment figures, but several authors conclude that these treatment goals may not be as applicable in the Indian sociocultural context (Kakar, 1989; Ramanujan, 1983; Carstairs & Kapur, 1976). Effective therapeutic work with Indian American families requires a sensitivity to spiritual embedding, hierarchical organization, and interdependency issues transformed over the life cycle.

REFERENCES

Almeida, R. V. (1990). Asian American Mothers. *Journal of Feminist Family Therapy* (Special Issue), 33–40.

Anant, S., Rao, S. V. R., & Kapoor, K. (1986). *Women at work in India.* New Delhi: Sage.

Ananth, J., & Ananth, K. (1996). *East Indian immigrants to the United States: Life cycle issues and adjustment.* East Meadow: Indo-American Psychiatric Association.

Arnold, F., Minocha, U., & Fawcett, J. (1987). The changing face of Asian immigration to the United States. In J. Fawcett & B. Carino (Eds.), *Pacific brides: The new immigration from Asian and the Pacific Islands* (pp. 105–152). Staten Island: Center for Migration Studies.

Basham, A. L. (1996). *The wonder that was India.* Calcutta: Rupa.

Bassa, D. M. (1978). From the traditional to the modern: Some observations on changes in Indian child-rearing and parental attitudes. In E. J. Anthony & C. Chiland (Eds.), *The child in his family: Children and their parents in a changing world* (pp. 333–334). New York: Wiley.

Brody, E. B. (1973). *The first ones.* New York: New York International University Press.

Brown, R. H., & Coelho, G. V. (1986). *Tradition and transformation: Asian Indians in America.* Williamsburg, VA: College of William and Mary Press.

Bumiller, E. (1990). *May you be the mother of a hundred sons: A journey among the women of India.* New York: Random House.

Carstairs, G. M., & Kapur, R. L. (1976). *The great universe of Kota.* Toronto: Clarke Irwin.

Chandrasekhar, S. (1982). *From India to America: A brief history of immigration, problems of discrimination, admission and assimilation.* La Jolla, CA: Population Review.

Chin, J. L. (1994). Psychodynamic approaches. In L. Comas-Díaz & B. Greene (Eds.), *Women of color: Integrating ethnic and gender identities in psychotherapy* (pp. 194–222). New York: Guilford Press.

Das, A. K., & Kemp, S. F. (1997). Between two worlds: Counseling South Asian Americans. *Journal of Multicultural Counseling and Development, 25*(1), 23–33.

Dasgupta, S. D. (1986). Marching to a different drummer? Sex roles of Asian Indian women in the United States. *Women and Therapy, 5*(2–3), 297–311.

Derne, S. (1995). *Culture in action: Family life, emotion, and male dominance in Banaras, India.* Albany: State University of New York Press.

Frawley, D. (1994). *The myth of the Aryan invasion of India.* New Delhi: Voice of India.

Gupta, U. (1991, June/July). Out of India. *New York Woman,* pp. 46–47.

Guzder, J., & Krishna, M. (1991). Sita-Shakti: Cultural paradigms for Indian women. *Transcultural Psychiatry Research Review, 28,* 257–301.

Hutnik, N. (1986). Patterns of ethnic minority identification and modes of social adaptation. *Ethnic and Racial Studies, 9*(2), 150–167.

Ibrahim, F., Ohnishi, H., & Sandhu, D. S. (1997). Asian American identity development: A culture specific model for South Asian Americans. *Journal of Multicultural Counseling and Development, 25*(1), 34–50.

Jayakar, K. (1994). Women of the Indian subcontinent. In L. Comas-Díaz & B. Greene (Eds.), *Women of color: Integrating ethnic and gender identities in psychotherapy. (pp. 161–181). New York: Guilford Press.*

Jiobu, R. M. (1988). *Ethnicity and assimilation.* Albany: State University of New York Press.

Juthani, N. (1990). *Differences between Indian and American families.* Paper presented at the Scientific Meeting of the Indo-American Psychiatric Association, Washington, DC.

Kakar, S. (1978). *The inner world: A psycholanalytic study of childhood and society in India.* Delhi: Oxford University Press.

Kakar, S. (1982). *Shamans, mystics and doctors.* Delhi: Oxford University Press.

Kakar, S. (1989). *Intimate relations: Exploring Indian sexuality.* New Delhi: Viking Press.

Krishnamurthy, J. (Ed.). (1989). *Women in colonial India: Essays on survival, work, and the state.* Delhi: Oxford University Press.

Krishnaswamy, S. (1988). Female infanticide in contemporary India: A case study of the Kallars of Tamilnadu. In R. Ghadially (Ed.), *Women in Indian society* (pp. 186–195). New Delhi: Sage.

Kristof, N. D. (1991, November 5). Stark Data on Women: 100 million are missing. *New York Times,* pp. C1, C12.

Kumar, R. (1993). *The history of doing: An illustrated account of movements for women's rights and feminism in India, 1800–1990.* New Delhi: Kali for Women.

Lee, J. F. J. (1991). *Asian American experiences in the United States.* Jefferson, NC: McFarland.

Lessinger, J. (1995). *From the Ganges to the Hudson: Indian immigrants in New York City.* Boston: Allyn & Bacon

Lévi-Strauss, C. (1966). *The savage mind.* Chicago: University of Chicago Press.

Liddle, J., & Joshi, R. (1986). *Daughters of independence: Gender, caste and class in India.* London: Zed Books.

Luthra, R. (1989). Matchmaking in the classifieds of the Indian immigrant press. In Asian Women United of California (Eds.), *Making waves: An anthology of writings by and about Asian American women* (p. 344). Boston: Beacon Press.

Madan, T. N. (1987). *Non-renunciation: Themes and interpretations of Hindu culture.* New Delhi: Oxford University Press.

Maitri. (1997). *The Maitri Quarterly, 2*(2), 2.

Manavi. (1992). *Newsletter: An Organization for South Asian Women, 4*(1), 1.

Mandelbaum, D. G. (1986). *Women's seduction and men's honor: Sex roles in North India, Bangladesh, and Pakistan.* Tuscon: University of Arizona Press.

Misra, S. S. (1992). *The Aryan problem: A linguistic approach.* New Delhi: Munshiram Manoharlal.

Mitter, S. S. (1991). *Dharma's daughters.* New Brunswick, NJ: Rutgers University Press.

Nandy, A. (1980). Women versus womanliness in India: An essay in social and political psychology. In R. Ghadially (Ed.), *Women in Indian society* (pp. 69–80). New Delhi: Sage.

Obeyesekere, G. (1977). The theory and practice of psychological medicine in the Ayurvedic tradition. *Culture, Medicine and Psychiatry, 1,* 155.

Pandey, B. N. (1991). *A book of India.* Calcutta: Rupa.

Passano, P. (1995). Taking care of one's own: A conversation with Shamita Das Dasgupta. *Manushi Magazine, 89,* 17–26.

Patel, S. P., & Gaw, A. C. (1996). Suicide among immigrants from the Indian subcontinent: A review. *Psychiatric Services, 47*(5), 517–521.

Patel, V. (1988). Sex determination and sex preselection tests: Abuse of advanced technology. In R. Ghadially (Ed.), *Women in Indian society* (pp. 178–185). New Delhi: Sage.

Phinney, J. S., & Chivera, V. (1992). Ethnic identity and self-esteem: An exploratory longitudinal study. *Journal of Adolescence, 15,* 271–281.

Rajaram, N. S. (1993). *Aryan invasion of India: The myth and the truth.* New Delhi: Voice of India.

Ramakrishna Vedanta Centre. (1972). *Women saints of East and West.* London: Author.

Ramanujan, A. K. (1982). On women saints. In J. S. Hawley & D. M. Wulff (Eds.), *The divine consort* (pp. 316–324). Boston: Beacon Press.

Ramanujan, A. K. (1983). The Indian Oedipus. In L. Edmunds & A. Dundes (Eds.), *Oedipus: A folklore casebook.* New York: Garland Press.

Ramu, G. N. (1988). *Women, work and marriage in urban India.* New Delhi: Sage.

Roland, A. (1989). *In search of Self in India and Japan.* Princeton, NJ: Princeton University Press.

Rosenthal, D. A., & Feldman, S. S. (1992). The nature and stability of ethnic identity in Chinese youth: Effects of length of residence in two cultural contexts. *Journal of Cross-Cultural Psychology, 23,* 214–227.

Saran, P. (1985). *The Asian Indian experience in the United States.* Cambridge, MA: Schenkman.

Sethi, R. R., & Allen, M. J. (1984). Sex-role stereotypes in Northern India and the United States. *Sex Roles, 11*(7–8), 615–626.

Siddique, C. M. (1977). Structural separation and family change: An exploratory study of the immigrant Indian and Pakistani community of Saskatoon, Canada. *International Review of Modern Sociology, 7,* 13–34.

Singh, A. (1990, November). The plight of the girl child. *India Today,* pp. 2–3.

Skultans, V. (1991). Women and affliction in Maharashtra: A hydraulic model of health and illness. *Culture, Medicine, and Psychiatry, 15,* 321–359.

Sodowsky, G. R., Kwan, K. K., & Pannu, R. (1995). Ethnic identity of Asians in the United States. In J. G. Ponterotto, J. M. Casas, L. A. Suzuki, & C. M. Alexander (Eds.), *Handbook of multicultural counseling* (pp. 123–154). Thousand Oaks, CA: Sage.

Sodowsy, G. R., & Carey, J. C. (1988). Relationships between acculturation-related demographics and cultural attitudes of an Asian-American immigrant group. *Journal of Multi-Cultural Counseling and Development, 16,* 117–133.

Sue, D. W. (1981). *Counseling the culturally different.* New York: Wiley Press.

Takaki, R. (1989). *Strangers from a different shore.* Boston: Little, Brown.

Talageri, S. G. (1993). *Aryan invasion theory and Indian nationalism.* New Delhi: Voice of India.

Thapar, R. (1966). *A history of India.* New York: Penguin Press.

U.S. Bureau of the Census. (1980). *1980 census of population.* Washington, DC: U.S. Government Printing Office.

U.S. Bureau of the Census. (1990). *1990 census of population.* Washington, DC: U.S. Government Printing Office.

U.S. Commission on Civil Rights. (1992). *Civil rights issues facing Asian Americans.* Washington, DC: U.S. Government Printing Office.

Violence against Women Act. (1990). *Hearing before the Committee on the Judiciary,* S. Rep. No. 545, 101st Cong., 2nd Sess.

Wakil, S. P., Siddique, C. M., & Wakil, F. A. (1981). Between two cultures: A study of socialization of children of immigrants. *Journal of Marriage and the Family, 43,* 929–940.

5

Filipino American Families

JULIANA SUSTENTO-SENERICHES

This chapter discusses the cultural background and attributes of the Filipino American. I first describe life in the Philippines and then go on to explore the unique aspects of the acculturation process and how it affects Filipinos in their adaptation to their new country. Finally, I describe the implications of their cultural background on the assessment, diagnosis, and treatment of Filipino Americans who seek help.

THE NATIVE COUNTRY

The Philippines is a tropical archipelago consisting of 7,107 islands, many of which are habitable, covering a land area slightly larger than the state of Nevada. Two-thirds of the population of 64 million people live in poor, rural agricultural areas, often isolated from one another by geography, lack of decent transportation, and limited communication facilities. With thousands of miles of coastline, it is also a land of many natural disasters, including typhoons, volcanic eruptions, earthquakes, tidal waves, and droughts. It has many natural resources, including rich volcanic soil, fishing grounds, timberlands, and such mineral deposits as gold, copper, iron, chromite, manganese, limestone, shale, coal, petroleum, and uranium.

The archipelago setting of the Philippines has had an enormous impact in creating pockets of strong regionalism and different cultural values. The relative isolation of the islands as a whole and many regions on the bigger islands encourages the need for extended families, the emergence of dominant clans, and the existence of about 75 ethnolinguistic groups speaking more than 111 different dialects (Igacnio, 1991). Examples of regional groups are the Tagalogs from Manila and surrounding areas, the Visayans from the middle islands, and the Ilocanos from the northern part of Luzon island. Dominant clans include prominent names like the Lopezes, the Elizaldes, the Coquancos, and the Ayalas. The isolation has paved the way for such cultural tendencies as the propensity to feel shame (hiyâ) when one's actions are seen as deviant by the close-knit community, as well as the powerful need of the family to present a good, respectable front to others. The stigma against mental illness is therefore very strong.

This geographical setting encourages family members to migrate to neighboring islands for economics, trading, and educational advancement. Although people may leave their home island, they maintain close economic and emotional ties to their family.

The Philippines has been subjugated by many colonial powers, including the Spanish, the Americans, and the Japanese. These colonizations affected the cultural traditions in the country and also contributed in a major way to the "colonial mentality," a sense of inferiority to and suspiciousness of the colonizer. The culture was also influenced by neighboring Chinese, Asian Indians, Indonesians, and Arabs (who came in 1380).

The Philippines is the only Catholic country in the whole of Asia, a testimony to the more than 300 years of Spanish domination (from 1521 on). The 83% of the population who are Catholic interpret their religion with rituals and a simple faith that influences most aspects of their lives.

The Americans, who arrived at the end of the 19th century, developed a system of free public education, thus making the country the most literate of all Asian countries. As a result, the Filipinos have a high regard for education. English is the predominant language of instruction in schools and is spoken throughout the country. When Filipinos emigrate to the United States, they have a much greater knowledge of English than those coming from most other Asian countries.

Political upheavals, as well as corruption within the government, have created economic disasters, which have helped to encouraged emigration to other countries.

MIGRATION HISTORY

The first Filipino arrived on American soil about a century or so after the Mayflower landed (Espina, 1981). The year was 1763 and Spain had started the galleon trade from the ports of Manila and Cebu, passing through

Mexican and American waters on its way to Europe. Filipino slaves and workers were recorded (Cordova, 1983) to have jumped off the galleon vessels in Mexico and Louisiana. "Manilamen," as they were called, became the first wave of Filipino migration to the United States. Three more immigrant waves followed.

The second immigration wave (1906–1934) consisted of farmworkers (derogatorily nicknamed Pineapples) initially recruited to work the pineapple fields of Hawaii and various farms on the West Coast. These immigrants later worked in the canneries and fishing boats in Alaska. They were mostly single men who were not allowed to own properties or marry interracially. They lived substandard lives and were subjected to racial discrimination (another derogatory nickname was little brown monkeys). Because there were virtually no Filipino women, a number of these men (*manongs,* or older brothers) remained single, without families, living out their final years close to the farmlands they used to till (Urban Associates, 1974).

The third wave of immigrants (1945–1965) were Filipino servicemen (who fought side by side with the Americans during the Japanese occupation) and their families.

The fourth immigration wave came after the lifting of the Tydings–McDuffie Act and its accompanying immigration quota (1965 and on). The 1960s saw the influx of the "brain wave," as doctors, nurses, and engineers came for further training or better employment. Between 1970 and 1980, the Filipino American population increased by 113% as a result of the country's downward financial spiral and political oppression from the Marcos dictatorship. Thus, a vast majority of this Asian group are new immigrants. Many have legal immigration problems, causing such situations as "buying an American citizen spouse" to get a green card.

FILIPINO AMERICANS TODAY

Currently, the Filipino Americans constitute the second largest Asian group in the United States. Numbered at 1.4 million (U.S. Bureau of the Census, 1990), 45.8% of them settled in the San Francisco Bay Area, where they are the state's largest Asian American group (Bouvier & Martin, 1985; U.S. Census, 1990). It is projected that by the year 2000, the Filipino American population will reach 2.1 million and will then be the largest Asian group in the whole country (Bouvier & Agresta, 1987). Most are first-generation immigrants. The 1991 census showed that the annual income per worker for this group is lower than that of their Chinese, Japanese, Asian Indian, and Korean counterparts. Many of the 74.2% who have at least a high school education are underemployed and underpaid. It is worth noting that Filipino women have the highest participation rate in the work force among Asian American women (Gardner, Robey, & Smith, 1989).

THE TRADITIONAL FAMILY AND VALUES

The Extended Family

The Filipino concept of family is not limited to the nuclear family members. It includes the clan and the community, even the island, the town, or the province. This is a distinctly Filipino version of the extended family. Indeed, a Western observer noted that a Filipino in the Philippines is born to about 280 family members, including aunts, uncles, and cousins, once, twice, and three times removed. Kinship is further enlarged by religious rites such as baptism, confirmation, and marriage. These rites establish godparents who become *kumares* and *kumpadres* of the parents. The Catholic church confers much meaning and obligations to such religious membership in the clan. In-laws, friends, neighbors, town mates, and province mates (*kababayans*) also have special bonds of kinship: mutual expectations of recognition in times of honor and aid in times of need.

The first-generation immigrant re-creates this extended family system in his or her new country. If job opportunities are available, he or she tends to settle near other members of the clan. When immigrants come to this country alone, they diligently plan to sponsor all of their immediate family, one by one, no matter how long it takes. In the meantime, it is not unusual for immigrants to be invited to stay with a relative or a province mate until they can afford their own residence. The man is called uncle by the children or *kuya* (older brother) by the younger members of the family. If there are no clan members around, the new immigrant begins forming his or her own by designating newfound friends as, for example, *ate* (older sister), or auntie, and so forth.

The Filipino American household is very extended. Different roles are given to different members. The regional or clan groups developed into extensive organizations in the United States, including hundreds of associations such as the Iloilo Circle, the San Miguel Association, the Antiquenos, and so on. Like the many religious associations, including the Santo Niño group, the charismatic movement, and the Black Nazarene group, these groups provide solid sources of emotional support for the Filipino immigrant.

In their native country, Filipinos are used to having lots of company. For the visitor or new immigrant, the most common complaint is loneliness.

Male and Female Roles

The Filipino father–mother dyad is unlike the stereotypical version of the all-powerful father and the silent, subservient wife in Asian families. From the pre-Hispanic times, Filipino men and women have functioned side by side in an equal fashion. Documentation of the pre-Hispanic era shows many well-respected women *barangay* (community) chieftains and lawmakers. Moreover, women were among the first recognized healers in the community.

When the Spaniards arrived, they brought with them the concept of male *machismo*. Men were seen to have sexual supremacy and were encouraged to have concubines (*queridas*). Nowadays, rich and powerful men in the Philippines still have *queridas*. Similar to the Hispanics, wives who may be holding powerful jobs themselves can still accept their husband's philandering "because they are men." The husband has a strong sense of duty to financially support his wife, children, and mistress. This arrangement has been strongly challenged by the younger generation and by new Filipino American immigrants. Moreover, it has been difficult to maintain in the United States, given often more limited financial resources and societal support or sanction.

Outward presentation to the community is important. The husband may be deliberately presented as the head of the household, in keeping with the tradition of male *machismo*. Yet the reality may be quite different; most major family decisions are a consensus between husband and wife. The wives traditionally hold the purse strings. Studies show the wives to feel largely responsible for maintaining family equilibrium. Within the extended family and the community, the women feel pride for their ability to help out with the family's finances. For both men and women, the sacrifice of traveling to a foreign country for a job beneath their status (e.g., a nurse becoming a household helper in Saudi Arabia) for the good of the family's welfare is socially sanctioned. The rest of the family then helps out by taking care of the nuclear family members left behind.

Family Hierarchy

The family structure is distinctly hierarchical, based on respect and responsibilities. Seniors are accorded much respect for their age and wisdom and much gratitude for their past sacrifices for the family. The older brother and sister, called *kuya* and *ate,* are also shown much respect. If younger members of the family do not speak with respect to their parents and elders, they bring deep shame upon the family. *Hô* and *pô* are respectful Tagalog words used in every sentence when addressing an older family member. Because sensitivity to losing face, especially in public leads to deep narcissistic hurt and shame, clinicians dealing with Filipino families should do their best to show respectful recognition and deference to the older family members. This abiding respect and patience for the elderly make the Filipino Americans very good caretakers in the many nursing homes they own. Not unsurprisingly, formal recognition of one's status (as a doctor, club president, or relative of an important figure), especially in public, is important as well.

Traditional Values

Filipinos' communication style is predicated on maintaining this hierarchy of respect, as well as on making sure relationships are harmonious. Rather than through direct statements, or confrontation, Filipinos communicate through actions, insinuations, euphemisms, and jokes. In contrast to the restraint of Japanese Americans, Filipino Americans express themselves with exuberance, smiles, and many broad gestures. The need to be pleasant makes it hard for the traditional Filipino to say "no" or to disagree openly.

Filipino Americans harbor values unique to their culture. These values are found especially in first-generation Filipino Americans, but they are also incorporated by other generations. These values present themselves in a host of attitudes, such as a strong sense of family; an adherence to an authoritarian hierarchy; a sense of taking things personally; a powerful adherence to religion; a reaction to colonialism, which often takes the form of deep rooted inferiority and suspiciousness; and adaptability. New immigrants tend to take things personally, to try to protect themselves from the inherently discomforting feelings of colonial subserviency, and such attitudes can color their communication style and perception of others. Enriquez (1987) identified some basic Filipino traditional commitments: interaction with concern as one equal with others (*pakikipagkapwa*), sensitivity, and regard for others.

Other cultural traits include a propensity to feel *hiyâ*, or shame; a *bahalana*, or a fatalistic attitude ("Leave it to God," or "Come what may"), which some attribute to the resignation of a people to a history of repeated colonializations and recurrent natural disasters. Filipino Americans also have a child-like, fun-loving side which also helps them in the face of adversity. Their approach to life may also be a result of childrearing practices that encourage a leisurely maturation, which takes the form of a relaxed attitude toward weaning; no rigid, systematic toilet training; and allowing the child to be a child for as long as it is tolerable. In rural areas, it is not uncommon for a mother to allow a toddler to suckle on her milkless breast to soothe and bond with the child. The extended family system, and the many men and women who help raise the child, allows for this kind of childrearing.

One of the most important traits is what is known as *utang na loob,* which refers to an abiding and eternal debt of gratitude for favors extended to a member of the family. This attitude pulls the clan members more closely together.

EFFECTS OF CULTURAL TRANSITION

The majority of Filipino Americans currently living in the United States are first-generation Americans. They have been dealing with the necessity of acculturation and its accompanying difficulties.

The same cultural traits that can be helpful in the face of adversity can also create psychological and emotional difficulties during the process of acculturation. For example, the fact that this group takes slights very personally can make the group members vulnerable. In addition, their extreme family and group orientation can make it more difficult for them to find ways to be involved in the new culture. Their strong sense of shame and colonial mentality, along with the loss of familiar support networks, status, and so forth, can add to their already vulnerable state. Like any new immigrants, their ignorance of legal and educational systems and any legal immigration problems can create additional difficulties.

In my own practice, I have tried to categorize the problems my Filipino American clients have brought to the consultation room (Sustento-Seneriches, 1991). Most of my patients were diagnosed with adjustment disorders. I would list a number of factors as precipitants to these adjustment disorders: (1) losses experienced in the immigration process, including loss of status and financial security (with underemployment and reports of discrimination), loss of the extended family, and so forth; (2) changes in the traditional male–female roles; (3) discrepancy in acculturation between first-generation and American-born later generations; (4) shame-evoking situations in the workplace; (5) ignorance of the country's laws or cultural norms; and (6) illegal immigration status. Losses and conflict during the immigration process often culminate in depression, which is a basic problem among first-generation Filipino Americans in the San Francisco Bay Area. In one study, close to 30% of Filipino Americans in a Bay Area community showed signs of depression (Tompar-Tiu & Sustento-Seneriches, 1995).

At the same time that some of these cultural traits can prove to be detrimental to adjustment, they can also mitigate the effects of the stress of coming to the United States. The presence of a supportive family, relatives, or friends; a social or church network; a personal sense of spirituality and connectedness; and a fulfilling sense of sacrifice for the common good of the family system are all helpful in times of stress.

It is important to understand traditional Filipino beliefs about the causation of illness. These beliefs will have a strong bearing on the ways in which therapists can make their interventions more helpful. The traditional Filipino believes illness is an interweaving of different physical, mental, spiritual, and psychological components. As in many other aspects of their lives, Filipinos blend the cultures that have passed through their islands into the original belief system. They recognize interconnecting causations. In rural and urban Philippines, people believe that illness are caused by germs (73%); inadequacy of nutritious foods (66%); such natural elements as rain, cold, and heat (57%); God's will (15%); evil spirits (5%); and witchcraft (3%) (Tan, 1987). Among Filipino Americans surveyed in Los Angeles, illnesses have been blamed on overeating or delayed eating, viruses, pollution, tension, body abuse, combining of incompatible foods and temperatures, and divine punishments for sins.

One patient sought treatment for depression. She harbored a mystical belief that a curse by an elder for past disrespect had caused the illness. She also held a personal belief that a recently dead grandparent was "longing" for her. Along with these two beliefs, she felt that exposure to the cold evening dew caused a sense of fatigue. This patient was taking antidepressants, so on some level she also believed that the disease was physiologically based (a naturalistic belief).

ASSESSMENT, DIAGNOSIS, AND TREATMENT

The assessment and diagnostic process needs to take into consideration all the different influences on the patient who comes to treatment. When taking a history, it is important to consider the patient's acculturation status, asking questions such as: How long has he been in this country? How much does she associate with the dominant culture? With other cultures? Which part of the Philippines did he originally come from? Was this a rural or an urban setting? The therapist could then move on to questions regarding the social support network: Who constitutes her support system in this country—her immediate family? extended family? Who remains behind in the home country, and is she still communicating with them? What dialect does she speak at home? In the workplace?

An interpreter can be very useful when the patient speaks English but needs help in being understood (see Chapter 32). Sometimes it can also be extremely useful to involve an outside therapist with a deeper knowledge of the Filipino culture to help with the initial intake. Even though the Filipino American immigrant may be able to speak English, talking about emotional issues can be very difficult when the immigrant is not using his or her native tongue. The therapist may sometimes need to refer the patient to a Filipino-speaking therapist.

The history taking should also include questions about why the patient came for help at this particular time. Psychiatry and mental health are new in the Philippines and the stigma of mental illness is very powerful in communities in which everyone is interrelated. Thus, Filipino Americans do not seek help unless they have compelling reasons to do so. In addition, a person may wait until he or she is in dire straits before coming in for help. This culture tolerates a high level of regression; thus it is very important for the assessor to be on the lookout for the underlying crisis.

An assessment of the client's extended family system is essential in understanding the problems facing the client and mapping out an effective treatment plan. Questions include: Who brought the client in? Who are the respected family or clan elders? To whom does the client listen? Sometimes this person can be tapped later for help (e.g., in using behavioral techniques for the chronically ill). It may be that the most influential family member is located somewhere else in the world. Nevertheless, the therapist may want to consider consulting this person at some point or at least considering his or her role in the treatment plan.

The initial engagement phase in therapy may be the most difficult. Because Filipino Americans hold the medical profession in high regard, clients and their families usually look up to the clinician and harbor preconceived expectations. The traditional healer or doctor gives medications or herbs and may prescribe rituals and incantations or even direct advice regarding lifestyle or attitudinal changes. In the Philippine rural setting, the patient "drops in" any time to the doctor's office. Coming in on time or ending the session on time can be problematic. Of course, acculturation changes old-country behavior. The clinician is also incorporated into the extended family hierarchy, and personal questions—such as asking whether you are married or where you come from—should be regarded as ways in which the client wants to bond with the clinician.

Given the lack of exposure to Western mental health practices, psychoeducation is critically important for clients and their families. In addition, ongoing exploration of the client's and family's understanding of their treatment allows therapists a clear picture of the process the family is undergoing. At times, indigenous healing practices, along with psychotherapy or medication, are very helpful.

In regard to psychoactive medications, most clients will be wary of taking medications, fearing addiction or side effects. Indeed, studies show that Asian groups in general require a smaller dose than do their Western counterparts (Chien, 1989).

Finally, the therapist may be called on to help with many practical aspects of the immigrants' life. Indeed, the trials of living may be first on the agenda: referrals to immigration lawyers, working through the local social security office, even basic fundamentals, such as a map of the subway system.

Two case examples demonstrate cultural aspects in the diagnosis and therapeutic interventions.

CASE EXAMPLE 1

A couple in their 30s, along with their young son, recently migrated to the United States. The wife, a nurse, was recruited to work in a convalescent home as an aide. The husband, a practicing lawyer in their hometown, decided to study and take the bar exam. The wife was also studying for the nursing licensure exam. Both came from the same hometown and have extensive family systems. In the Philippines, they had had a caretaker for their son (a *yaya*), a maid, a car, and a chauffeur (the latter provided by the husband's father), plus an endless array of relatives and childhood friends.

In their new home, all of this changed. Both had to do the household chores and take care of the son. They had no extended family or even province mates close by. The husband was very isolated and had made no new friends; the wife had made friends with some of her coworkers, some of whom were from the Philippines.

When the husband failed his bar exam twice and his wife passed her exam, he grew despondent, slept a lot, gained weight, and did not take baths for days. He was so irritable that he actually struck his wife. Although he was remorseful afterward, he felt endlessly dispirited. His wife begged him to see a psychiatrist, a suggestion to which he reacted with horror. He relented only after she called his father who in turn called him from the Philippines exhorting him to seek treatment. Later, in therapy, he divulged that he had noted his wife confiding in and probably falling for a male coworker. This was another reason he finally relented and sought help. His presenting symptoms were physical. The clinician addressed each one of them, even ordering some laboratory work, in addition to taking the husband's vital signs. When the therapist introduced the possibility of taking antidepressants, she carefully explained to the husband that depression was a physical illness brought on by stressors. The husband found this very helpful. Because the narcissistic hurts came from changes in the traditional male–female roles and his failures in the bar exams, it was important that the clinician showed him respect and acknowledged his obvious strengths, including his decision to seek help. Involving his wife in the initial psychoeducation also emphasized the marital bond. The therapist helped the wife confirm her commitment to her husband.

Because both were suffering from real losses in their support systems, they were encouraged to help the husband develop some activities and friendships outside the home. He found a group of Filipinos who played basketball and occasionally went bowling. Finding some new friends and taking part in athletics helped him to regain a sense of "being a man." Both the husband and wife got involved with the local Catholic church and joined the Filipino church neighborhood group; they were also able to get involved with a cooperative babysitting group. Continued psychoeducation about mental health and stress were necessary for this patient. Gradually he got better and his symptoms disappeared.

CASE EXAMPLE 2

A 27-year-old single Filipina, a 5-year immigrant living in a large American city, was seen in the emergency room of the city hospital. She was frightened and incoherent and had a painfully stiff neck. She was talking loudly in her native Ilocano dialect and occasionally in English. Her brother and cousin were holding her and trying to calm her down. She was also accompanied by her three sisters, her mother, and an uncle. The brother served as the interpreter and explained that she was speaking loudly because there were invisible dwarves and spirits from the backyard anthill who were following her around and trying to torture her. The stiff neck was attributed to her sitting in one position for hours on end. It was acute and created the rapid escalation of the client's fears. Having family members around her in a private interview room seemed to calm the client rather than talking to her alone. (The issue of confidentiality must be carefully weighed against the client's degree of interdependency with the family. A signed release form may be obtained if necessary, although this release must be introduced carefully as the new immigrant may not understand the necessity for it.)

The history was pieced together through the combined accounts of everyone who came with the client. All were apparently concerned and caring. The older brother was the original immigrant to this country. He sponsored all of his sisters as well as his mother. His mother and the two single sisters were living with him, his wife, and their infant son. The client was the last one to come because she had needed more documents. She had been diagnosed as mentally retarded when she was in the sixth grade in the local school. Her mother had been sickly while she was pregnant with the client. Having a retarded family member was considered good luck to the family, whose members, in turn, pampered her and closely looked after her welfare. She did household tasks under supervision and took great pride in her work. She had been treated very well by her extended family and even by the local teachers, who had allowed her to pass through the early grades.

She handled her first years in the new country fairly well. She had been seen by a psychiatrist as a requirement for her entry into the country.

At that time, she was given a fairly clean bill of health and was allowed to stay with her family. During the past year, her two sisters married and moved out of the house. Most of the day, the client was alone in the house with her mother, who was busy taking care of the baby. Unlike in her hometown, the neighborhood was not conducive to allowing her to go out and mingle with neighbors. For the previous 3 months, she had been getting cranky and had short bursts of temper. The family was extra patient with her, even scheduling weekend visits to her married sisters. The mother prayed the novena for her and a Filipino *hilot,* or masseur, did some therapeutic massaging "to put her uterus back it proper place." When she had insomnia for several nights and was talking to the spirits, her cousin next door volunteered some leftover medications that his wife had had. The medication had been prescribed to his wife by a family doctor in the Philippines when she had terrible insomnia after the birth of her child. The family had given the patient this medication in the few hours before she was brought to the hospital. As it turned out, the medication (Stelazine, a major tranquilizer with strong extrapyramidal side effects) had caused the stiff neck that had precipitated the emergency room visit. The family members said that they had never thought of bringing the patient to a psychiatrist, explaining that "craziness does not run in this family."

Treatment consisted of prescribing an antidote to the Stelazine and a minor tranquilizer to relieve the pain, anxiety, and insomnia. After a few hours in the emergency room, the patient was sent home in the care of her family with specific instructions for outpatient follow-up. With the constant involvement of her family, the client was eventually introduced to a nearby sheltered workshop where she was able to earn her own money.

REFERENCES

Bouvier, L. F., & Martin, P. (1985). *Population change and California's future.* Washington, DC: Population Reference Bureau.

Chien, C. (1989). *Culture, ethnicity, and psychopharmacology.* Paper presented at the annual meeting of the American Psychiatric Association, San Francisco.

Cordova, F. (1983). *Filipinos: Forgotten Asian Americans.* Dubuque, IA: Kendall Hunt.

Enriquez, V. G. (1987, April 27). *The structure of Philippine social values toward integrating indigenous values and appropriate technology.* Paper presented at the Symposium on Social Values and Development in the Third World Countries, University of Hong Kong.

Espina, M. E. (1981). *Collected writings and research on the history and folklore of Americans of Filipino ancestry in Louisiana.* Earl K. Long Library, University of New Orleans, Somorana.

Gardner, R. W., Robey, B., & Smith, P. C. (1989). *Asian Americans: Growth, change, and diversity.* Washington, DC: Population Reference Bureau.

Ignacio, T. (1991). *Tagalog versus Filipino.* Paper presented at the Conference of the C. E. Smith Museum of Anthropology and the Center for Philippine Studies, California State University at Hayward.

Sustento-Seneriches, J. (1991). *Comparison of diagnoses among Filipino patients seen in private practice, Philippines and the United States.* Paper presented at the Fifth Pacific Rim College of Psychiatrists Meeting, Los Angeles.

Tan, M. (1987). *Usug, Kulam, Pasma: Traditional concepts of health and illness in the Philippines.* Quezon City, Philippines: Alay Kapwa Kilusang Pangkalusugan.

Tompar-Tiu, A., & Sustento-Seneriches, J. (1995). *Depression and other mental health issues; the Filipino American experience.* San Francisco: Jossey-Bass.

Urban Associates. (1974). *A study of selected socioeconomic characteristics of ethnic minorities, based on the 1979 census* (Vol. 2). Arlington, VA: Author.

U.S. Bureau of the Census. (1990). *1990 census of population.* Washington, DC: U.S. Government Printing Office.

6

Japanese American Families

REIKO HOMMA-TRUE

HISTORICAL BACKGROUND

Japanese immigration into the United States began more than 100 years ago when farmworkers and laborers were first brought in as alternatives to Chinese laborers in the 1880s. At the time, the Chinese were perceived as an increasing economic threat and their immigration was sharply curtailed by the enactment of the Chinese Exclusion Act in 1882. The timing coincided with major sociopolitical changes taking place in Japan, which was aggressively trying to transform itself rapidly into a modern, industrialized nation at great financial cost to its people. Poverty was rampant, particularly among the tenant farmers, who saw the opportunity to send their sons to work overseas as a way to get out of heavy debt (Takaki, 1989).

The peak period for Japanese immigration occurred between 1880 and 1920, during which time nearly 400,000 men and women entered the United States. Unlike the Chinese, who were originally reluctant to bring their wives to the new country, the Japanese government actively encouraged the emigration of women to become wives of the laborers, thinking their presence would prevent prostitution, gambling, and other undesirable activities. Many women came as picture brides without knowing the men they were to marry. Despite the hard labor expected of Japanese men and women under harsh conditions, as well as persistent anti-Asian discrimination, many survived and began to set roots in their chosen communities (Kikumura, 1981).

As they began to establish themselves in the United States, they also became the target of mounting hostility from the general American public. When World War II broke out, anti-Japanese sentiment reached a level of hysteria and resulted in the U.S. government's internment of all West-coast Japanese, including the U.S.-born Japanese Americans, into concentration camps in remote desolate desert areas in such states as California, Arizona, and Idaho (Kitano, 1969b). The traumatic experience of being uprooted from their own homes, losing most of their hard-earned possessions, and being subjected to subhuman conditions was devastating for the Japanese Americans. Although Japanese Americans have struggled to rebuild their ruined economy and lives, many families still suffer from the psychological scars left by the experience (Nagata, 1990).

When Japanese immigration resumed after World War II, many of the new immigrants were women, who are often referred to as war brides because of their marriage to U.S. servicemen. Unlike the earlier immigrants, who settled primarily on the West Coast, war brides settled in diverse parts of the country, often isolated from other Japanese Americans. Although some of them were accepted by their husbands' families, others were rejected by them as well as by their own families for breaking the cultural taboo against interracial marriages. Many marriages ended in divorce, which left these women in desperate conditions in their adopted country (Kim, 1977). When the focus of the U.S. military moved from Japan to other parts of Asia in the 1960s, the influx of Japanese war brides also stopped and was replaced by brides from other Asian countries such as Korea, the Philippines, and Vietnam.

Improved economic conditions in Japan as well as the quota system for new immigrants has reduced the influx of Japanese into the United States to a trickle compared to other Asian groups, such as Chinese, Koreans, Filipinos, or Southeast Asian refugees. However, a significant number of Japanese businessmen and their families are sent to the United States to conduct business on behalf of Japan-based parent companies. They stay for a few years and constitute a visible presence in many major U.S. cities.

CURRENT STATUS OF THE JAPANESE AMERICAN COMMUNITY

Demographics

Japanese Americans now number approximately 850,000 and are mostly concentrated in Hawaii and West Coast states (U.S. Bureau of the Census, 1993). Although the majority of other Asian Americans are foreign born, 67.6% of Japanese Americans are born in the United States, with only 17.7% having arrived from Japan between 1980 and 1990. The median age for Japanese Americans is 36.3 years, which is considerably older than the total Asian population of 30.1 years, or the U.S. total of 32.9 years. The proportion of families maintained by married couples is 83.1%, somewhat higher than the Asian average (81.6%) and the national average (78.6%). The percentage of female-headed households is 12.3, which is slightly higher than the Asian average (11.9%) but considerably lower than the national average (16.5%) (U.S. Bureau of the Census, 1993).

The educational level for Japanese Americans is relatively high. The percentage of high school graduates is 89.9 for males and 85.6 for females, which is highest among Asians for both males and females. However, at the college level or higher category, they are in the sixth place, considerably lower than Asian Indians, who have the highest attainment at 65.7% for males and 48.7% for females, compared with 42.6% for males and 28.2% for females for the Japanese. The rates for total United States and Asians are 23.3% and 43.2% for males and 17.6% and 32.7% for females, respectively (U.S. Bureau of the Census, 1993).

Contrary to the stereotypical perception of Asian and Japanese women as housewives, many Japanese American wives are in the labor force, supplementing their husbands' income. Perhaps because of this double income, coupled with their relatively high educational level, their median family income at $51,550 is the highest among all Asian groups and is significantly higher than the U.S. median level of $35,225. The poverty level is also low for the Japanese, with persons in poverty at 7%, whereas the figures for Asian total and U.S. total are at 14.0% and 13.1%, respectively (U.S. Bureau of the Census, 1993). However, behind this picture of relative affluence, there are subgroups (e.g., war brides abandoned by husbands and elderly widows) who are isolated and struggling to survive with declining health and meager resources.

Subgroups

There are several subgroups within current Japanese American communities. The oldest immigrant generation is popularly called *Issei,* which means "the first generation" in Japanese. Although most *Issei* are now deceased, those surviving are now in their 80s and 90s and the majority are widows. Subsequent generations of Japanese Americans are called *Nisei* (second generation), *Sansei* (third generation), and *Yonsei* (fourth generation). There is also a subgroup of *Nisei,* called *Kibei,* which literally means "returned to the United States" and refers to those *Nisei* who were born in the United States but were sent to Japan for a variety of reasons and were unable to return until after World War II. Although most of them escaped internment in the United States, they endured trauma and discrimination both in Japan, where they were labeled as American sympathizers, and in the United States, where they were perceived as not loyal enough (Kitano, 1969b).

The more recently arrived immigrants, although relatively small in number, are sometimes called newcomers, to distinguish them from the older *Issei*, and include the previously mentioned war brides, extended families of earlier immigrants, immigrants with technological know-how, and businessmen and their families. In comparison to the U.S.-born Japanese Americans, they are frequently confronted with the stress of adjusting to a new environment (e.g., language, cultural, and lifestyle differences).

Another group, which is emerging in recent years, comprises those who marry outside their community and choose interracial partners. Although interracial marriages were initially taboo both in Japan and among the Japanese Americans, the barrier is rapidly disappearing in recent years. Initially, the war brides from Japan broke the taboo, but it is now the U.S.-born *Sansei* and *Yonsei* who are choosing to marry partners of other races in increasing numbers. The issues faced by the offspring of these marriages, biracial or multiracial Japanese Americans, are complex and include questions of identity and their impact on the future survival of Japanese American communities (Iwasaki-Mass, 1992; Kitano & Kikumura, 1973).

Traditional Family Organization and Value Orientation

The traditional family organization first brought by Issei was patriarchal, in which the father was the supreme head of the family and the decision maker for all family members. The values emphasized by the *Issei* were strongly rooted in the philosophical and moral principles established by Confucius in China and adopted by the Japanese during the seventh century. They stressed the need for respect for social order, respect for elders and superiors, maintenance of interpersonal harmony, and male supremacy over females and discouraged individual autonomy and competitiveness (Uba, 1994).

The survival of the family, rather than the fulfillment/satisfaction of individual needs, took priority in the family system. To preserve the family honor, each family member was expected to persevere under adverse circumstances and not bring shame, *haji*, into the family. The Japanese word *gaman*, meaning perseverance and endurance, is frequently brought up among Japanese American families as a reminder of surviving under difficult circumstances. Other terms derived from the Confucian tradition, such as *oyakoko* (filial piety), *giri* (social obligation to be fulfilled), *on* (a debt of gratitude, a favor to be repaid in future), and *enryo* (diffidence, modesty, not being a burden on others), are terms that are still often repeated among Japanese American families to honor some of the important cultural legacies related to personal and family duties and interpersonal relations. Also, certain values such as hard work, education, and achievement correspond to the values emphasized by the dominant Judeo-Christian society and were helpful for the Japanese Americans to succeed in academic and occupational fields (Connor, 1974; Kitano, 1969b).

As the succeeding generations of Japanese Americans became more acculturated, the family organization and values gradually changed. For example, in her observations of Seattle Japanese American families, Yanagisako (1976) noted that the originally patriarchal, male-dominated family network was gradually replaced during the Nisei generation by women, who began playing more central roles in keeping the family network together and making family decisions.

It is generally agreed that following the deeply painful wartime discrimination experienced by Japanese Americans, many *Nisei* parents tried to disassociate themselves and their children from Japanese cultural tradition and to become model Americans in the Anglo-Saxon tradition. By making this effort, they hoped to eliminate discrimination directed against themselves. However, such efforts were often made at a considerable personal and psychological cost, alienating them from their cultural roots. In spite of their effort, however, the racism directed against them has not been eliminated completely and still persists in many areas (Hosokawa, 1969; Nagata, 1990).

Language and Communication Patterns

With the exception of *Issei* and more recent immigrants, the majority of Japanese Americans are English-speaking and are educated in the United States. Although one might expect them to have adapted to the dominant style of communication in the United States, many have retained certain characteristics which are rooted in the Japanese cultural tradition. When compared with white Americans, they are often judged to be more reserved in their communication style, less extroverted, and less expressive of their emotion and affection, and to rely on more subtle and indirect, nonverbal cues (Hsu, Tseng, Ashton, McDermott, & Char, 1985; Hieshima & Schneider, 1994). Some of the factors involved include continued cultural emphasis on deference to authority, which discourages individual opinions, assertion, or arguing; the presence of well-defined expectations of social behavior and roles, requiring less verbal communication; the lingering impact of the trauma from wartime discrimination; and the residual cultural value for self-effasiveness and control of emotion even among family members (Uba, 1994). This tendency is particularly strong among *Nisei* and often leads to conflicts with the younger generation, who expect their parents to behave like other American parents, encouraging active flow of communication and greater expression of affection and feelings.

Religion

Although Buddhism and Shintoism played historically dominant roles in Japan, Shintoism was mostly dropped by the Japanese Americans. Instead, many of them adopted the dominant religion of the adopted country, which was mostly Protestant in the areas they settled. In most Japanese American communities, both Buddhist and various Protestant churches play significant roles as part of the community institutions in the area. However, like the experience of other immigrant groups, succeeding generations are becoming less involved with established religion and churches, preferring to be independent and free of the church's influence.

CLINICAL CONSIDERATIONS

When attempting to engage Japanese American families in treatment, it is important to bear in mind that they perceive treatment as an embarrassment. Moreover, to most Japanese Americans, mental health treatment or psychotherapy is a foreign concept and the possibility that one might be mentally ill evokes deep-rooted fear. Mental illness in Japan historically was viewed as the result of evil spirits or a curse, and the identified mentally ill were stigmatized and castigated by the community. Japanese Americans are still influenced by this fear and are still reluctant to seek outside help (Kitano, 1969a).

Despite the cultural stigma that discourages utilization of mental health services, many Japanese Americans are experiencing personal crisis and stresses which could benefit from timely therapeutic interventions. Through exposure to information about mental health services, an increasing number, especially among the younger generation, are beginning to seek help during crisis (Nishio & Murase, 1983). Although data on the reasons that bring them into treatment are limited, the survey cited by Nishio and Murase (1983) provides a glimpse into some of the problems they present, which include serious mental illnesses as well as personal relationship problems; anxiety and depression; substance abuse problems, especially among the younger generation; intergenerational and marital/family problems; isolated problems of elderly people; problems related to racism and cultural conflict; and desire for personal growth.

Currently, most Japanese Americans seeking treatment are seen in individual therapy sessions (Furuta, 1981). Utilization of family therapy as a treatment modality among Japanese Americans is still limited. Some of the reasons for this may be such factors as therapists' lack of skill, absence of a reimbursement mechanism for family therapy, family reluctance because of the traditional fear or shame, and geographic distances among family members. However, considering the importance placed on family relationships and togetherness in the community and the potential benefit to be gained, therapists should make a greater effort to consider the applicability of family therapy. Reports by those who were able to engage families in therapy are encouraging not only for the individuals in distress but for other family members as well (Furuta, 1981; Nagata, 1991).

When involving Japanese American families in treatment, a therapist needs to carefully weigh the relevance of the traditional diagnostic formulation against the cultural influence in the family's various stages of transition in the United States (Landau, 1982). For this purpose, Lee's (1982) framework for understanding Chinese American families is useful for Japanese American families as well. Therapists not acquainted with Japanese American families should consult an expert if one is available or do considerable research into the background of Japanese Americans relative to the position of the client family. For example, the problems faced by an elderly Japanese *Issei* farmer and his wife are very different from those of the *Nisei* family in urban areas, *Sansei, Yonsei, Kibei,* war brides, or the more recent immigrants.

Following are two case illustrations which provide some under- standing of the problems experienced by Japanese American families and the therapeutic approaches that can be used to assist each of the families. The first case illustrates a family whose dysfunctional relationships spilled over into their child's difficulties at school. The second case illustrates a Japanese and Chinese American couple whose relationship problems were related to their divergent cultural backgrounds. To ensure confidentiality for the families, fictional names have been used and some of the factual information was altered.

CASE EXAMPLE 1

Mike was referred to the clinic because of his behavioral problems at school. He was 6 at the time and was living with his father, who worked as a gardener, his mother, and his 4-year-old sister. Mike was described by his teacher as hyperactive and assaultive to other children, speaking in incomprehensible English, which made the teacher believe he was autistic. When he was evaluated, Mike was judged to be above average in intelligence but hyperactive and undisciplined. It turned out that his speech, which had a strange singsong quality and intonation, was exactly like his mother's Japanese, which was characterized by the pronounced accent of a rural province. Assessment of his parents' background indicated that they were both bright and reasonably well educated but frustrated in this country because of limited employment opportunities. It appeared that causal factors for Mike's problems included an overly demanding, punitive father; a non-limit-setting, indulgent mother who tried to compensate for his father's negative treatment; the social isolation of Mike and his family; serious marital problems between the parents; and the teacher's lack of understanding of the cultural problems faced by Mike and his family.

The therapist concluded that the relationship between Mike's parents was dysfunctional and that there was a strong alliance between the mother and Mike. Although Japanese mothers are known to be indulgent with children, especially with their sons (Doi, 1973), this mother's overinvolvement with her son was creating deep family strains and also interfered with the boy's chance for becoming more independent and forming outside peer relationships. It should be noted that when they left Japan, the family also lost the support of their extended family, which was not replaced with a substitute support system within their adopted community, thus creating an added source of strain. The importance of the interdependence of the extended family system is one of the issues identified by practitioners of the multigenerational school (Boszormenyi-Nagy & Spark, 1973; Bowen, 1978) as a factor to be included in developing intervention strategies.

In working with the family, the therapist tried to capitalize on the parents' shared concern for the child. They were given guidance on cultural differences in childrearing practices, relationships with school personnel, and peer relations in Japan and the United States. To reduce the level of the family's isolation, the mother was encouraged to become more involved with the neighborhood families and school activities and to provide more freedom and opportunities for Mike to play with other children in the neighborhood. She was also encouraged to be more active in limit setting. The parents were also seen for couple therapy, where they could begin to communicate more openly about their sources of frustration and disappointments, which were often rooted in the social and cultural barriers they faced in the United States but were misplaced on each other. The father was able to recognize his own frustration and sense of failure in this country and how he was displacing it onto Mike or trying to drown it by drinking. As his wife became more effective in limit setting and less obsessed with Mike, the father was able to reduce his unreasonable demands and expectations of Mike.

In addition to traditional therapeutic work to deal with the dysfunctional family relationships, it was necessary, as it is with many other Asian American families, to make considerable environmental interventions (Nishio & Murase, 1983). The therapist provided consultation to the school to reassure officials that Mike was not autistic but needed considerable support and guidance to become better socialized with his peers and special help to improve his English. School personnel were also encouraged to reach out to the mother to involve her more in school activities.

CASE EXAMPLE 2

Bob and Mary were seen for couple counseling because Bob was unhappy with Mary and was considering breaking off his relationship with her. Bob was a Japanese American *Sansei*; Mary was a second-generation Chinese American. Both had graduate training as professionals and had successful careers in two unrelated fields. Although they had dated each other exclusively for 3 years, they had begun to have many disagreements. Bob was frustrated at work and was considering dating other women. Mary was dismayed and could not understand what part she played in the deteriorating relationship with Bob.

Bob's parents met in a concentration camp in Arizona, where both their families were sent during World War II. Both parents worked to support themselves during the difficult postwar period and managed to complete their college education before getting married. Despite college degrees, employment opportunities were limited for Japanese Americans at the time, and both Bob's parents had to accept lower-level government jobs to support their growing family of three children. All the children were encouraged to be self-sufficient, to not complain, and to *gaman* (persevere) through difficult times. Unlike many Japanese American families, which do not encourage communications among family members, Bob's parents encouraged open and active communication within the family. However, like many other *Nisei* parents, they placed strong emphasis on the acquisition of a financially secure, practical profession and discouraged Bob from pursuing his considerable artistic interests, which they considered as irrelevant and self-indulgent.

On the other hand, Mary's father had a well-established professional business in his community so that he could afford to support his wife and two children in a comfortable lifestyle. Mary's mother devoted all her life to the welfare of her family and was overprotective and intrusive in her relationship with her children. Mary did not question her mother's intrusiveness and even depended on her mother to do her chores. This dependence extended to her relationship with Bob, on whom Mary depended a great deal. As her father was a man of few words, the communication in her family was limited and dominated primarily by her mother. Although intelligent, Mary, like her father, was not verbal, and she was quite shy in expressing her thoughts with Bob or in social situations. This was a source of much frustration for Bob, who missed the free and open dialogue in his family.

Through mutual exploration of their own family backgrounds and their interaction, they were able to recognize that some of the causes for their conflicts were rooted in their family and life experience differences: dependence/independence needs, communication patterns, parent–child relationship, and social relationships. Through couple therapy, they were able to renegotiate their relationships to be more mutually considerate and to not blame each other for being insensitive. For example, Mary recognized her need to become more independent not only from her parents but from Bob as well. She made a concerted effort to set limits with her mother and to develop personal interests and social relationships independent from Bob. Bob learned to understand the impact of his parents' stoic lifestyle on himself, to accept that Mary's interdependence with her family was not necessarily a sign of her inadequacy, and to be more supportive of her effort to change. In lieu of the significant amount of time they were spending with Mary's family, they also made an effort to find other couples who shared their interests and to socialize with them more. In addition, Bob was able to rid himself of guilt feelings about his artistic interest and was able to develop a comfortable balance between his professional life and creative, fun activities.

SUMMARY

The experience of Japanese Americans in the United States is quite unique and different from that of other Asian Americans and includes being herded into concentration camps based solely on ethnicity without due process. There are several subgroups among Japanese Americans each representing different stages of cultural transition and integration. Although their attitude toward psychotherapy and family therapy is tinged with the cultural stigma and reluctance to ask for outside assistance, there is increasing recognition of this need because of the current pressures on families and the erosion of the traditional family support system.

REFERENCES

Boszormenyi-Nagy, I., & Spark, G. (1973). *Invisible loyalties: Reciprocity in intergenerational family therapy.* Hagerstown, MD: Harper & Row.

Bowen, M. (1978). *Family therapy in clinical practice.* New York: Jason Aronson.

Connor, J. W. (1974). Acculturation and family continuities in three generations of Japanese-Americans. *Journal of Marriage and the Family,* 36, 159–165.

Doi, T. (1973). *The anatomy of dependence.* Tokyo: Kodansha.

Furuta, B. S. (1981). Ethnic identities of Japanese-American families: Implications for counseling. In C. Getty & W. Humphreys (Eds.), *Understanding the family* (pp. 200–231). New York: Appleton Autum.

Hieshima, J. A., & Schneider, B. (1994). Intergenerational effects on the cultural and cognitive socialization of third- and fourth-generation Japanese Americans. *Journal of Applied Developmental Psychology, 15,* 319–327.

Hosokawa, W. (1969). *The quiet Americans.* New York: Morrow.

Hsu, J., Tseng, W-S., Ashton, G., McDermott, J., & Char, W. (1985). Family interaction patterns among Japanese-American and Caucasian families in Hawaii. *American Journal of Psychiatry, 142,* 577–581.

Iwasaki-Mass, A. (1992). Interracial Japanese Americans: The best of both worlds or the end of the Japanese American community? In M. Root (Ed.), *Racially mixed people in America* (pp. 265–279). Newbury Park, CA: Sage.

Kikumura, A. (1981). *Through harsh winters.* Novato, CA: Chandler & Sharp.

Kim. B. L. (1977) Asian wives of U.S. servicemem: Women in shadows. *Amerasia Journal, 4,* 91–116.

Kitano, H. (1969a). Counseling and psychotherapy with Japanese Americans. In A. J. Marsella & P. B. Pedersen (Eds.), *Cross-cultural counseling and psychotherapy* (pp. 228–242). New York: Pergamon.

Kitano, H. (1969b). *Japanese Americans: The evolution of a subculture.* Englewood Cliffs, NJ: Prentice Hall

Kitano, H., & Kikumura, A. (1973). Interracial marriage: A picture of the Japanese American. *Journal of Social Issues, 29,* 66–81.

Landau, J. (1982). Therapy with families in cultural transition. In M. McGoldrick, J. K. Pearce, & J. Giordano (Eds.), *Ethnicity and family therapy* (pp. 522–572). New York: Guilford Press.

Lee, E. (1982). A social systems approach to assessment and treatment for Chinese American families. In M. McGoldrick, J. K. Pearce, & J. Giordano (Eds.), *Ethnicity and family therapy* (pp. 527–551). New York: Guilford Press.

Nagata, D. (1990). The Japanese American internment: Exploring the transgenerational consequences of traumatic stress. *Journal of Traumatic Stress, 3,* 47–69.

Nagata, D. (1991). Transgenerational impact of the Japanese American internment: Clinical issues in working with children of former internees. *Psychotherapy, 28,* 121–128.

Nishio, K., & Murase, K. (1983). *Characteristics of psychotherapists and their clients in Japan and psychotherapists and their Japanese American clients in the U.S.* Paper presented at Conference on Japanese culture and mental health, East–West Center, Honolulu, HI.

Takaki, R. (1989). *Strangers from a different shore: A history of Asian Americans.* Boston: Little, Brown.

Uba, L. (1994). *Asian Americans: Personality patterns, identity, and mental health.* New York: Guilford Press.

U.S. Bureau of the Census. (1993). *We the American Asians.* Washington, DC: U.S. Government Printing Office.

Yanagisako, S. (1976). Women-centered kin network in the Seattle Japanese-American community. In *Asian American women.* Palo Alto, CA: Stanford University Press.

7

Korean American Families

SUNG C. KIM

Koreans are one of the fastest growing ethnic groups in the United States. Recent Korean immigrants constitute the vast majority of the Korean American population. This chapter thus focuses on recent Korean immigrant families. Only recently has there been a systematic attempt at understanding and describing the Korean American family; the effects of immigration on their adjustment, adaptation, and acculturation; and the status of their mental health. This chapter highlights findings from relevant studies, rather than observational data or anecdotal impressions, on aspects of Korean American families and their psychological functioning.

HISTORICAL BACKGROUND

As a peninsula located in the heart of northeastern Asia, Korea's geography provided a cultural link between China and Japan. Confucianism and Buddhism, along with other aspects of the arts and culture, were introduced to Japan through Korea. In spite of the strong cultural influence of their neighbors, Koreans have nonetheless managed to maintain their own unique cultural identity in terms of their language, art, customs, and belief in a common historical destiny (Choy, 1979).

Korea's turbulent national history has been the story of its struggle to maintain independence from external interference (Choy, 1979). The wars and conflicts over Korea among its three neighbors (China, Japan, and the Soviet Union), as well as post-World War II superpowers, have caused much suffering and hardship for the Koreans. In this century alone, Korea was colonialized by Japan for 36 years until Japan was defeated in World War II. Korea was then divided into North and South Korea. Shortly after, the Korean War (1950–1953) erupted. Since the early 1960s, South Korea has launched itself on the path of modernization, industrialization, and economic independence.

MIGRATION HISTORY AND DEMOGRAPHICS IN THE UNITED STATES

The first wave of immigrant Koreans consisted of 7,226 Koreans who immigrated to Hawaii between 1903 and 1905 and 1,100 picture brides who joined them. Between 1905 and 1945, students, intellectuals, and political exiles came to the United States. The second wave of Koreans arrived in the United States between 1951 and 1964 and consisted of some 37,000 Korean wives of U. S. servicemen, war orphans, and students. The third wave, constituting the vast majority of Korean Americans, are immigrants who have arrived in the United States since 1965. The 1965 Immigration Act allowed 20,000 Koreans a year to enter the United States. In 1970, about 70,000 Korean Americans lived in the United States. The 1980 Census registered 357,393. The 1990 Census registered approximately 800,000. In the early 1970s, occupational immigrants, mostly professionals, and their families constituted the majority of Korean immigrants. However, the majority of Korean immigrants admitted over the last 10 years have come to this country by virtue of their relationships to those already here.

A large percentage of Korean immigrants (43.4%) live in the western region of the country, and approximately 30% are located in California (U. S. Bureau of the Census, 1983). The rest of the Korean population is evenly scattered throughout other parts of the country, with a strong tendency to settle in large metropolitan cities. Except for "Koreatown" in Los Angeles, Korean immigrants do not maintain nonterritorial ethnic communities by way of ethnic organizations, informal networks with kin members, alumni, and friends. In addition, various ethnic church and professional or recreational associations constitute the backbone of social activities for Korean immigrants (Min, 1988).

The primary reasons for the Korean migration are better economic opportunities in the United States, followed by better opportunities for children's education and political and social insecurity in South Korea (Hurh & Kim, 1984; Min 1988). Kim's (1978) study in Chicago showed that Koreans have stronger family ties than do other Asian groups and that family unification is the leading reason for the immigration of Korean women and the elderly.

Underemployment is a major problem in Korean immigrants' occupational adjustment. Whereas more than 90% of Korean adult immigrants were engaged in white-collar occupations in Korea, the 1980 Census (U. S. Bureau of the Census, 1984) indicates that only 47% of them are in white-collar occupational categories. The Korean group records the highest self-employment rate among 17 recent immigrant groups classified in the 1980 Census. Some 25–30% of Korean households own at least one business. A typical Korean business is a small family business, usually operated by the husband and wife.

TRADITIONAL FAMILY ORGANIZATION AND VALUE ORIENTATION

Family Characteristics, Patterns, and Roles

Historically, Korea was heavily influenced by the Chinese culture, especially Confucianism, which permeated the daily life and consciousness of Koreans. Confucianism, as applied to the Korean family system and social life, demanded children's one-sided obedience to and respect for parents and other adult members (Min, 1988). Confucianism emphasized a clear role differentiation and behavioral expectations between the husband and wife and parents and children. This principle helped to establish a rigid form of patriarchy and hierarchy in Korea. In the traditional Korean society, the husband was the breadwinner and decision maker and exercised authority over his wife and children. The wife was expected to obey her husband, serve him and his family members, and produce children. Older brothers or sisters were allowed to exercise a moderate level of authority over younger ones.

Perceptions about the proper role for women and children in the family and society, the language they use, and expected behavior are beginning to change in Korean society. In spite of the modernization in Korea, the traditional conjugal role differentiation has not been significantly modified (Min, 1988). The immigration of Koreans to the United States has led to many changes in the traditional Korean family system and structure, one of which is the disruption or at times reversal of this conjugal role differentiation. The 1980 Census shows that 56% of immigrant Korean married women are in the labor force, primarily because the wife's work is necessary for economic survival, especially for self-employed families.

Language and Communication Patterns

Koreans speak the same language, Korean, with relatively little regional variations. *Hangul*, based on a simple phonetic alphabet, is the official written language and is often combined with Chinese characters.

Two aspects of the Korean language are related to the nature of social relationships. One aspect is called the honorific humble system (Chang, 1988). Each honorific designation has different nuances of respect, distance, intimacy, and other interpersonal considerations. The skillful use of the system has traditionally been considered a highly valued personal and social asset, which often reveals the quality of one's upbringing, emotional stability, and other qualities. The principle underlying the honorific humble system is identical in Korea and Japan but is little developed in China (Chang, 1988). The other aspect is the use of different levels of speech (polite–formal, polite–informal, plain, and intimate style). The rules governing the choice of style in conversation derive from the art of knowing the complex sociocultural fabric of Korea.

Unique Value Orientation

Koreans emphasize education as the main avenue for social mobility. This is, in part, because the "civil service examination" stemming from Confucianism historically provided a major outlet for upward social mobility. Education is thus a viable means of success, and social distinction is reinforced by this Confucian value.

Influenced by their historical background, Koreans are noted for their endurance and resiliency under the most adverse conditions. Kim (1981) studied Korean immigrants in New York City and found that the Korean War experience and the sociocultural milieu of South Korea created a personality profile strong in survival instincts, opportunity seeking, and materialistic ambition.

In addition, Koreans adhere to family-centered Confucian ethics and adapt the ethics of self-discipline and dedication to work. Long work hours and sacrifices for the sake of family unity and well-being characterize many immigrants' lives.

Religion

Although only 25% of the population in Korea is Christian, about 60% to 70% of the new immigrants attend Korean ethnic Christian churches in the United States. The phenomenon of such a great number of Koreans attending ethnic Christian churches has not been found among other ethnic groups. Many Korean immigrants may be attracted to the church because they feel isolated and the ethnic church provides social and psychological support in addition to religious functions (Hurh & Kim, 1988). The church serves the role of extended family for many immigrant Koreans.

Special Life Cycle Rituals

According to Korean tradition, the 100th day after the birth of a baby was an occasion of great celebration because it signified the survival of the baby in early times. The two most important birthdays in the life of a Korean are the first and the 60th, *hwan-gap*. The 60-year cycle symbolizes the completion of a full cycle in life. Weddings are another rite of passage with great ceremony. Traditional funerals are also ceremonies of great meaning to the family and involved elaborate rituals and reflected the concern for the departed, the cornerstone of the traditional Confucian family system.

EFFECTS OF CULTURAL TRANSITION ON THE FAMILY SYSTEM

Special Stresses and Strengths

On the one hand, the Korean American family system represents a relatively stable and secure environment for Korean children as they adjust to life in the United States. Many Korean American children are exposed to their parents' firm belief about the value of education, hard work, adaptability, discipline, self-confidence, and pride in their ethnic identity. Compared with the national average, Korean have fewer single-parent families and a lower divorce rate. (However, recent Korean immigrants show a five to six times higher divorce rate than does the general Korean population [Min, 1988], which suggests a breakdown in the traditional family system.)

On the other hand. Korean immigrants' occupational adjustment in small businesses, particularly women's necessary involvement in the work force, has caused many parents to work long hours and to be away from the home. This may contribute to such emerging concerns among Korean American children as truancy, alcohol abuse, and psychological problems. It may also lead to a significant modification of the traditional marital-role differentiation.

Adaptation and Acculturation

"Critical phases" in the "adaptation process" (Hurh & Kim, 1990) of Korean immigrants provide a useful framework to understand structural and situational contexts of migration process and adjustment. This framework hypothesizes that an immigrant Korean would go through various critical phases of adaptation. The first is called "exigency" (1-2 years of the resettlement), which can be characterized by problems of language barrier, unemployment, underemployment, social isolation, and culture shock. Exigency is redressed through the second, or "resolution," stage (2 to 10-15 years) and the immigrants' life satisfaction may reach its peak (the "optimum" stage). In the next stage, "social marginality," the stagnation in life satisfaction occurs, reportedly because of an identity crisis stemming from feelings of relative deprivation and marginality. The last stage involves being resigned to "marginality acceptance" or developing a "new identity."

A study of this model (Hurh & Kim, 1990) essentially confirmed the hypothesized critical phases and indicated that (1) the immigrant's mental health is most vulnerable at the early stage of migration, or the exigency stage; (2) as length of residence extends, the degree of an immigrant's well-being increases; and (3) the rate of increase in the immigrant's mental well-being tends to stagnate after the resolution stage, thus confirming the marginality hypothesis.

An example of the differential rate of acculturation is the division that exists between traditional parents and their rapidly acculturating children. Parents often believe that their children should simply follow the narrow range of alternatives that make up the parents' value system and tend to use authoritarian parenting strategies. Their well-entrenched Korean values frequently set them against those values of their children, especially in the areas of dating, sex, and interracial marriage.

In a major study, Hurh and Kim (1988) also found sex differences in the mental health correlates among Korean immigrants. Work-related variable, such as job satisfaction, occupation, and income, are strongly correlated with the male respondents' positive mental health. On the other hand, female respondents' positive mental health is more related to family life satisfaction, ethnic attachment variables (e.g., Korean church affiliation, kinship contact, and reading of Korean newspaper), and some variables of Americanization (driver's license, English proficiency, and American friends). Of interest was a finding that as a result of immigrant life conditions and the persistence of the traditional gender-role ideology (woman as a homemaker), most of the employed wives carry a double burden of performing the household tasks and working outside the home. The traditional ideology of conjugal-role differentiation persists in the Korean immigrant community and the double roles give Korean immigrant working wives additional stresses.

Coping Strategies

Hurh and Kim (1990) distinguished two kinds of coping strategies. Marginality acceptance is a negative coping strategy, that is, a passive acceptance of the immigrant's precarious place as the Korean minority in American (resignation). In contrast, a positive coping would be the creation of third identity—the Korean American ethnicity, which yet to be defined.

Hurh and Kim (1984) also noted a pattern of "adhesive or additive mode of adaptation" of the immigrants. In this pattern, the immigrants do not resist acculturation but rather seek to adopt the new culture without necessarily discarding or weakening the old. The model probably has the greatest applicability to first-generation immigrants. For later-generation Korean Americans, "biculturality" is more applicable and needs to be further developed, because there is no current model of Korean biculturality.

Functional and dysfunctional coping strategies were addressed by a study on Korean American elderly (Kiefer et al., 1985). In this particular study, adjustment was positively related to education, length of residence in the United States, and multigenerational immigrants who were better educated and hence more resourceful in learning English and as a result able to take a more responsible and active role in the family. Elders living in two- and three-generation households often had problems of crowding, overwork, and strained social relationships, yet they tended to exhibit more positive morale and better self-concept than those who lived alone or alone with a spouse. The "low adapted group" had a strong tendency to express their maladjustment and emotional difficulties somatically (particularly through depression).

Common Presenting Mental Health Problems

No systematic epidemiological studies have been conducted on the prevalence rates of mental or emotional disorders among Korean Americans in the U. S. In the absence of data for Korean Americans, recent psychiatric epidemiological data obtained at the community level in Korea can be cited as baseline information and a point of reference. Lee (1988) found that the overall lifetime prevalence rate of psychiatric disorders in Korea was about 13.5%. When alcohol abuse or dependence and tobacco dependence were added, almost 40% of the subjects were found to have at least 1 of 20 diagnoses according to the third edition of the *Diagnostic and Statistical Manual of Mental Health* (American Psychiatric Association, 1980). The prevalence rates for alcohol abuse or dependence were 22%. For drug abuse or dependence the rate was 0.7%. The lifetime prevalence rates were as follows: 0.46% for schizophrenic disorders, 5.4% for affective disorders (with major depression, 3.37%; manic episode, 0.42%; and dysthymia, 2%), and 9.5% for anxiety disorders. Information on Korean immigrants seeking mental health care at a community mental health-based service in San Francisco indicated the same wide range of mental health problems (Kim et al., 1989). However, the Korean data may have limited generalizability for Korean immigrants. If any, the prevalence rates for psychological disorders among Korean immigrants may be higher than those for Koreans in Korea because of additional adjustment stress in the United States. Korean wives of the U.S. servicemen, who have "doubly marginal" status, and Korean elderly populations are, for example, particularly vulnerable to emotional problems.

Another index of the stress of Korean Americans can be found in Kuo's study (1984) on the prevalence of depressive symptoms among Asian Americans in Seattle. His Korean sample exhibited the highest depression scores in comparison with those of Chinese, Japanese, and Filipino Americans. Structural and situational factors seemed to account for the finding: shorter length of residence, higher rates of underemployment (higher educational status but lower-prestige jobs), limited ability in English, and higher concentration in small businesses located in high-risk districts.

CLINICAL CONSIDERATIONS

Conceptualization of Mental Illness and Emotional Difficulties

From the traditional perspective, mental illness is regarded as a supernatural intervention, an affliction caused by evil or vengeful spirits, or a result of hereditary weakness, character weakness, physical and emotional strain, or imbalance within the body of *yin* and *yang*. Stigma and shame are attached to mental illness, and all members of a family share in its impact.

Help-Seeking Behavior and Mental Health Service System in Korea

Many patients who visit a mental health practitioner have already attempted various folk-healing methods. In a survey of 100 psychiatric patients in Korea, Rhi (196) found that 66% of them had previously tried Eastern healing methods, including shamanistic sessions, faith-healing endeavors, and Chinese medicine in various combinations, and that the more chronic the disorder, the greater the variety of remedies sought by patients.

A study of Koreans utilizing a mental health service in San Francisco found that they severely underutilized the service in spite of active outreach efforts (Kim et al., 1989). In addition, only 9% of the referrals were self-made. Korean patients in general sought mental health help only as a last resort when they were severely disturbed or in an acute crisis. Most of them tried herbal medicine, acupuncture, Christian religious counseling, and medical help before they sought Western psychological treatment modality.

Expectations of Treatment

When Koreans were asked about effective treatment for the mentally ill, they responded that isolation, rest, prayer, and penitence were key ingredients of therapy (Ahn & Rhi, 1986). Many families prefer to place their mentally ill members in mountaintop prayer centers, temples, locked religious facilities, or "Christian asylums" for the mentally ill rather than psychiatric hospitals (Kim, 1992). Quite often, folk-healing methods in

Korea combine elements from diverse healing traditions. For example, folk therapies may include rare organic food, herbs, ceremonial purification of ancestral spirits, chanting, hymning, and prayer. Faith healing, religious counseling, fasting, and special prayer groups are often used for the mentally ill.

Perception of Professional Roles

It is often necessary for the therapist to assume multiple roles, especially in working with patients who present with severe problems stemming from several hardships. The work may necessitate coordination, advocacy, case management, and psychoeducation and requires time and active involvement of the therapist. In addition to the challenging process of working with the difficult-to-engage patient, the therapist typically needs to work with significant others of the patient.

Effective Therapeutic Techniques

The fundamental premise in beginning treatment with Korean American patients is to accept their inner reality and world view as valid. Patients must feel that the therapist understands them and accepts their concerns and fears (e.g., shame and stigma of being emotionally imbalanced) as reasonable and valid.

The engagement process is the most challenging because of strong cultural injunctions against seeking mental health. Shame of exposing one's own or one's family's problems in public and fear of being stigmatized as being "crazy" are major cultural obstacles that discourage Koreans from seeking mental health services.

Clinicians need to develop ways of encouraging Korean Americans to stay in therapy. Some studies have discussed structural and strategic elements useful in working with Korean American families (Kim, 1985). For example, addressing the family of the social and power hierarchy as prescribed by the Korean culture would be the safest way to begin the family therapy. This is in keeping with the understanding that the structure of the Korean language is generally not conducive to conducting family therapy in an egalitarian, open, direct, and conjoint fashion. "Protecting the parent's face" is important, at least until the therapist has gained the necessary and sufficient "authority" and trust in the parent's eyes and until the therapeutic relationship is strong enough to withstand a confrontation in sessions. Reframing may be very effective with the Korean American family because relabeling what people do in a positive way saves face and encourages change. For example, the shame related to having to seek therapy can be countered by pointing to the kind of unrecognized strength that transcends the cultural injunction and is in keeping with restoring the good family name. Also, it is advisable to conduct separate (rather than conjoint) interviews initially for couples and family members (Kim, 1985). The function of the therapist as a "go-between" can bridge the culturally induced gap in power and communication among family members.

Goal setting may best be stated in terms of situational change or external resolution (as opposed to internal resolution, such as emotional expressiveness, self-assertion, and insight acquisition). Long-term goals may best be broken down into a series of visible, achievable, interrelated short-term goals which are renegotiable with the family. Such an approach is not intended to minimize the importance of insights, dynamics, or emotional expressiveness but rather to engage the family in therapy.

Kim et al. (1989) have identified some of the therapeutic elements that respond specifically to Korean cultural/psychological needs. They include (1) structuring (recognizing the perception of the therapist as the authority, high initial anxiety, and the lack of knowledge about how psychotherapy works); (2) educating the client about the therapeutic process, obstacles, and outcomes; (3) being willing to give culturally congruent directives (given the cultural expectation for direct answers, if not guidance); and (4) allowing a safe environment for catharsis (recognizing long suppressed emotions and secrets in most clients).

CONCLUSIONS

Korean Americans are largely recent immigrants who face multiple stresses related to the processes of their immigration, adjustment, and acculturation. Understanding the Korean American family requires consideration of the sociocultural, structural, and situational contexts of their immigration.

Although there seems to be universality of presenting concerns and the kinds and range of emotional disorders, qualitative differences exist between Korean Americans and others related to variables such as help-seeking pattern, engagement, and roles of the therapist. The differences, stemming from different world views held by Korean Americans, necessitate a need to alter our concept of what constitutes "good" psychotherapy. If we are to equate good psychotherapy with insight and process orientations, as valid as they are, we may be denying many Korean Americans the opportunity to benefit from mental health care. Therapists need to conceptualize psychotherapy in a larger context that goes beyond theoretical provincialism, and be open-minded and flexible in providing culturally relevant and sensitive mental health services to Korean Americans.

REFERENCES

Ahn, D. H., & Rhi, B. Y. (1986). Community leaders' reactions to mental disorder. *Seoul Journal of Psychiatry (Korea), 11*(4), 281–293.

American Psychiatric Association. (1980). *Diagnostic and statistical manual of mental disorders* (3rd ed.). Washington, DC: Author.

Chang, S. C. (1988). The nature of the self: A transcript view. *Transcultural Psychiatric Research Review, 25*(3), 169–203.

Choy, B. Y. (1979). *Koreans in America.* Chicago: Nelson-Hall.

Hurh, W. M., & Kim, K. C. (1984). *Korean immigrants in America.* Cranbury, NJ: Fairleigh Dickinson University Press.

Hurh, W. M., & Kim, K. C. (1988, June). *Uprooting and adjustment: A sociological study of Korean immigrants' mental health.* Final report to the National Institute of Mental Health. Macomb, IL: Western Illinois University.

Hurh, W. M., & Kim, K. C. (1990). Adaptation stages and mental health of Korean male immigrants in the United States. *International Migration Review, 24.*

Kiefer, C. W., Kim, S. C., Choi, K., Kim, L., Kim, B. L., Shon, S., & Kim, T. (1985). Adjustment problems of Korean American elderly. *The Gerontologist, 25*(5), 477–482.

Kim, B. L. (1978). *The Asian Americans: Changing patterns, changing needs.* Montclair, NJ: Association for Korean Christian Scholars in North America.

Kim, L. (1992). Mental health of Korean Americans. In A. Gaw (Ed.), *Culture, ethnicity, and mental illness.* Washington, DC: American Psychiatric Press.

Kim, I. S. (1981). *New urban immigrants: The Korean community in New York.* Princeton: Princeton University Press.

Kim, S. C. (1985). A strategic–structural approach for Asian American families. *Psychotherapy, 22*(2), 342–348.

Kim, S. C., Lee, S. U., Chu, K. H., & Cho, K. J. (1989). Korean American and mental health: Clinical experiences of Korean American mental health services. *Asian American Psychological Journal,* pp. 18–27.

Kuo, W. H. (1984). Prevalence of depression among Asian-Americans. *Journal of Nervous and Mental Disease, 172.*

Lee, C. K. (1988). *Psychiatric disorders in the Republic of Korea.* Paper presented at Scientific Annual Convention of American Psychiatric Association, San Francisco.

Min, P. G. (1988). *The Korean American family.* In C. H. Mindel, R. W. Habenstein, & R. Wright (Eds.), *Ethnic families in America: Patterns and variations.* New York: Elsevier.

Rhi, B. Y. (1976). Analysis in Korea with special reference to the question of success and failure in analysis. In G. Adler (Ed.), *Proceedings of the Fifth International Congress for Analytic Psychology.* New York: Putnam's Sons.

U.S. Bureau of the Census. (1983). General social and economic characteristics. In *1980 census of population* (Vol. 1). Washington, DC: U.S. Government Printing Office.

U.S. Bureau of the Census. (1984). Detailed population characteristics. In *1980 census of population* (Vol. 1). Washington, DC: U.S. Government Printing Office.

8

Laotian American Families

LAURIE JO MOORE
KHAM-ONE KEOPRASEUTH
PAUL K. LEUNG
LOO HANG CHAO

The degree and intensity of suffering of the Laotian people as a result of the Indochinese war have been no less dramatic than that of the Khmer and the Vietnamese. The exodus of Laotians began shortly after the fall of Saigon in 1975. During the past two decades, 243,374 Laotians have been forced to flee their homeland (Haywood, 1995). In the United States, Laotians account for nearly one-fourth of the 1.5 million Indochinese refugees. Laos has historically supported and maintained more than 68 different distinct ethnic populations. Of these ethnic populations, the Laotian refugees have primarily been members of the lowland ethnic Lao and the highlander tribespeople, chiefly the Hmong, Mien, Kmu, Tai Dam, and Lao-Theung.

HISTORICAL BACKGROUND

The recorded history of Laotian people extends several thousand years into the past. It documents periodic invasions of the area and conquests by neighboring countries. Unfortunately, most Laotian historical records were destroyed during the years of the Burmese and Thai invasions in the 1700s (Viravong, 1964). Through access to Chinese chronicles, remnants of ancient relics, and oral history, scholars have been able to piece together some knowledge of the formation of the Lao Kingdom. The establishment of the modern Lao government in the 14th century was the product primarily of the lowland ethnic Lao. This occurred at the zenith of their civilization as the feudal states with their tribal and indigenous populations were united as a nation (Coedès, 1959). The Lao migrated from their ancient homeland of Nong Sae (the present-day provinces of Szechwan and Yunan in southern China). King Khun Borom (A.D. 729) established the first formal state, called Muong Soua. Muong Soua became the ancient capital now called Luangprabang. King Fa Ngum later renamed the country Anajak Lan Xang (the Land of Million Elephants) in 1353.

Recent archaeological findings dating back 5,000 years produced evidence of 35 kings who ruled this land before King Khun Borom. They revealed the existence of the Ban Chiang civilization in northeastern Thailand (Labbe, 1985; Bhamorabutr, 1988). This was a rice-growing civilization whose people have survived but scattered and assimilated into different ethnic groups as a result of the ravages of wars with neighboring powers. In the 19th century the Laotians were overtaken by the French colonial powers. After years of unsettled dispute over the claim of this area between Laos and Thailand, the French negotiated the settlement in favor of Thailand. The country of Laos and its people have suffered repeated devastation during almost 100 years of war that began with the French, continued during the Japanese invasion in World War II, and extended over four decades during the war in Indochina.

TRADITIONAL LAOTIAN CULTURES

Lao culture has been influenced by Hindu traditions and has inherited rich resources of Hindu literature and philosophy, including an intellectual perspective on life that encourages a pursuit of harmony with the environment and nature. Many Lao rituals and cultural practices are reminiscent of the Hindu tradition of Brahmanism, an ancient healing practice that involves appeasing the soul and spirit world. The intent of many Lao spiritual ceremonies is to empower people to address the demands made on them by spiritual entities or deities.

In the 14th century, Buddhism was introduced as a state religion by King Fa Ngum. Other religious practices were forced underground for centuries to come. The Theravadan Buddhist sect emphasizes individual pursuit of enlightenment. The virtues of Theravadan Buddhism have been integrated into Lao beliefs, healing practices, and patterns of conflict resolution. This includes beliefs such as reincarnation and placing great value on selflessness and freedom from attachment to worldly possessions.

The cultural diversity of Lao society has provided a strength and a resiliency that has helped sustain the nation despite the destruction wrought by the ravages of war. The highland tribes such as the Hmong and Mien are autonomous tribal societies with separate and distinct language and customs that date back 3,000 years (Vang, 1976). The Hmong and Mien tribes have patrilinear family clan systems of organization. They have survived throughout their history as highland farmers, sometimes cultivating opium as a cash crop. They have been successful in shielding their society from the domination and impact of urbanization partly by virtue of their isolation in high and relatively inaccessible mountainous terrain. They have been able to preserve their cultural identity, including their entirely oral language tradition and family values (Iwata, Sakamoto, & Halpern, 1960). The only documents of their intellectual and cultural practices are written in Mandarin Chinese and these are largely the domain of the shaman. Some Chinese texts are available as resources to heads of the family. The traditions of these tribes suggest a strong influence by the Chinese culture, which is reflected in folk-healing practices and philosophical views of the world.

In the past 50 years, the sociopolitical turmoil in Laos has dramatically affected the Mien and Hmong tribes due to their direct involvement with Central Intelligence Agency operations. Politically these tribes were especially vulnerable to persecution by the communists. They suffered severe casualties during the war and were subjected to decades of atrocities leading to the loss of their homeland.

In the contemporary societies of the Hmong and the Mien in America, the most pressing issues are no longer basic survival as younger-generation professionals have gained a foothold in the work force and are thriving economically (Vang 1976; Yang 1995). Although traditional animistic and humanistic religious beliefs have been kept intact, family tragedy, major illnesses, or unremitting suffering has led some people to give up their faith for the monotheistic worship of Christianity in the hope that their plight will be assuaged.

THE TRADITIONAL FAMILY

Laotians are peaceful people. They have coexisted in a multicultural society for generations and they share a diverse heritage that they deeply cherish and appreciate. Lao may appear shy and subdued because of their tradition of respect for elders, politeness, and tolerance of strangers (Phommasouvanh, 1976). Underneath the facade, behavioral conditioning, and emotional discipline, however, lies a strong sense of character and self-determination with common aspirations rooted in their spiritual beliefs and the long history of the lush and abundant tropical jungle that is their homeland.

Traditional Laotian societies are based on a system of family hierarchical power and extended kinship. Lowland Lao tend to be more urbanized and adapt more easily to Western conventions. They are likely to be more familiar with health care services and the use of Western medications. Rural Lao families tend to be more reliant on traditional healing methods and sacrificial remedies performed by shaman. Others may use rituals when it is convenient. Some of these practices involve offering food and drink to appease the spirits of ancestors or deities. Conditions that cannot be corrected by using these practices are eventually referred to Western medical practitioners. Emotional or psychological conditions may often be considered spiritual problems. By the time a Lao patient has presented to the Western medical caregiver, the family has tried everything within its knowledge and has exhausted its local ethnic community resources. So the family turns to Western medical providers with a mixture of extreme reservation and high anxiety.

Roles of the Old and the Young

The hierarchy of power in a Lao family is structured from the top down, from the elders to the multigenerational offspring who constitute the extended family unit. The relationship is built on the Theravadan Buddhist concept of a life as a circle: birth, growth and development, aging, illness, and death (Luangpraseut, 1987). Parents and grandparents are devoted to raising their young with the hope that the children and grandchildren will perform their duties and fulfill their obligation toward their elders according to family teaching throughout the cycle of family life and their journey through time.

Roles of Husband and Wife

Men are the head of the household in Laotian culture and they make all important decisions and take responsibility for providing for the well-being, growth, and development of family members. The family may include more than one generation and distant relatives both by blood and by marriage. In the male-dominant society, Lao women are trusted with the responsibility of handling money and they are expected to pattern their lifestyle and interests to augment their husband's career or business. Traditionally, a woman's role is the care of the children and the home (Phommasouvanh, 1976).

Roles of Son and Daughter

As part of growing up in Lao families, children learn to put their self-interests second to those of the family, group, or nation. The notion of independent decision making is not highly valued during childhood. Interdependence and subordination to one's elders are revered. The Theravadan Buddhist virtues of self-negation and modesty are part of the essence of being Laotian. Becoming an adult means achieving these virtues and fulfilling one's obligations to the family. Once these skills are accomplished a young person is able to move toward independence and a career that involves assuming a role as head of a household for men or motherhood for women. Family loyalty and a sense of obligation toward younger siblings are expected as well as helping with household chores and being responsible for self-care. Boys are assigned heavy outdoor types of chores under the supervision of the male adults in the family, who could be either the father, uncle, older sibling, or grandfather. These chores include activities such as farmwork, tending livestock, drawing water from wells or streams, repairing homemade equipment, making household repairs, building, and producing crafts or pottery for sales. Girls are given household duties such as cooking, cleaning, tending the garden, weaving, or manufacturing silk clothing or crafts for sale in the home-based cottage industry.

THE FAMILY IN TRANSITION

Life in the United States has been a mixed blessing for Laotians. Over the past 20 years, traditional families have gone through a full revolution of the circle of life: A new generation has been born and the older generation is passing their prime. Lao families find themselves struggling to preserve life as they know it in the context of a rapidly changing and challenging American culture that determines what options are available for their development in school, work, social, recreational, and community settings.

The First Immigrants

Following the escape from their homeland, the first immigrants to America came with whatever they could preserve of their family unit. Often parents came alone, as a couple, or with young children who were born in Laos or in the refugee camps. The early years of resettlement demanded that individuals, both male and female, make a rapid adaptation to learning English and obtaining job skills. It was necessary for women and young people to assume important roles in the family as breadwinners and communicators. This was in direct conflict to traditional Lao values, and this dynamic became another stressor that upset the family already overwhelmed with losses and the demands of acculturation.

Changes in the Family Structure

Adapting to American culture has required major transformations in the cognitive and behavioral aspects of family functioning. Work and financial security have become the central focus of family life. Employability and ability to speak English have created parent–child role reversals that are deeply problematic. Children quickly learn to assimilate to the perceived norms of their peers and relate to their parents with a sense of entitlement. Their defensive stance may even imply the threat of child abuse accusations. Parents feel their authority in their traditional role as caregivers is being undermined and they feel precariously defensive around their children and neighbors. Traditional disciplinary measures (corporal punishment and the threat of harsh treatment of any degree) are no longer acceptable or legal.

The family encounters a paradigm shift in its sense of morality. There is little left to the sanctity of the old laws of *karma* (reincarnation) and spiritual principles of daily living that would normally encourage young people to strive for harmony and happiness under the spiritual guidance of their parents. The five precepts (no killing, no lying, no stealing, no sexual misconduct, and no use of intoxicants) seem of no consequence to the second generation of some youth. Parents find it increasingly difficult to relate these principles to their children and they find it difficult if not impossible to prevent the shame or disgrace that results from the mischevious behavior of their children. The traditional authority of the elders is no longer recognized in the eyes of the police or the courts of law.

In these situations a traditional Lao person may feel the only option is to resist change. This resistance essentially blocks the family's process of acculturation and leaves confused or insecure persons in a position of doubting their self-esteem and their identity in relation to the ethnic community. These internal family conflicts disrupt the family's ability as a group to perform tasks and be productive. These conflicts can also ruin any opportunity for the kind of quality time and nourishment that traditionally support a Lao family. For some people, there is no such thing as family time. Spare time such as it is has dwindled down to the time between work and sleep. Many family members are working two jobs and overtime to make ends meet. Individuals are thus forced to face all the complications of acculturation in a new society without the support or nurturance of their family. It is easy to see how young people become dissatisfied, angry, and disenfranchized with family and material acquisitions and thereby become more vulnerable to physical or emotional distress.

The New Family Roles, Identities, and Cultural Conflicts

Once family members become established on a career path and economically and socially integrated into mainstream culture they can begin to feel some hope that they will be able to resurrect their ideal traditional family life. When economic survival is addressed the family can turn its attention to accommodating to other cultural stresses such as learning English and new social values. This endeavor varies for individuals and families. People may find themselves anywhere on the spectrum between being very traditional and acculturated and being Americanized. An acculturated person has been described as someone who has learned the sociocultural skills to survive as an independent and self-sufficient, bicultural/bilingual person (Khoxayo, 1993). However, when different family members find themselves at different places on this spectrum, this leads to a sense of dysphoria and value conflict in family dynamics.

In a study of lowland Lao in Oregon, health problems and physical pain were found to significantly affect mental and the general physical health. The level of acculturation was a predictor for the subjective experience of well-being. The more proficient a person was in the English language, the fewer mental health symptoms he or she had. People with intact social support systems (e.g., married people) had fewer mental and physical health symptoms than those who were divorced, widowed, or separated (Vandiver, Jordan, Keopraseuth, & Yu, 1995; Vandiver & Keopraseuth, in press).

TREATMENT CONSIDERATIONS

Resistance to Seeking Help

When the threshold of tolerable family stress is exceeded, emotions flare and expectations run wild; communication breaks down and depression and anxiety may set in. The Breakdown of the family system might be expressed, for example, by incidents of child abuse, spouse abuse, an increase in substance abuse, and/or possibly legal difficulties. In a family with an intact natural support system, a scenario such as this would be appropriately handled in a private and formal conflict resolution process directed by the elders of the family, group, or clan. In families lacking adequate support or in situation in which this intervention proves unsuccessful, most Lao families would be reluctant to seek help from the Western-designed system of care (e.g., individual/couple/family counseling or clinical psychological/psychiatric services). This reluctance may be the result of the stigma associated with mental illness. It could also be the result of a lack of information or understanding of the helping process.

In some cases in which discord has escalated to the breaking point and violence has occurred, involvement with the criminal justice system forces the family into the care system by virtue of its need for emergency medical treatment. People who respond well to initial contact with the treatment system are likely to be convinced that they are on the right course and are likely to ask for more help. They may be willing to explore therapeutic services for self-development as well as to learn skills to cope with life changes. They may even be receptive to biological and chemical interventions. Most Lao people know how to adjust the level of service they require to the minimum. The severely ill with chronic major mental disease, however, tend to be shy and disorganized as a result of poor social skills and impaired judgment and need much more direction and support.

The Therapeutic Alliance

It takes a long time to develop a trusting therapeutic relationship with a client from this population. Most Laotian people do not understand the significance of medical specialists and relate to mental health professionals as they would to general medical healers. They are preoccupied with discussing their concerns about physical aches and pain. These physical symptoms may be urgent and access to adequate health care providers with professional interpretation may be limited so that the person feels compelled to take advantage of the opportunity for getting help. As immediate health concerns are addressed, people may begin to discuss family issues and other emotional problems. This may be the first chance the person has had to discuss very sensitive and troubling feelings and symptoms that are confusing and frightening. It is important to listen and facilitate communication in a genuine, empathic and nonjudgmental manner.

The Communication Process

Some clients understand English but possess a limited speaking ability. It is important to speak to the client directly and encourage him or her to speak English as much as possible. It is important to allow adequate time to understand what a person wants to communicate. Most people do not feel comfortable sharing intimate problems with people they do not trust. Communicating across a cultural barrier requires patience and kindness. It may take months or years to understand what might otherwise be communicated in a short visit. People need to know that the clinician is committed to helping them no matter how long it takes or how confusing it is. This helps clients feel connected and may allay some of their frustration at not being able to get the help they need.

Interpretation and translation services ought to be structured so that a minimal amount of time is spent on translating or speaking two languages. Instead, interpreters or translators should attempt to convey the optimal information and encourage direct communication between the caregiver and the client while the interpreter quietly assists with difficult words or technical expressions or issues important to clarify the accuracy of medical inquiries. If the interpreter is working as a regular team member, he or she can gather most of the basic information and then facilitate the interview by directing the caregiver to the areas of most important concern. If no interpreter is involved, caregivers must be very cautious because patients may not really understand what is being said and they may feel compelled to respond in a gracious, deferential manner that may be completely misleading clinically.

Medical and psychiatric symptoms are often intermixed with substance abuse issues (Tung, 1985; D'Avanzo, 1994). Clinical symptoms may be the result of culture-bound syndromes and practices of rituals based on a magico-religious beliefs such as *phii* (genii) or deities (Suwanlert, 1979; Westermeyer, 1979). As succinctly put by Luangpraseut (1987), that mystical relationship between a person's sense of self and his or her belief about the causes of ill health has a controlling and healing power over many aspects of human life.

High Prevalence of Mental Illnesses

Lao, Mien, and Hmong refugee populations have been noted to present to health care settings with a high prevalence of somatic or bodily complaints. When no physical cause for such complaints can be found, these symptoms can be described as somatization, a presumed phenomena whereby psychological problems are expressed or experienced as physical problems. Lin (1983) found that 42.7% of Southeast Asian refugees presented to primary care settings with somatization. Westermeyer has reported that with time and acculturation, depression and somatization became less evident but anxiety, hostility, and paranoia changed very little. (Westermeyer, 1989). Mollica et al. (1990) found that among Indochinese refugees, the Lao and Hmong had the least reduction in depressive symptoms and in fact had an increase in anxiety and somatic complaints over time.

Kroll et al. (1989) found an 80% prevalence rate among the Hmong of major depression in a mental health clinic, the highest rate of the four Southeast Asian ethnic groups.

Kinzie et al. (1990) found that in Southeast Asian patients presenting to a psychiatric clinic, the prevalence of posttraumatic stress disorder

(PTSD) was underestimated even when doctors and counselors were well trained in working with people who had been severely traumatized. In this population, depression was frequently recognized. But especially in the hill tribes people, the diagnosis of PTSD was frequently missed. Varying estimates have been made about the prevalence of depression and PTSD in refugee populations depending on the population being studied.

Both Mien and Lao psychiatric patients experience high prevalence rates of physical pain (Moore & Sager, 1997). In a study with 59 Mien and 30 Lao psychiatric patients suffering from depression and PTSD, 95% of people complained of chronic pain. When these patients were examined by a rheumatologist, 88% had a rheumatological diagnosis, including predominately myofascial pain syndromes, fibromyalgia, osteoarthritis, perathritis, and carpal tunnel syndrome. In addition, 56% of the Mien and 48% of the Lao had unexplained pain or paresthesias. Approximately 93% of people had unexplained pain and paresthesias in combination with a diagnosable rheumatological disorder.

These findings are consistent with studies that correlate functional somatic symptoms with anxiety and depression (Lader & Marks, 1971; Katon, Reis, & Kleinman, 1984). Pain is a common symptom accompanying depression, with authors reporting rates from 27% to 100% (Moore & Sager, 1997). At the same time, when people experience more than one pain site there is an increased risk of depression: 8.96% prevalence with two sites of pain; 11.96% with three sites (Dworkin, Von Korff, & LeResche, 1990).

Given this information, it is prudent to carefully evaluate Lao, Mien, and other hill tribes people for the presence of depression and PTSD. It is also important to perform a thorough medical history and examination to identify treatable medical conditions that might be contributing to depression and anxiety. Any screening of refugee patients for depression and PTSD ought to be done with a counselor or translator specifically trained in mental health.

It is not acceptable to presume that somatic complaints are somatization without an adequate assessment. Medical conditions that may be contributing to psychological symptoms need to be diagnosed and treated.

It is wise to remember that PTSD may remain hidden despite a thorough initial history. Patients may be reluctant to discuss something so traumatizing with a clinician they hardly know. Psychogenic amnesia may play a role. However, patients who have been treated for as long a 10 years may suddenly be able to discuss a history of trauma that completely changes the clinician's understanding of their suffering. When working with people who speak another language, it is always wise for caregivers to keep an open mind and to consider their understanding of the patient's condition as relative and incomplete.

CASE EXAMPLE 1

MV was a 36-year-old ethnic lowland Lao woman who had been married for 7 years and lived with her husband and four children. She came to the United States in 1980. She was first seen in 1981, complaining of an 8-year history of headaches. Upon further questioning she reported that she had also been depressed for 8 years. The depression had become worse in the last 3 months after she had a tubal ligation. MV reported poor sleep, decreased appetite with a 40-pound weight loss, loss of pleasure and interest in life, and thoughts of suicide.

Family History

MV was the oldest of two children. She grew up in Laos. Her father died in 1975 and she left her mother and brother in Laos when she moved to the refugee camp where she remained for 6 years. While she was in the camp two of her children, ages 16 and 6, died.

Assessment and Diagnosis

MV was felt to be suffering from major depression and she was started on imipramine, an antidepressant. She was seen individually every 4 to 6 weeks and responded to the support with resolution of her symptoms.

Two years later, MV presented with rapid speech reporting that she heard the voice of her deceased grandfather. She reported seeing his portrait, which no one else could see. She was not oriented to her environment and her judgment was impaired. An antipsychotic was added to her imipramine. Her family then moved to another state and when they returned a year later she had stopped taking her medications. Her symptoms were exacerbated with more psychosomatic complaints.

Her medicines were reinstituted and she continued taking them until 1985 when the antipsychotic was discontinued. Two months later she reported seeing ghosts and feeling very angry. On further questioning it was learned that she had separated from her husband for financial reasons. He was unable to support the family. In order to survive, MV needed to apply for general assistance.

Treatment Course

Her treatment continued without unusual events until August 1986, when she presented with paranoia and inappropriate laughter. She said that her heart was swinging like a pendulum. The shaking of her heart was associated with shortness of breath, sweating, tingling in her extremities, shaking, and fear of impending doom. She was having daily attacks like this that lasted 5 to 6 hours. She seemed to be suffering from panic disorder and propranolol was added to her medicines. She did well until October 1986.

In October, MV began hearing voices. She was also disturbed by a sensation of numbness in her legs. She told us that at the age of 31 she had been paralyzed for 2 years and had been unable to walk. She experienced a gradual ascending paralysis over a 4-day period associated with loss of sensation in her legs. She was very worried that the paralysis would recur. A neurological examination was arranged and was completely normal so no follow-up was pursued.

After being in treatment for more than 6 years with the same doctor and ethnic counselor, MV reported in December 1987 that she was being possessed by her ancestor's spirit. She had been drinking and had stopped taking her medication. Her husband reported that she was disorganized and angry. In the Portland area at this time several robberies had resulted in the murder of a Cambodian family. These events had been extremely disturbing to MV.

MV reported that her spirit possession had begun when she was 30 years old. Two cousins and a niece were also channels for their ancestor's spirits. One cousin had died as a result of possession. MV was fearful that her third child was showing signs of disturbed behavior, such as seeing ghosts, attacking MV, thinking that MV was a ghost, and talking irrationally. MV felt that this child had already been chosen to be a channel for her ancestors' spirits, *phii-xeua*.

In June 1988, MV reported for the first time that she was having nightmares, startle reactions and intrusive memories of traumatic experiences she had experienced in Laos. Upon further questioning it was clear that she was suffering from PTSD.

At a subsequent group meeting, MV became disorganized and saw the ghost of her mother trying to take her back to the dead. (We discovered later that she had received bad news from her family regarding an older cousin who was a channel and who had become very ill and needed to be restrained in chains). MV was able to reconstitute herself and did not want hospitalization. However, at the next group meeting she reported receiving a call from a community member harassing her for her involvement in the mental health system. She was paranoid, disorganized, and incoherent and threatened to cut her throat. She required hospital care.

Following this admission the family decided to take her to Laos for spiritual exorcism with a spirit master, *maw phii*. MV needed to perform special ceremonies that involved the consumption of large amount of alcohol, which Lao women do not usually consume. It took over a year, but finally, in November 1989, MV traveled alone to Laos for the exorcism. The exorcism seemed to provide initial relief but by March 1990 MV had become depressed again.

MV continued to have a variable clinical presentation that was punctuated by dramatic episodes with psychotic and severe dissociative symptoms in addition to depression and anxiety. We discovered that she was actually consuming large amounts of alcohol on a regular basis and while intoxicated her behavior was more bizarre and disruptive. Every exacerbation of her behavior was related to some family conflict or bad news she received from Laos. She felt so untrusting of the community that she did not want to attend any group treatment activities. Despite all these difficulties she remained a loving and attentive mother and an extremely excellent seamstress, making clothes without patterns.

CASE EXAMPLE 2

CM was a 60-year-old Mien woman who came to the clinic in 1984 with a 2-month history of somatic complaints including headaches, back pain, knee pain, and an upper respiratory infection. She had had these pains for more than 3 years. She had been sleeping an average of 1 to 2 hours a day over the last 2 months. On further questioning she had had a decrease in appetite, fatigue, poor concentration and thinking, and feelings of sadness and depression. She was preoccupied with the loss of her children and husband and felt hopeless about her future. She had begun to believe that life was not worth living.

Past Psychiatric History

CM reported similar feelings 16 years ago when her husband died as well as 14 years ago when her son was killed in battle during the Indochinese War.

Family History

CM was born and raised in rural Laos. Her family were highland farmers. She had no formal education and could not read or write. She married at an early age and had six children. Her oldest son died in battle; her husband and a young child died of illness. She came to the United States with one son and three daughters. The three daughters married and moved to California. Her son, who would have traditionally cared for her, was having trouble supporting his family and she had to live with a friend from the church. She had converted to Christianity after coming to the United States.

Medical History

Later in 1984, CM was hospitalized with disseminated miliary tuberculosis. There was a great concern that she would not survive. That same year she was also hospitalized for treatment of a bleeding ulcer. Shortly after this, she was hospitalized a third time with a renal stone and a kidney infection. She also required treatment for asthma. Over the next 2 years CM continued to be very depressed and preoccupied with dying. At the end of 2 years she was able to stop her antituberculosis medications but she continued to believe that she would die of a cancer that her doctors knew about but would not discuss with her.

Treatment Course

In 1987, CM began to participate in the Mien Women's Socialization group and received some comfort from this. Late that year she reported symptoms of panic attacks. Her daughter wanted her to move to California, and making this decision was very stressful for her. Finally, CM decided to remain in Portland. It was in the middle of the next year that we discovered that CM was suffering from the full syndrome of PTSD. In late 1988 she received a letter from her sister in a refugee camp stating that the rest of the family had not been selected to come to the United States and would be sent back to communist Laos. For months after this, CM's symptoms of PTSD were markedly increased. Early in 1989 her symptoms were again exacerbated by reports of a burglar in the neighborhood.

In March 1991, CM felt unable to care for herself at home and assistance from her grandchild was authorized by her treating physician as a means of providing daily care. A physical examination in May 1991 failed to reveal any specific etiology for her condition but in October 1991 she presented with unusual symptoms. She felt faint, complained that her nose was congested, and said she had been vomiting all day. Her blood pressure seemed to be fluctuating widely. A discussion ensued as to whether she needed to be hospitalized immediately and during this discussion she began to ask about whether opium smoking was something that could be treated or cured. Seven years into her treatment, CM revealed to us that she had had a problem with smoking opium for more than 15 years.

In the following weeks we discussed hospital detoxification and the initiation of an opiate antagonist, naltrexone. CM successfully completed treatment with the continued support of her family and much reassurance. Over the following 3 years, CM remained on monitored naltrexone and showed dramatic improvement in her mood and well-being. She became a strong advocate of treatment for other people in the community and continued to receive help from participation in the socialization program.

CM's history demonstrates a complex intermixing of medical and psychiatric symptoms. It took many years to uncover the diagnosis of PTSD and yet again as many years to establish CM's problem with opium

addiction. CM's symptoms clearly reflected the current psychosocial
trauma in her life and were directly related to exacerbation of her PTSD.
As approximately one-third of Mien people have done, CM abandoned
her traditional spiritual practices in an attempt to find relief of her
suffering.

CONCLUSIONS

In working with Southeast Asian refugee patients, it is important to
understand that it may take an extended period of time to really understand what is occurring. Complex social and cultural issues may be
involved in creating symptoms. Medical and psychiatric symptoms may
often be intermixed. In addition, substance abuse problems may be
contributing to both medical and psychiatric problems without the awareness of the caregiver.

A dramatic increase in physical as well as psychological symptoms
may be present whenever there is intense family or social distress. Patients
may not offer this information spontaneously. It is important to take an
active role in interviewing. Whenever a new or increased physical or
psychological complaint is mentioned, family and social stressors should
be reviewed.

Psychosocial stressors play a dominant role in the lives of Southeast
Asian refugees. Some of these may be hidden from the caregiver's
awareness. The stresses placed on a family system may be extreme.
Multiple family members may have been traumatized, killed during the
war, or left behind on different continents. Financial pressures can be the
cause for further separation of families within the United States. The
process of acculturation adds further confounding chaos to the devastating losses sustained by refugee families. The pressures of adapting to a
new society disrupt traditional values and polarize young and older
generations at a time when family is the central source of support and
identity.

Community attitudes toward mental illness may have dramatic effects
on a patient's willingness to come for help and to accept treatment. It is
essential to remember that Southeast Asian patients are involved in
multiple care systems, including Asian physicians, traditional spiritual
healers, herbal/folk practitioners, religious communities, and occult
groups.

Perhaps the most important thing caregivers can learn from this
chapter is that whatever assistance they may be able to provide really
matters. That someone is concerned enough to try to help matters more
than that the caregiver has a full understanding of what is occurring.
People are often caught in the most impossible and unbelievable situ-

ations, where their cultural, medical and or psychiatric conditions severely compromise their ability to cope and solve problems. Having survived profound losses and horrible traumas, it is difficult to integrate these experiences and have the will to go on with life, to love, and to participate in any community. Understanding that someone cares and is trying to help can make all the difference in the world.

REFERENCES

Bhamorabutr, A. (1988). *Ban Chiang: The unexpected prehistoric civilization in Thailand.* Bangkok: Department of Corrections Press.

Coedès, G. (1959). An introduction to the history of Laos. In R. de Berval (Ed.), *Kingdom of Laos* (pp. 19–23). Saigon: France-Asie.

D'Avanzo, C. E. (1994). The Southeast Asian client and alcohol and other drug abuse: Implications for health care providers. *Substance Abuse, 15*(2).

Dworkin, S. F., Von Korff, M., & LeResche, L. (1990, March). Multiple pains and psychiatric disturbance. *Archives of General Psychiatry, 47,* 239–244.

Haywood, M. (1995, Spring). *The channel.* Chicago: National Association for the Education and Advancement of Cambodian, Laotian and Vietnamese Americans.

Iwata, K., Sakamoto, H., & Halpern, J. (1960). *Laos project.* (Paper No. 16: Minority Group in Northern Laos. Especially the Yao). University of California.

Katon, W., Reis, R. K., & Kleinman, A. (1984, March/April). The prevalence of somatization in primary care. *Comprehensive Psychiatry, 25*(2), 208–215.

Khoxayo, P. (1993). *Issues in counseling Southeast Asians in an educational setting.* Paper presented at the 14th annual conference on Indochinese Education and Social Services, Des Plaines, IA.

Kinzie, J. D., Boehnlein, J. K., Leung, P. K., Moore. L. J., Riley, C., & Smith, D. (1990). The high prevelance rate of PTSD and its clinical significance among southeast Asian refugees. *American Journal of Psychiatry, 147,* 913–915.

Kroll, J., Habenicht, M., MacKenzie, T., Yang, M., Chan, S., Vang, T., Nguyen, T., Ly, M., Phommasouvanh, B., Nguyen, H., Vang, Y., Souvannasoth, L., & Cabugao, R. (1989). Depression and posttraumatic stress disorder in Southeast Asian Refugees. *American Journal of Psychiatry, 146,* 1592–1597.

Labbe, A. J. (1985). *Ban Chiang: Art and prehistory of Northeast Thailand.* Bangkok: Bowers Museum.

Lader, M., & Marks, I. M. (1971). *Clinical anxiety.* New York: Grune & Stratton.

Lin, T. (1983). Psychiatry and Chinese culture. *Western Journal of Medicine, 139*(6), 862–867.

Luangpraseut, K. (1987). *Laos culturally speaking.* San Diego: San Diego State University Press.

Mollica, R. F., Wyshak, G., Lavelle, J., Truong, T., Tor, S., & Yang, T. (1990). Assessing symptom change in Southeast Asian refugees and survivors of mass violence and torture. *American Journal of Psychiatry, 147,* 83–88.

Moore, L. J., & Sager, D. (1997). *Somatic pain and rheumatological disorders in Lao and Mien psychiatric refugees.* Manuscript submitted for publication.

Phommasouvanh, B. (1976). *Bridging cultures.* Indochinese Refugee Action Guide. National Indochinese Clearinghouse, Center for Applied Linguistics.

Suwanlert, S. (1979). Phii Pob: Spirit possession in rural Thailand. In W. P. Lebra (Ed.), *Culture-bound syndromes, ethnopsychiatry, and alternate therapies* (pp. 68–73). Honolulu: University of Hawaii Press.

Tung, T. M. (1985). Psychiatric care for Southeast Asians: How different is different? In T. C. Owen (Ed.), *Southeast Asian mental health: Treatment, prevention, services, training, and research* (pp. 5–40). Rockville, MD: National Institute of Mental Health.

Vandiver, V. L., Jordan, C., & Keopraseuth, K. O., & Yu, M. (1995, Summer). Family empowerment and service satisfaction: An exploratory study of Laotian families who care for a family member with mental illness. *Psychiatric Rehabilitation Journal, 19*(1), 45–54.

Vandiver, V. L., & Keopraseuth, K. (in press). Community response to refugee plight: Impact of substance use on acculturation and trauma with Laotian residents—A Community Health Survey. Portland, OR.

Vang, T. F. (1976). *Bridging cultures.* Indochinese Refugee Action Guide. National Indochinese Clearinghouse, Center for Applied Linguistics.

Viravong, M. S. (1964). *History of Laos.* New York: Paragon Books.

Westermeyer, J. (1979). Folk concepts of mental disorder among the Lao: Continuities with similar concepts in other cultures and in psychiatry. *Culture, Medicine and Psychiatry, 3,* 301–317.

Westermeyer, J. (1989). Psychosocial adjustment of Hmong refugees during their first decade in the United States: A point prevalence study. *American Journal of Psychiatry, 145,* 197–202.

Yang, K. Y. (1995, Spring). *Hmong women redefining success? The channel.* Chicago: National Association for the Education and Advancement of Cambodian, Laotian and Vietnamese Americans.

9

Vietnamese American Families

PAUL K. LEUNG
JAMES K. BOEHNLEIN
J. DAVID KINZIE

HISTORICAL BACKGROUND

Between 1975 and 1992, more than 500,000 Vietnamese were admitted into the United States. Most of them were refugees (Kinzie & Leung, 1993). Since then, many studies have focused on health (Muecke, 1983a, 1983b; Strand & Jones, 1983) and mental health (Kinzie et al., 1988; Kinzie & Manson, 1983; Pennsylvania Department of Public Welfare, 1979; Vignes & Hall, 1979) problems of Vietnamese refugees. Several authors have discussed the practice of folk medicine and its impact on acceptance of contemporary medical treatment (Golden & Duster, 1977; Kinzie & Leung, 1993; Ladinsky, Volk, & Robinson, 1987; Muecke, 1983b). Other studies have repeatedly pointed out that the Vietnamese underutilize mainstream mental health treatment resources, even though the prevalence rates of various mental health problems for the Vietnamese are higher than in the general U.S. population (Gong-Guy, 1987; Nguyen, 1985). We have also seen the coming of the American Vietnamese in large numbers beginning in the early 1980s (Boehnlein, 1987; Kinzie et al., 1990; Kinzie & Leung, 1993). Subsequent studies have revealed certain unique problems this group faces in contrast to the others (Chanon & Ness, 1981; Kelly, 1977).

As the early refugees settled into the host society, they began to sponsor family members left behind to come to the United States. This reunification has allowed for the regrouping of the fundamental element of Vietnamese society, the family, which is in most aspects similar to other Asian cultures. However, in the many studies about the Vietnamese since 1975, the focus has rarely been on the family, although many authors have pointed out the importance of involving the family in the process of treatment (Kinzie & Fleck, 1987; Lee, 1988) and the forming of "pseudo-family" (Lin, Tazuma, & Masuda, 1979) by unrelated individuals for the purpose of mutual support and survival. This chapter examines the traditional Vietnamese family as it is in its native environment, as well as the changes that have been brought about as the family has been "transplanted," largely not by choice, to a different culture. We also address the unique problems facing the Vietnamese American family. Several case histories at the end of the chapter highlight the issues discussed.

THE TRADITIONAL FAMILY

The culture and history of Vietnam have long been influenced by China (Frieze, 1986). In the middle of the 10th century, Vietnam became an independent sovereignty but maintained close ties with its much bigger and richer northern neighbor—China. Scholars, mandarins, merchants, and people from all walks commonly traveled between the two countries. These people ensured a steady stream of mutual influence on the two cultures. Vietnam adopted Chinese Confucianism with open arms, and this code of conduct has governed its society for centuries. In a larger sense, Confucianism demands the reverence of heaven, earth, emperor, parents, and one's teacher. On the individual level, one is to submit to the larger needs of the family. In the interpersonal area, loyalty and forgiveness are emphasized. The "self" is always insignificant and is discouraged from unnecessary outward expression.

In a family, ancestors occupy a critically important position. Ancestor worship is practiced in Vietnamese society even among Catholic and Protestant converts. On important anniversaries or significant dates or during festivals, gifts or foods are offered or significant dates or during festivals, gifts or foods are offered to ancestors as the first act of celebration. This offering is usually made by the elderly figures in the family with active involvement by the younger members. Children are constantly reminded that one never commits an act that would shame the ancestors.

Confucianism teaches respect for the order that separates the young from the old. The traditional Vietnamese society behaves similarly to the other Asian cultures in that the elders are to be respected and not to be openly disagreed with. Those in the family and in the neighborhood are often called on to help with resolving conflicts and crises among young couples. The younger ones are often reminded to remain quiet when in the midst of elders. Married persons may speak their minds but need to select their words carefully. Elders deserve and demand total support from their family. In this area the practice of filial piety is upheld to its utmost. A person may easily become an outcast from his or her clan and community if he or she demonstrates unwillingness to support elderly parents.

Certain rules of etiquette govern the relationship of husband and wife in the traditional family. The couple may have married each other by arrangement of their respective parents. It is important for the parents to see to it that the two families about to enter into this relationship are compatible in terms of social status, cultural backgrounds, and religious beliefs. The bond of marriage is regarded as unbreakable except when the woman (not the man) commits adultery.

Prior to World War II, it was exceedingly rare to have divorce among couples in Vietnamese society. However, it was acceptable for a man to take on a second or third wife, or a mistress. This situation changed somewhat after World War II, with laws that forbid polygamy, but the practice of men "entertaining" or "enjoying" themselves in the "leisure-oriented environment" is still quietly accepted. A wife usually does not comment on the subject as long as her position in the extended family is secure and the man continues to fulfill his obligation to her and their children.

Regarding financial issues, the man usually sees himself as the provider for his family but does not discourage his wife from engaging in a small family business, thereby supplementing the family's financial needs. Before the fall of Vietnam it was common for men to work in an office environment or to hold a job with the government. Women, however, operated the shops, restaurants, open markets, and vending businesses.

In the traditional setting children were regarded as the property of their parents, although the control exerted on children has loosened to a large extend as the country became more Westernized after World War II. Parents have the responsibility of providing for their children and being accountable for their children's actions. Children are expected to follow their parents' advice in every aspect of their lives, including the selection of future mates and career paths. It is the children's responsibility to fulfill the dreams of the parents, often presented in the name of the "family." As the children grow and become financially self-sufficient, they are expected by society to demonstrate their gratitude to their parents by assuming the responsibility to provide for them. Anyone failing to do so is treated as an outcast of the community. Examples of conflicts between the two generations are abundant, but the matters are always handled with great care, in silence, and out of the sight of the public.

The first born of a family always holds a special position, and that is especially true for a son. Sometimes the eldest sibling can assume the position of leadership among the children in the absence of the father, who generally is regarded as the head of the household. He or she is expected to provide a role model for the rest of the siblings and takes the blame for wrongdoings in that generation. Parents most likely favor the eldest child but also expect to be cared for by him or her, and they take pride in announcing that. The eldest child, especially the son, also is expected to carry on the good name of the family.

HISTORICAL REALITIES

The disruption of the Vietnamese family system really has its roots prior to the Indochinese conflict. As early as before World War II, the struggle to gain independence from the French colonial government had already pitched members of families against each other because of differences in political ideology. In 1954, two Vietnams were created by the signing of the Geneva Agreement, with a plan to reunite the country under an elected government by 1956. However, South Vietnam refused to agree to this reunification. Instead, the separation brought about an exodus from the north of people fearful of communist rule. As a result, many family members did not see each other for the next 20 years or so. The years of the Indochinese conflict continued to see the breaking up of family units, the destruction of communities, and the disruption of society due to the very nature of continuous war. However, the Vietnamese family was able to hold on to its basic integrity through all of these toils because it could still draw the support from its own natural cultural environment. However, the uprooting process that was greatly accelerated in 1975 has had a major effect on the integrity of the traditional Vietnamese system.

Not all those who have come to the United States since 1975 have been fortunate enough to arrive with an intact family unit. Traumatic deaths occurred on the high seas or in detention camps in Asia while people awaited permission to come to America. Many would not see their loved ones for more than a decade, or still may not be reunited. For many Vietnamese, April 30, 1975, the day Saigon was lost to the North Vietnamese, began the destruction of a way of life that they had embraced since birth, a life that treasures harmonic living among people related by blood or marriage.

The following case history of Mr. Pham illustrates the sad reality of an ordinary family.

Mr. Pham is a 55-year-old man who served in the South Vietnamese military. He was sent to a reeducation camp for 7 years, and a year after his release he escaped with his youngest son, Tuan, to Malaysia. He was allowed to come to America in 1984. He left behind his ailing wife and three grown children who had their own families. Shortly after arriving in the United States he was diagnosed with a severe stomach ulcer and diabetes, which rendered him unable to work. He is now relying on public assistance. His son, Tuan, became involved in a local Vietnamese gang. In 1989, during a shootout at a gambling house, Tuan was shot to death. In the meantime, Mr. Pham received news that his eldest son had made it safely to Hong Kong and hoped that Mr. Pham could sponsor him in the United States (or else he faced repatriation). Because Pham has no financial ability, the Immigration and Naturalization Service has not responded to the application for 4 years. At this time, Mr. Pham has begun to accept the fact that he probably will never see his family again.

Mr. Pham represents those who left Vietnam with a dream that sometime in the distant future their family would be united in a new homeland, only to see the shattering of this hope due to the unforeseeable harshness of reality.

TREATMENT CONSIDERATIONS

The Indochinese Psychiatric Program of Oregon Health Sciences University has 15 years of experience with delivering mental health care to Indochinese patients. A major problem in the Vietnamese family, as with the other Indochinese groups, is the parent–child relationship. In a study conducted among the clinic patients in regard to family functioning, Vietnamese patients have consistently outnumbered the others in reporting problems with their children (Boehnlein et al., 1993). Their problems fall into the categories of communication, personal behaviors, school performance, social behaviors, and antisocial behaviors. Vietnamese parents often present the problems in the context of the loosening of parental authority. They frequently comment that these problems would never have arisen if they were living in Vietnam. Nguyen and Williams (1989), in their study of Vietnamese refugee families, noted that Vietnamese parents continue to strongly endorse the traditional family values regardless of the length of time they have been living in America, and they have ambivalent views of the rights and privileges of their adolescent children. In the same study, however, the authors found that adolescents increasingly expressed disagreement with the parents' traditional family values as their time in the United States increased.

Ms. Tran is a 52-year-old divorced Vietnamese woman who was abandoned by her husband shortly after they arrived in the United States 12 years ago. She has raised her three children by relying on a grant from the local welfare agency. She came to the clinic 7 years ago to seek treatment for her chronic headaches and was diagnosed as having a chronic dysthymic disorder. She has been receiving medications and therapy to deal with the symptoms. For the last 2 years she has been struggling with her 17-year-old daughter who has been bringing boyfriends home overnight. Ms. Tran is unable to stop that behavior and yet she cannot bring herself to "kick my own daughter out of the house." Her 16-year-old boy is skipping school and involved in breaking into cars and stealing stereos. He has threatened his mother when she tries to admonish him. Her depression has been getting worse and there is no additional help she can obtain due to the limitation of appropriate resources.

Westermeyer (1991) has elaborated on the work of others (Dunnigan, 1982) in pointing out that the structures, functions, and histories brought over by refugee families could impede the adaptation of family members if they are applied rigidly in the United States. In the particular area of sex roles, as a result of the many changes forced on the Vietnamese family, we have witnessed frequent conflicts. Surviving in America often means the need for both spouses to engage in employable activities outside their home. This need has created a mutual partnership between the couple regarding the financial responsibility for the family. In recent years we have noticed an increase in open demands from Vietnamese women to be treated as equal partners with their husbands rather than assuming the traditional submissive role. Indeed, this has brought about a new conflict which the family is ill-prepared to resolve. After a long day of work, the female spouse is still expected to tend to the needs of the children, husband, and often the elderly in-laws, leading to disharmony in the family and sometimes the dissolution of the marriage.

Mrs. Dam is a 57-year-old mother of four young adult children with two boys still living at home. She came to the United States in the late 1970s with her husband and children. Her 72-year-old mother-in-law joined them about 3 years ago. Mrs. Dam was admitted to the psychiatric service with a complaint of "extreme sadness, and I don't want to go on." After 10 days of hospitalization she requested that the doctor talk to her husband and children in order to "help them to understand my problems. . . . I cannot be expected to cook for everyone after a long day working as a seamstress and then help to bathe my mother-in-law. Please tell my husband to stop scolding me for not being able to finish the housework." She also asked the doctor to tell her husband that she wants to "live a separate life, although I will stay in the same house."

For many Vietnamese Americans, it is a matter of honor and responsibility to bring relatives from Vietnam, and especially parents, in order to reunite the family. The media often produce special features that record the long ordeal of a certain family or individual in sponsoring the rest of the family from Vietnam and suggest that a happy life has thus been secured. In fact, many of these individuals and families who sponsor others must struggle to readjust to life all over again. Suddenly, they are faced with the cruel reality of helping loved ones to survive in an ultra-modern society so drastically different from the one they have just left. Younger siblings are expected to go to school to learn a new language, find jobs in a hurry, or have the continuous ability to deal with the day-to-day problems of living in a different society. In addition, the needs and costs of supporting elderly parents from overseas are often not considered carefully prior to their arrival, and this later produces conflict in the family. The harsh reality remains that the financial burden of medical care for the elderly parents who are not yet eligible for public assistance is tremendous. The spouse who is either unfamiliar with Eastern values or does not care any longer about traditional Vietnamese culture may not want to care for the elderly parents as he or she would be expected to do if they were all still in Vietnam.

> Mrs. Le is a 36-year-old woman who came to America in 1975. She met her husband when they were both working as assembly-line technicians and married him in 1979. The couple was able to buy their home, improve their standard of living, and better their education by working very hard to realize the "American dream." In 1989 the husband was able to sponsor his mother and four of his siblings to come to this country. In 1992, after her family doctor had unsuccessfully treated her for multiple aches and pains for 1 year, he referred Mrs. Le to a psychiatrist. Mrs. Le was diagnosed as having major depression and was started on an antidepressant. In the course of treatment with the psychiatrist she admitted to a long list of resentments directed at her husband's family. She was specifically disturbed by the lack of motivation of the younger in-laws to look for employment or advance through education. In addition, the medical costs for her ailing mother-in-law are staggering. The additional financial burden has brought their plan to move to a bigger house to an indefinite halt. The couple has stopped communicating about this matter after a few attempts that resulted in heated arguments.

Over the past decade and accumulated body of data has revealed high levels of distress and psychiatric disorders among refugees, especially those from Southeast Asia (Gong-Guy, 1987; Kinzie et al., 1990; Lin et al., 1979). Clinical studies of this group have shown that depression and posttraumatic stress disorder (PTSD) are the most prevalent disorders (Kinzie et al., 1990; Kinzie & Manson, 1983; Mollica, Wyshak, & Lavelle, 1987). A study involving nonpatient Southeast Asian high school students has shown a high prevalence of depression and PTSD (although the study focused on Cambodian youths and used a relatively small sample) (Kinzie & Sack, 1991). Furthermore, several authors have noted that parents with mental illness can adversely affect the development of interpersonal skills in their children, as well as foster a sense of distrust of the outside world (Anthony & Cohler, 1987; Freyberg, 1980; Westermeyer, 1991). When working with refugee families, including the Vietnamese, practitioners should always keep in mind the effect of mental illness, as well as the distress of being a refugee, on the integrity of the family. For example, a middle-age father who is accused of verbally abusing his children may well be suffering from depression. Or, young children who cannot catch up in school and get into trouble may not be well supervised at home by a mother who cannot deal with the trauma of losing her husband during the war. A young bride who is unwelcome in her husband's family could have become an outcast because of the family's discovery that she was raped repeatedly by pirates during her escape from Vietnam. Many more of these countless examples could be recorded.

CONCLUSION

Providing mental health care for Southeast Asian families continues to pose tremendous challenges to professionals for a number of reasons. These challenges include bridging languages, the differences in cultural perspectives resulting in different expectations, and simply the severe shortage of providers with adequate training in the field. The development of human resources in the fields of health, mental health, and social work; improving government policy toward refugees at the local and national levels; and teaching appropriate cultural sensitivity and knowledge remain the most urgent needs if we want to be effective in reaching and serving the ethnic families. Working with families of a different ethnicity is a relatively new subject in professional writing and demonstrates the potential to be a rewarding path for researchers.

REFERENCES

Anthony, E. J., & Cohler, B. J. (Eds.). (1987). *The invulnerable child.* New York: Guilford Press.

Boehnlein, J. K. (1987). A review of mental health services for refugees between 1975 and 1985 and a proposal for future services. *Hospital and Community Psychiatry, 38,* 764–768.

Boehnlein, J., Tran, H., Riley, C., Tan, S., Vu, K. K. C., & Leung, P. K. (1993). *A*

comparative study of family functioning among Vietnamese and Cambodian refugees.
Manuscript in preparation.

Chanon, D. W., & Ness, R. C. (1981). Emotional distress among Vietnamese adolescents. *Journal of Refugee Settlements, 1,* 7–15.

Dunnigan, T. (1982). Segmentary kinship in an urban society: The Hmong of St. Paul, Minneapolis. *Anthropological Quarterly, 55,* 126–134.

Freyberg, J. (1980). Difficulties in separation–individuation as experienced by offspring of Nazi holocaust survivors. *American Journal of Orthopsychiatry, 50,* 87–95.

Frieze, R. (1986). The Indochinese refugee crisis, in the price of freedom. In J. Krupinsk & G. Burrows (Eds.), New York: Pergamon Press.

Golden, J. M., & Duster, M. C. (1977). Hazards of misdiagnosis due to Vietnamese folk medicine. *Clinical Pediatrics, 16,* 949–950.

Gong-Guy, E. (1987). *The California Southeast Asian's mental health needs assessment* (California State Department Mental Health Contract #85-7628-2A-2).

Kelly, G. P. (1977). *From Vietnam to America: A chronicle of the Vietnamese immigration to the United States.* Boulder, CO: Westview Press.

Kinzie, J. D., Boehnlein, J. K., Leung, P. K., Moore, L. J., Riley, C., & Smith, D. (1990). The high prevalence rate of PTSD and its clinical significance among Southeast Asian refugees. *American Journal of Psychiatry, 147,* 813–917.

Kinzie, J. D., & Fleck, J. (1987). Psychotherapy with severely traumatized refugees. *American Journal of Psychotherapy, 41,* 82–94.

Kinzie, J. D., & Leung, P. L. (1993). Psychiatric care of Indochinese Americans in culture, ethnicity, and mental illness. In A. C. Gaw (Ed.), *Culture, ethnicity, and mental illness* (pp. 281–304). Washington, DC: American Psychiatric Press.

Kinzie, J. D., Leung, P. K., Bui, A., Rath, G., Keopraseuth, K., Riley, C., Fleck, J., & Marie, A. (1988). Group therapy with Southeast Asian refugees. *Community Mental Health Journal, 24,* 157–166.

Kinzie, J. D., & Manson, S. (1983). Five years experience with Indochinese refugee psychiatric patients. *Journal of Operational Psychiatry, 14,* 105–111.

Kinzie, J. D., & Sack, W. (1991). Severely traumatized Cambodian children: Research findings and clinical implications, in refugee children, theory, research, and services. In F. L. Ahearn Jr. & J. L. Athey (Eds.), *Refugee children theory, research, and services.* Baltimore: Johns Hopkins University Press.

Ladinsky, J. L., Volk, N. D., & Robinson, M. (1987). The influence of traditional medicine in shaping medical care practices in Vietnam today. *Social Science and Medicine, 25,* 1105–1110.

Lee, E. (1988). Cultural factors in working with Southeast Asian refugee adolescents. *Journal of Adolescence, 11,* 167–169.

Lin, K. M., Tazuma, L., & Masuda, M. (1979). Adaptational problems of Vietnamese. *Archives of General Psychiatry, 26,* 955–961.

Mollica, R. F., Wyshak, G., & Lavelle, J. (1987). The psychosocial impact on war trauma and torture on Southeast Asian refugees. *American Journal of Psychiatry, 144,* 1507-1572.

Muecke, M. A. (1983a). Caring for Southeast Asian refugee patients in the USA. *Public Health, 73,* 431–438.

Muecke, M. A. (1983b, December). In search of healers—Southeast Asian refugees in the American health care system, in cross-cultural medicine [Special issue]. *Western Journal of Medicine, 139*(6), 835–840.

Nguyen, N. A., & Williams, H. L. (1989). Transition from East to West: Vietnamese adolescents and their parents. *Journal of the American Academy of Child and Adolescent Psychiatry, 28*(4), 505–515.

Nguyen, S. D. (1985). Mental health services for refugees and immigrants in Canada. In T. C. Owan (Ed.), *Southeast Asian mental health: Treatment, prevention, services, training, and research.* Washington, DC: U.S. Department of Health and Human Services.

Pennsylvania Department of Public Welfare. (1979). *National mental health needs assessment of Indochinese refugee population.* Bureau of Research and Training, Office of Mental Health.

Strand, P. J., & Jones, W., Jr. (1983). Health service utilization by Indochinese refugees. *Care, 21,* 1089–1096.

Vignes, A. J., & Hall, R. C. W. (1979). Adjustment of a group of Vietnamese people in the United States. *American Journal of Psychiatry, 136,* 442–444.

Westermeyer, J. (1991). Psychiatry services for refugees' children: An overview in refugee children, theory, research, and services. In F. L. Ahearn Jr. & J. L. Athey (Eds.), *Refugee children: Theory, research, and services.* Baltimore: Johns Hopkins University Press.

Part II

Developmental and Life Cycle Issues of Asian Americans

10

Asian American Children

WAI CHUNG

Little has been written about clinical work with Asian American preschool to school age children. The need for research is reflected by statistics showing the increasing numbers of Asian American children attending school in major urban areas around the country. As the first part of this book has shown, the Asian American population is a very complex group, each subgroup being unique in its own political, socioeconomic, migration, and acculturation history. All these variables have affected the family in its adjustment to the larger society and, in turn, have determined its children's success and failure in developing a positive self-image. As a clinician with some specialty in working with Chinese American children of immigrant background in an outpatient setting in San Francisco, I offer the reader some of my own clinical experiences in this chapter with the hope that they will serve as a "map" for working with this particular group. Of course, this guide is neither an exhaustive nor an in-depth analysis but rather a quick survey of the landscape.

CULTURAL AND FAMILY CHARACTERISTICS

The previous section has described in some detail the characteristics of Asian American families. In this chapter, I highlight some of the factors that have particular relevance for children. Some of the more common traditional cultural values shared by Asian Americans are obligation and obedience to parents, respect for elders, loyalty to the group, humility and unwillingness to draw attention to oneself, industriousness, suppression of negative feelings, avoidance of expression of any emotion, maintenance of interpersonal harmony at all cost, deference to authority, strict disciplining, and overprotectiveness of children. In traditional Asian American families, major decision making is vested in the father followed by the older male. The oldest son receives preferential treatment from the family and is expected in return to perform more responsibilities for the family. The mother is the nurturer, caring primarily for her husband and children. Female children have less status in the family. Because children represent the future for the family, failure to meet the expectations of the family brings extreme shame and loss of face to both the children and their parents. Parents do not express affection or praise their children, fearing that this will encourage laziness. The value of education is strongly emphasized at home.

DEVELOPMENTAL ISSUES

There is more than one theory on the psychosocial development of children. According to Erik Erikson's theory of psychosocial development, children of early childhood and latency experience four stages: basic trust versus mistrust, autonomy versus shame and doubt, initiative versus guilt, and industry versus inferiority (Erikson, 1963). The following section highlights Erikson's four stages and the tasks that each Asian American child has to work through to become a sociable and productive person. Cultural factors in childrearing are also considered. Each culture has its own rationale for its childrearing norms which play a very important role in complementing the hierarchical functions of that society. When there are broad differences in the cultural norms between the mother country and the host country, a parent's continuous practice of those traditional norms creates profound confusion and ambivalence for the child.

Basic Trust versus Mistrust (First 18 Months)

At this stage, a mother who is in tune with her infant will be able to instill a sense of security and worthiness in the infant. She accomplishes this by her picking up the right cues in knowing how her infant will behave when he or she is hungry, wet, curious, and frightened. Trust will be established in the infant as long as the caring is carried out consistently and continuously by the primary caretaker and supported by each significant family member (e.g., father, siblings, and grandparents). In Asian American families, the coming of the baby is celebrated with close friends and relatives. For those Asian American parents whose culture is rooted in countries such as Japan and China, which have upheld patriarchalism for centuries, the value of a male child over that of a female child still continues to dominate their attitude toward their newborn. In addition, families of immigrants from Southeast Asia who have gone through wars, lived in refugee camps, and lost a male member in the family such as a father or a son will place great value on a male infant for the purpose of continuing the name of the family as well as remembering the loss of a loved one. Such a male child will be showered with gifts and attention. In a country such as China, government policy allows its citizens to have only one child in each family. Thus, when a family has a male child, the parents and the grandparents give to him unconditionally and sometimes even beyond their financial ability and emotional strength. As a result, this male child may later develop a narcissistic or dependent personality. In contrast to the preferential treatment of the male infant in some Asian American families, a female infant is more apt to be neglected and rejected emotionally by her parents, especially in families in which an attempt to have a male child has failed. Such behavior will affect the female infant's sense of trust in her environment and the value of her own femininity. However, this attitude of preference toward a male is rapidly changing, especially with the second-generation Asian Americans who are more influenced by the Western and feminist cultures in America.

Autonomy versus Shame and Doubt (18 Months to 3 Years)

A toddler learns many tasks during this period. For example, a toddler in the process of letting go of part of himself (the feces) receives in return praises and approval from his parents. Simultaneously, the toddler can also retain the need to eliminate, giving himself a sense of inner self-control. A parent who is able to be flexible and nurturing toward a child who is ready to be toilet trained will strengthen the child's ability to achieve autonomy without a sense of shame and doubt. Some Asian American families (e.g., recent immigrants living together with grandparents or grandparents close by) tend to toilet train their children in a more traditional way. Such immigrants generally toilet train their children at a much earlier age, usually 1 year old, frequently bringing the child to a toilet throughout the whole day. Parents sometimes use shaming to motivate the child to cooperate. This rigid and strict structure in toilet training is also extended to other areas of childrearing, such as feeding and helping the child to cope with his environment. Asian American children who grow up in this type of environment may benefit later in school by being able to conform to the structures in the classroom, but they may have some difficulties in being as confident and assertive as their Western counterparts.

Initiative versus Guilt (4 to 5 Years)

At this stage, a child is fascinated by his own mobility, language capability, and sexuality. A boy may compete with his father for his mother's affection and a girl may compete with her mother for her father's affection. Boys and girls are curious about each other's body parts. The fantasy and the curiosity that arise here offer ways for a child to rehearse his or her future role as father or mother. The structure of an Asian American family promotes very clear-cut sexual roles. A boy is encouraged to dominate and is reminded of his resemblance to his father. A girl is encouraged to be more ladylike and submissive. In some traditional Asian American families, parents still maintain a protective attitude toward their children, providing them with few opportunities to develop the initiative to dress themselves, feed themselves, sleep by themselves, or explore their environment.

Industry versus Inferiority (6 to 12 Years)

Failing to do well in school not only will cause a child to become regressive but also is very detrimental to his self-esteem. Most Asian American families, because they look on education as the key to success for their children, value teachers highly. Asian American parents want the teacher both to impart knowledge and to "teach" their children how to be a "person" (i.e., to teach morals, values, and proper conduct). As a result, Asian American children learn to take pride in their achievements at school. At the same time, the parents tend to put too much pressure and shame on their children when they fail to get good grades in school, yet they fail to acknowledge their children's weakness and strength in certain subjects and their effort to succeed. Their insensitivity causes their children to become anxious, obsessive–compulsive, and depressed when they have problems in learning.

Common to many immigrant children from different countries, some Asian American children whose parents are not literate in English experience additional stresses at this stage because they cannot get any help from their parents. Moreover, they have to become their parents' spokesperson in their adjustment to the host country. Their parents' anxiety and paranoia about the differences between the host and the mother country often get transferred onto them, sometimes making it difficult for them to handle conflicts with other children or to seek help from their teachers.

INTERVENTION AND TREATMENT

There have been a growing number of studies on clinical work with Asian Americans as a group. These studies show that Asian Americans have always underutilized the mental health services provided through either the public or private sectors. Data presented by Sue (1997) revealed that significantly more Asian Americans (over 50%) dropped out of treatment after one session compared with Caucasian Americans (about 30%). The reasons for such a high dropout rate are clear. The concept of psychotherapy places a high value on the expression of feelings as a way of healing emotional wounds from the past and allowing the development of self to go forward. This concept creates extreme conflict, anxiety, and guilt for those Asian American families that still practice very traditional values. Asian American children are seldom referred to mental health services by their parents, schools, or physicians because they are, in part, being stereotyped as the model students: quiet, shy, and well-behaved. Their parents only seek help for them in a crisis. However, resistance to such services may be gradually lessening, largely because the more recent immigrants have to cope with extra stressors due to the economic decline in the United States, giving rise to increased racial tension, scarcer job opportunities, unsafe neighborhoods, inequality in education, and an easy availability of drugs to children. Because they do not have the structure of an extended family as easily available to them as it is in their mother country, they become more open to seek support and resources from mental health and social services agencies.

The following sections discuss specific issues in working with Asian American children and their families in relation to (1) the initial engagement of the parents in supporting treatment for their child, (2) the therapist's sensitivity to the social and cultural factors affecting a client and his or her family, and (3) the advantages and disadvantages of specific treatment models. Vignettes highlight the discussion on each topic.

Initial Engagement of the Family

When an Asian American family with traditional values and norms comes into contact with the mental health system, the family is usually overwhelmed with confusion, shame, and guilt. The family may still believe that mental health services are primarily for "crazy" people. In most Asian countries, even those that are more urbanized, therapy is still not widely used as a way to resolve emotional problems. In general, Asian culture is dominated by the concept of shame. Shame is used as a powerful tool by parents to motivate their children to achieve success in school and in life. Parents disdain the concept of emotional problems in children, seeing it as a way of avoiding responsibility, hard work, and becoming strong.

With this awareness of Asian American parents' cultural attitude toward mental health, a therapist's first step in engaging the family is to provide an extensive education about the concept of mental health. A therapist can compare similarities between mental health and physical health as to their separate but equal significance in enhancing mastery of the environment. Parents should be encouraged to discuss their fear of loss of authority and loss of their children's respect should they "buy" into trying therapy. The second step that a therapist should take is to reassure the parents that the child's therapy will be kept confidential. Most Asian American families come from closely knit communities and fear the shame of exposure in their communities. The third step is to have parents share their perspectives on the causes of their children's problems. Often, Asian American families blame their children's emotional problems on physical factors or fate. For example, an Asian American parent might attribute a child's learning problem to a fall that happened when the child was an infant even though the child's medical records have shown no neurological damage.

It is important for the therapist not to dispel those beliefs because this line of explanation is less threatening to Asian American parents, more logical, and more culturally relevant than facing the prospect that they may have failed somewhere as parents. The therapist should be formal and yet empathic, addressing the parents by their last name as well as sharing with them some personal information such as his or her country of origin, length of residency in the United States, and educational background.

Case Example

Vicky is a 5-year-old second-generation Chinese American who had been attending a Chinese bilingual and bicultural preschool for 6 months. Both her parents were originally from China. They moved to Hong Kong during their young adult years and then immigrated to the United States in their mid 30s. Both had a high school education and blue-collar jobs. Vicky was to start kindergarten in another 3 months. The staff of the preschool was concerned that Vicky was extremely shy, tended to isolate from children as well as adults, and did not communicate verbally. Instead, she used nonverbal gestures such as nodding. The staff put a lot of pressure on Vicky's mother to take her to a clinic for treatment. The therapist assigned to this case was a female, also first-generation Chinese American and in her early 30s. In talking with Vicky's mother on the phone, the therapist discovered that the staff of the preschool had pressured Vicky's mother to take Vicky for treatment in front of other parents. This, in turn, made Vicky's mother feel very ashamed. The therapist empathized with the mother's struggle as an immigrant and as a working mother and with the guilt as well as shame that she experienced when her child's problems were pointed out to her in front of other parents. The therapist suggested that she would mediate for this mother by letting the center know of her intention to seek help once she could rearrange her hours at her job. She also educated the staff of the preschool on how to introduce a referral sensitively to parents and how to interpret parents' resistance to service. After the pressure was lifted from Vicky's mother, she felt better about the staff of the preschool and was able to seek therapy for Vicky a month later.

Therapist's Sensitivity to Cultural Factors

Therapists need to be aware of their own countertransference in terms of thoughts evoked by their client's ethnic and cultural background. They should remain nonjudgemental and respectful of their client's values. Having the same ethnic identity as the Asian American parent can be a valuable asset for the therapy process in building trust between the parent and the therapist.

Case Example

Ken is a 40-year-old first-generation Chinese American from Taiwan, divorced with one child, age 9. He is an adopted child who immigrated to the United States in his early 20s, studied very hard in college, and graduated with a degree in chemistry. He holds a respectable position as a chemist in a large firm. His son, Jimmy, attended a very prestigious private school. He was very bright but displayed immature and defiant behavior in class. He was also socially isolated and into daydreaming. At times, when he was frustrated with his classwork, he would throw a temper tantrum and need to be consoled by his teacher. His mother had completely dropped out of his life after she divorced his father (when Jimmy was only 5 years old). There were ongoing problems, as Ken was extremely strict and rigid in his ways of disciplining Jimmy. However, Jimmy's behavioral problems became even more severe when his mother suddenly showed an interest in his life. Her reemergence brought to the surface a lot of Jimmy's repressed feelings of abandonment (e.g., confusion, disappointment, anger, and sadness). A Chinese American female therapist also in her early 40s was assigned to the case. She worked with Jimmy individually in play therapy and with Ken in collateral sessions. She was sensitive to Ken's difficulties in expressing his feelings of shame, loss, and anger toward his child's mother, who had taken the initiative to leave him as well as the child. These feelings were even more intensified by his earlier childhood experience of being abandoned by his own natural parents. At the beginning of treatment, the therapist was very careful not to probe into Ken's past history but focused on changing some of the ways he disciplined his son. As Jimmy made progress at school, Ken also regained some of his self-esteem as a father. From then on, he began to use his collateral session to work on his feelings in regard to his previous marriage. The therapist made minimal interpretations and always acted as a good listener and adviser.

Advantages and Disadvantages of Specific Treatment Models

Play Therapy

The concept of play therapy is quite difficult for most Asian American parents to accept. When they bring their children in for treatment, they think that the therapist is an expert who uses verbal techniques to convince their children to behave properly. It is, therefore, very important for the therapist to be patient in explaining the concept of play to Asian American parents. The therapist should emphasize play as a tool to communicate with the child. Children use symbols, fantasy and role play to express their viewpoints about their problems. Play cuts across all cultures, languages, and age barriers. The therapist also should be open to discuss the child's session, not in terms of details but in terms of impressions. This will reassure parents that the therapist wants their full participation in their children's treatment process. Asian American children respond very well to this medium. In the initial stage some of the children seem to shy away from activities that involve water, clay, paint, puppet, and sandtray. Such media encourage expression of feelings and creativity and are, therefore, more novel and threatening to some children because of their cultural background. However, with time, as they feel supported by the therapist and their parents, they will also begin to explore the use of these media. Other media, such as markers and pencils, scissor, board games, doll houses, and storytelling, are effective vehicles working with Asian American children to demonstrate socialization and problem-solving skills. With the therapist's support these children will be given opportunities to express their feelings in a safe way and to discover more appropriate and positive ways to relate to their peers.

Collateral Work with Parents

In working with Asian American families, it is important for the therapist to be aware and respectful of the family system. Because the father is still regarded as the major decision maker in most Asian American families, a real effort to involve or inform him, at least initially, about the treatment process of his child is highly beneficial and in alignment with the hierarchy of the family. Therapists also should see themselves as "educators" and "brokers" to help the families to gradually acculturate so that the gaps in values between the parents (the old culture) and the children (the new culture) can be bridged more easily (Spiegel, 1982). They should also negotiate with the children to carry on those cultural values which are extremely important to their parents, such as respect for the elders and group loyalty.

Case Example. June was a 12-year-old first-generation Chinese American from Vietnam. Escaping Vietnam as boat people, her family came to the United States when June was 5 years old. Although her parents were only in their early 40s, they had suffered tremendously both emotionally and financially. They had used up all their savings to leave their country, and had made a decision to leave June's younger sister behind with an adoptive family. They took June with them because June had diabetes and required a lot of attention. June also had severe learning disabilities, which resulted in her being more than 5 years behind her grade level. Her teacher at school found her to be very depressed and frustrated with her learning difficulties. Sometimes she had mild suicidal ideation and feelings of hopelessness. She had no friends and never joined in with the class to go on any field trips. The therapist assigned to this case made a real effort from the very beginning to involve both parents because they also showed symptoms of chronic depression and had difficulties in adjusting to the host country. She empathized with the parents' shame at receiving a government subsidy but praised them for their courage in adjusting to a new society for the future of their children. The therapist acted as June's advocate by helping her parents to let her try new experiences in school, such as going on field trips. She assured the parents that June would be safe. As June improved in her adjustment to school, both parents began to feel better about themselves and learned to become more resourceful in improving the quality of their life.

Preventive Model

Educational and socialization groups are useful models to provide support for Asian American parents in a culturally relevant way. The emphasis for these groups should be on education and networking for the parents. A wide range of topics can be addressed in these groups, including mental health, medical, legal, educational, and social issues. These types of groups often take the place of the close family network that is so treasured in most Asian American families and has been lost in some families due to migration.

SUMMARY

Though Asian Americans are fast becoming the largest minority group in this country, data continue to show that Asian American children have always underutilized mental health services. There is a lack of training and research on the culture of some Asian American subgroups and the trauma of their migration and acculturation process. This chapter has tried to highlight how Asian American children reach their developmental goals and the impact of their culture on their development. However, the material presented here is limited and more research into this field is greatly needed.

REFERENCES

Erikson, E. H. (1963). *Childhood and society.* New York: Norton.

Spiegal, J. (1982). An ecological model of ethnic families. In M. Mc Goldrick, J. K. Pearce, & J. Giordano (Eds.), *Ethnicity and family therapy* (pp. 31–51). New York: Guilford Press.

Sue, S. (1997). Community mental health services to minority groups: Some optimism, some pessimism. *American Psychologist, 32,* 616–624.

11

Asian American Adolescents

LARKE NAHME HUANG

Asian American adolescents are a diverse group, coming from different countries and social classes, speaking different languages with varying degrees of fluency, practicing different religions and cultural values, and establishing unique patterns of being "Asian American." As with many adolescents in general, they confront the complex tasks of identity formation and establishment of group affiliation. However, whether born in the United States or abroad, these adolescents straddle multiple cultures: the mainstream culture, the ethnic culture of origin, and the culture of adolescence. They confront the normal developmental tasks within each culture, with the added burden of integrating the sometimes conflicting values of these coexisting, occasionally competing, cultures. For some adolescents, the blending of cultures may be conflict-free; for others, this task of balancing and integrating disparate values, attitudes, and behaviors may be filled with conflicts. In this chapter, I attempt to delineate core developmental tasks for the Asian American adolescent, highlight the relationship of these tasks to clinical problems, present culturally sensitive approaches to assessment and intervention, and illustrate these issues with clinical case material.

DEVELOPMENTAL ISSUES

Identity Formation

A central task of adolescence is achieving a sense of identity, a subjective sense of continuity and sameness that provides a foundation for one's adulthood. Failure to establish a coherent, stable identity may lead to confusion and psychological distress (Erikson, 1968). Adolescence has been conceptualized as a period of psychosocial moratorium characterized by the opportunity for self-exploration and experimentation with various identities necessary for the development of a stable, consistent self-identity. Cognitively, the adolescent is increasingly capable of abstract thinking; thus the range of experimental roles and identities is dramatically expanded. The processes of adolescence are guided by the questions, "Who am I?" and "Where do I belong?" Inherent in this process of exploration is the gradual psychosocial separation from parents and family. Paradoxically, the socialization of American children is toward the objective of independence and autonomy; however, when this becomes imminent in adolescence, parents reflexively hold on to the child and restrain attempts at individuation. In spite of this circuitous path through adolescence, the generally agreed-on goal for good adjustment is a healthy sense of identity and belonging (Guisinger & Blatt, 1994).

In most Asian cultures, there is no developmental stage comparable to that of adolescence. Issues of individual identity formation and self-differentiation are minimized and have emerged only with increased contact with Western nations. This limited focus on individuation and identity is consistent with traditional Asian cultural values which diminish the importance of the individual in comparison to the family or the collective (Harrison, Wilson, Pine, Chan, & Buriel, 1990). The individual-centeredness of American society is in sharp contrast to the group-centered, extended family unit of Asian culture (Fry, 1995; Hsu, 1981). In Asian cultures, one derives a sense of identity from the family group identity and one's position in the family; a sense of belonging and affiliation is provided by the rigid boundaries of the kinship-based family network. Seeking a definition of self outside one's family is not encouraged and, in fact, is constrained by complex system of rules and obligations associated with various positions in the family. The achievements or setbacks of the individual are viewed in the context of the family system. Thus, the fame or notoriety one achieves outside the family is not conceptualized as an outcome of the individual's behavior but rather as a reflection on the family. High-achieving Asian American adolescents explained "their drive to excel in terms of the shame that can befall their parents should they fail, and the glory they bring to their families when they succeed" (Liu, Yu, Chang, & Fernandez, 1990, p. 110).

How are these contrasting value systems reconciled by the Asian American adolescent? Various researchers have proposed several different models of responding to cultural values conflicts (Tajfel, 1978; Berry & Kim, 1988) and to being a member of a minority group (Atkinson, Morten, & Sue, 1983; Parham & Helms, 1985; Cross, 1991). Phinney, Lochner, and Murphy (1990) summarize these patterns of behavioral and psychological responses and their associated mental health correlates under four strategies: (1) alienation/marginalization, which occurs when adolescents perceive their own culture negatively, develop a negative self-image based on societal reflections, become estranged from their own culture, and fail to adapt to the majority culture; (2) assimilation, which describes the response when the adolescents seek to become part of the dominant culture to the exclusion of ties within their own ethnic culture; (3) withdrawal or separation, which occurs when adolescents exclusively emphasize their ethnic culture and withdraw from contact with the dominant group; and (4) integration/biculturalism, which is evident when adolescents simultaneously retain their ethnic culture, its values, and its practices yet adapt to the dominant culture by learning the necessary values and skills. In this framework, integration/biculturalism is viewed as the coping pattern most associated with good psychological outcomes. Some empirical evidence indicates that maintaining one's ethnic traditions as well as contacts with the majority culture generates less stress than does withdrawal and separation (Berry, Kim, Minde, & Mok, 1987; Lang, Munoz, Bernal, & Sorenson, 1982; Szapocznik & Kurtines, 1980). Withdrawal and separation fail to prepare individuals for functioning in a bicultural context and often lead to maladjustment; similarly, alienation and marginalization often lead to feelings of hopelessness, low self-esteem, and more serious psychological disorders such as depression and suicide (Phinney et al., 1990).

The selected strategy of adaptation may be influenced by social context and parental identification. For Asian American adolescents who are ethnically isolated, race and ethnic identification may be an ever-present issue. In contrast, Asian American adolescents in homogeneously Asian communities may not experience race and ethnicity as important issues until they leave these communities. Adolescents in ethnically heterogeneous areas may confront these issues earlier in development.

Parental ethnic or racial identification may influence identity formation for the child (Huang & Ying, 1989; Ou & McAdoo, 1980; Uba, 1994) however, the direction of influence may not be predictable. For example, Asian parents who maintain a separatist strategy working and socializing within an exclusively Asian network, may have children who practice a similar strategy, or who actively reject this network and choose to be fully "Westernized" or "Americanized," or who learn to negotiate effectively in both cultures.

Acculturation Conflicts

Another developmental task specific to Asian American and other culturally different adolescents is the negotiation of acculturation conflicts. For
immigrant and even later-generation Asian American families, the rate of
adaptation and adjustment to the new, mainstream culture varies by
generation. Typically, the children in the family more readily acculturate
in comparison to the parents and older-generation members (Sluzki,
1979). Ironically, this older generation often benefits from the more rapid
acculturation of the children, who become interpreters and negotiators
for them within the new culture. Although parents may depend on the
youth to develop the skills and the language for becoming successful in
America, they are reluctant for the children to "become American." This
reluctance results in confusing messages for the youth and leads to
transgenerational conflict. For example, the parents may encourage the
child to learn English in order to succeed in American society but may
refuse to let them speak English in the home.

The Asian American adolescent, socialized by the school system and
peer group, is not immune to the generational conflicts characteristic of
parents and adolescents in mainstream American society. The appeal of
the peer group permeates the family boundaries and the Asian adolescent
is exposed to a wide range of adolescent behaviors. Depending on the
racial/ethnic composition and acculturation level of the peer group, the
Asian American adolescent may observe behaviors ranging from dutiful
compliance with parental expectations to autonomous strivings and family
distancing to total independence and rejection of parents. As the Asian
American adolescent becomes increasingly aware of identity issues and
the range of behaviors accompanying adolescence, the contrast between
the culture of origin and the mainstream culture also intensifies. Thus,
these youth are simultaneously confronted with acculturation and intergenerational conflicts.

The intensity and content of these developmental conflicts may be
quite variable. For example, American-born Asian adolescents may experience a certain vulnerability in their self-concept attributed to the lack of
fluency in their parent's language in conjunction with the American societal
perception that they are not native Americans. Foreign-born youth experience the inner turmoil associated with the clash of values between their
immigrant parents and their American peers (Liu et al., 1990).

PARALLEL ASSESSMENTS

In general, clinicians working with children and adolescents agree that
working with the family system and the school system facilitates effective

psychological intervention (Pothier, 1976; Reisman, 1973). An ecological approach to assessment provides multiple sources of data essential to a total picture of the youth. The relevant systems include the individual, the family, the school, and the peer group. Clinicians develop and refine their own standard approach to assessment. However, when evaluating culturally different youth, it is important to conduct not only the standard assessment but also an ethnocultural assessment. These are considered parallel assessments, with the former being the clinicians' standard mode of assessment and the latter focusing on specific sociocultural factors. These two parallel sources of data are essential for accurate construction of clinical hypotheses and conceptualization of the case material.

The categories of data used by clinicians in the standard assessment vary. Whatever the categories, however, it is important to be aware of the standard of reference for evaluating the clinical data. What may be considered pathological behavior in one culture, may be considered appropriate and acceptable in another. Table 11.1 outlines the categories of data in a parallel assessment.

TABLE 11.1. Parallel Assessment

Individual	Family	School	Peers
	Standard assessment		
Appearance	Composition	Demographics	Nature and degree of involvement
Speech	Subsystems	Philosophy re achievement	
Language	Role hierarchy		Values congruence
Affect	Communication patterns	Cohesiveness	Composition
Interpersonal relatedness	Affective expressiveness	Communication patterns	
Anxiety/defenses		Expectations of parent–school relationship	
Sexuality			
	Ethnocultural assessment		
Generational status	Migration history	History with cultural difference	Ethnicity, race
Level of acculturation	Level of acculturation	Ethnic/racial composition	Level of acculturation
Ethnicity and self-concept	Salience of ethnicity	Accountability versus blame	Place of origin
	"Generation gaps"		Salience of ethnicity
	"Acculturation gaps"		
	Home–school gap		

The Individual Person System

Standard Assessment

Age. Determining the accurate age of the individual, usually considered a routine, straightforward question, may be difficult in terms of immigrant and refugee youth. In some countries, age 1 starts with birth. Some youth do not come with accurate birth documents. For some refugee children, the age stated on official documents is several years lower than the child's actual chronological age as younger refugee children were usually given priority for food and shelter and would receive educational and welfare benefits for a longer period in the host country. After resettlement, however, this age deception may become problematic, especially for adolescents, as the 16-year-old in a class with 12- and 13-year-olds may feel socially and cognitively isolated and awkward (Nidorf, 1985).

Physical Appearance. For children and adolescence, conformity in appearance and behavior is highly valued and deviation from the norm is eschewed. For the Asian American adolescent, who differs in physical appearance and, depending on degree of acculturation, may also differ in dress, language, behavior, and mannerisms, this may be an area of conflict or sensitivity. In addition, the generally smaller physique of Asian American youth makes them especially vulnerable to the "heightism" prevalent in American society (Okie, 1988).

Speech and Language. Language spoken is probably one of the primary indicators of cultural affiliation and will vary according to degree of acculturation. Especially for immigrants, it is important to assess the degree of fluency in English and the native language, as this may affect competence in schoolwork. For the American-born adolescent, language may not be as critically related to academic and psychosocial competence. However, assessing its role in family dynamics may provide important clinical information. For example, the combination of monolingual parents with bilingual children may upset the traditional role configurations within the family. Or, the adolescent's refusal to speak the native language may represent a rejection of the culture of origin, much to the dismay of the parents and grandparents. Speech impediments may arise from different pronunciations schemes, leading to embarrassment and anxiety.

Affect. The value of displaying affect is quite different for Asian and Western cultures. In Asian cultures, expression of affect is not encouraged, especially in public situations. Suppression of emotions, particularly negative feelings, is highly valued and thought to be a reflection on one's upbringing. Thus, what may be considered excessively restrained or constricted affect in Asian American adolescents may in fact be culturally appropriate. This cultural value regarding affect often diminishes the effectiveness of clinical interventions based on the expression of difficult feelings. Facilitating the expression of "unacceptable" feelings for the Asian adolescent underscores a values conflict and often compounds the existing concerns regarding psychological intervention. Again, this may be related to degree of acculturation.

Interpersonal Relations. The quality of relatedness to peers and adults may be assessed for appropriate dependence, affection, closeness, and separation. In contrast to the "rugged individualism" characteristic of American society, interdependence and often prolonged dependence within the Asian family are encouraged. Acknowledgment of role relationships within and outside the family and the "proper" behavior associated with these roles contribute to a sense of formality and propriety, especially when adults are involved. In adolescence, this becomes especially problematic for the Asian American youth who needs to negotiate the competing pulls/tensions of an emerging peer group and the rigid expectations of the parents and family.

Anxiety and Patterns of Defense. The degree of anxiety, its manifestation, and its etiology are important to assess. With adolescents in general, and Asian American adolescents in particular, the earliest manifestations are often somatic concerns and complaints, sleep and appetite disturbances, and disruptions in school performance. Following this type of adolescent is a bimodal distribution of adolescents who cope with anxiety with either withdrawal or acting-out behavior disorders. In a study of Chinese American adolescents in New York City's Chinatown, Sung (1987) found that some teenagers cope with the loss of familial and kinship support by becoming gang members in an increasingly gang-organized Chinatown. In her study, the majority of gang members were foreign-born and from one locale, suggesting that a peer group identity in the form of a gang provides a sense of psychological security.

Sexuality. For adolescents, it is important to assess sexuality and its role in family dynamics. In many Asian American families, sexuality remains a taboo subject, not discussed across generations. However, a recent study of premarital sexual behavior among 500 Chinese college students in the United States indicated that more than 60% approved of premarital sexual intercourse when the partners were in a serious relationship, and the more acculturated the student, the more sexually permissive (Huang & Uba, 1992). The Chinese students were older when they first engaged in sexual intercourse compared to white and African-American college students, and 40% of the Chinese students as opposed to 73% to 83% of Caucasian students (Bauman & Wilson, 1974; Murstein & Holden, 1979) had engaged in premarital intercourse.

Ethnocultural Assessment

Generational Status and Level of Acculturation. Assessing generational status and level of acculturation is extremely important as it will affect the interpretation of data obtained throughout the assessment. A recent immigrant or refugee adolescent may be unfamiliar with American customs and values and may possess a distinctly Asian world view, with Asian values, traditions, and behaviors being the standards for this individual. In contrast, a third-generation, very Westernized adolescent may experience few cultural differences. English may be spoken in the home and values and behaviors may be very Americanized. Excessive attention to cultural explanations would be inappropriate in this situation. The bicultural child, somewhere in the middle range, incorporates both Asian and American values and behaviors. For some adolescents, being bicultural engenders stress, identity confusion, and occasionally psychopathology. Others, however, negotiate skillfully between the cultures, mastering both and competently employing situation-appropriate behaviors.

Immigration History. Age at the time of immigration and resettlement may influence the degree of acculturation and socialization to American society. Age and cognitive level also affect how the child or adolescent comprehends and copes with the emigration experience. Preschoolers and adolescents are in particular need of a stable, predictable environment as they undergo significant physiological changes and major psychological upheavals. Disrupted language patterns may confuse the preschooler and the identity-affiliation crisis of the adolescent may intensify (Le, 1983). Usually, younger children adjust with more ease than do older children, who may experience more difficulty learning the new language. Country of origin, socioeconomic status in that country, process of actual migration, status as refugee or immigrant, and persons accompanying the adolescent may also influence the ease of the transition and the adjustment of the adolescent. Many youth migrate with intact families, whereas many others are sponsored by relatives in the United States and are later joined by their parents. Some adolescents are separated from parents for prolonged periods. Readjustment to nuclear family life or to parents who are recent immigrants and unacculturated is often the source of much disharmony and conflict in the newly reunited family. Unaccompanied refugee minors from Southeast Asia were most at risk for disorders such as depression and posttraumatic stress disorders given their experiences of multiple and severe losses (Nidorf, 1985; Ahearn & Athey, 1992).

Although the immigration factor may not seem as critical for American-born Asian adolescents, it is important to understand the immigration history of their parents or grandparents. Many Asian parents emigrate to America for the futures of their children, undergoing much personal sacrifice in the process. This becomes a powerful dynamic in the family, and the burdens, responsibilities, and expectations placed on the children to justify the parents' sacrifices play an important role in the development of these youth.

Ethnic Identification. Asian American adolescents carve out different patterns of being an ethnic minority in American society. Incorporated in this process are feelings about oneself, stability of self-identification, self-esteem, sense of competence, manner of dealing with issues posed by one's ethnicity, and attitudes and decisions regarding being an ethnic group member in a pluralistic society. Many Asian American youth have experienced some sort of ethnicity-related insult, internal or external, to their sense of self. This insult may range from simple yet painful teasing at school to recurrent ethnic-derogatory comments by other significant persons to total denial of one's ethnicity (Huang, 1989; "Asian Immigrants," 1987). Although there are a variety of outcomes for youth in dealing with minority status, there is increasing empirical evidence that adolescents with an achieved ethnic identity show better psychological adjustment (Phinney, 1989) and higher self-esteem (Phinney & Alipuria, 1990). Accordingly, clinicians should be alert to the importance of enabling the adolescent to explore feelings and attitudes regarding their ethnicity.

The Family System

Standard Assessment

Clinical work with adolescents generally involves contact with the family. This contact may range from in-depth involvement and direct family intervention to more limited, periodic telephone contact. As adolescents are still active members of a family system, it is useful to conduct a family assessment as part of the overall ecological evaluation. There are several categories of assessment.

Composition and Subsystems. Family composition may be quite variable. Determining the actual members of the family household and the configuration of alliances generates useful clinical information. With Asian families, consideration of the role of the extended family is essential. A grandparent or family elder who does not reside in the adolescent's household may in fact be an instrumental member of the family and the family decision-making process. Furthermore, although one usually thinks of the extended family as visible and accessible, for many Asian refugees and immigrants, the extended family has become an inaccessible system as many members actually remain in the homeland. These members, psychologically present to the family, may have bearing on the daily functioning and adaptation of the migrant family (Harrison et al., 1990).

Role Relationships. Assessing the adolescent's role in the family is dependent on knowing the pattern of role relationships. Traditionally, Asian families were characterized by rigid role hierarchies based on gender and birth position. Duties, privileges, and responsibilities associated with each role were clearly delineated and inflexible. With migration to a new society, these rigid role structures are diluted and altered over the generations (Uba, 1994).

Patterns of Communication. Congruent with a rigid system of role relationships, patterns of communication were governed by the attributes of the parties involved. Within families, gender and age governed the degree of expression allowed, the initiator of conversation, the structure of the language used, and the topics to be addressed. Communication was often indirect or through third parties and direct confrontation was avoided. What may appear to be formal and stilted communication may actually be culturally appropriate. Communication is not democratic and free flowing and roles are not egalitarian. Thus, a reluctance to disclose family problems may not be "resistance" but culturally appropriate propriety and attempts to "save face." Shame and saving face are guiding principles of behavior and powerful motivating forces for conforming to societal or familial expectations (Shon & Ja, 1982).

Socioeconomic Status. Asian Americans span the entire socioeconomic range. Frequently, a household has multiple wage earners, sometimes including the adolescent children. If the adults are employed outside the home, adolescents may be responsible for child care and household duties. Data regarding social class may indicate the resources available to the family and may also shed light on the role arrangements within the family as they relate to occupational status. For recent immigrant and refugee families, traditional wage-earner relationships may be disrupted, generating disharmony within the family.

Ethnocultural Assessment

Level of Acculturation. As discussed earlier, Asian American families may experience "acculturation gaps" due to differential rates of adjustment among family members. This is a frequent source of disharmony, with adolescents occupying the most conflict-ridden positions. Differenti-

ating between generation and acculturation conflicts has important implications for intervention. Although the two conflicts are often intertwined,
different clinical interventions may be indicated.

Migration History. Sluzki (1979) delineates five discrete stages in the
process of migration, each of which is associated with different types of
family conflict and coping patterns. He suggests that evaluating the family
in regard to these stages yields important data about the presenting
disorder and its context. The first two stages are the preparation and
actual act of migration; the third stage, a period of overcompensation
characterized by a heightened level of activity focuses on survival and
primary needs. The fourth stage, a period of decompensation, is often
crisis-ridden as the family confronts the task of reshaping its new reality
and adjusting to the new environment. Family members reassess their
situation, disappointment may be acknowledged, and realization of the
losses associated with leaving their homeland begin to penetrate the
defense system that spawned the earlier period of overcompensation. The
fifth stage involves intergenerational and intercultural conflict. It is in
these latter two stages that families experience more difficulties and
contact mental health services.

The School System

A standard and ethnocultural assessment should also be conducted in
relation to the school system. Broader issues such as demographics of the
adolescent's class, philosophy regarding achievement, patterns of communication with teacher and administrators, and perceptions and attitudes
toward parents should be assessed when possible, as well as issues specific
to the adolescent, including academic performance, and social behavior
and integration (Slaughter, Nakagawa, Takanishi, & Johnson, 1990).

Ethnocultural factors such as racial/ethnic composition of the school
in general and the class in particular may generate important information:
Is the adolescent the only Asian American student in the class? American-
born or foreign-born? Is this of significance to the adolescent? For some
adolescents, it is isolating and intimidating. For others who maybe more
acculturated, it is of less consequence. The school's history with cultural
difference may be a predictor of how the school views the Asian American
adolescent. If the majority of students and staff are not Asian American,
there may be few models with whom to identify. If cultural difference is
denied and not explicitly valued, the Asian American adolescent may
avoid or deny the salience of ethnicity and attempt to blend in with the
majority or, conversely, may feel isolated and alienated. In multicultural,
multiracial schools, there is a tendency toward informal, self-segregation—
with white students grouping together, Asian American students together,

African American students, and so on (Youth News, 1983). Students from one ethnic group often do not know classmates from other ethnic groups, although, within ethnic groups, adolescents tend to have a very differentiated view of their classmates (Steinberg, Dornbusch, & Brown, 1992).

A significant group dynamic in interracial situations is the issue of *system accountability or victim blame.* In the adolescent–school interaction, where is the locus of responsibility? Does the school share in the responsibility for the student's performance or is this responsibility placed solely in the domain of the student? Studies of effective schooling indicate that schools that maintain an accountability for all students are more effective in terms of academic performance (Cummins, 1986; Lucas, Henze, & Donato, 1990). In addition, is the school's approach proactive or reactive, that is, do faculty reach out to culturally different students and their families or are they more crisis-oriented? Frequently, there are shared expectations between school and family but a misfit of approach. For example, immigrant parents may desire involvement in their child's schooling but may be uninformed about how to approach the school. Consequently, the school labels them apathetic and disinterested and the parents view the school as unconcerned and unresponsive.

The Peer System

The adolescent peer group is an influential force in development. Understanding the role of the peer group may reveal important data regarding the adolescent's clinical presentation (Huang, Leong, & Wagner, 1994). Standard inquiries include *composition of the peer group, age and gender breakdown, degree and types of involvement,* and *the congruence of values with family and school.* Ethnocultural factors include *ethnicity/racial composition, place of origin,* and *level of acculturation.* Understanding the processes of peer influence among minority youth may shed light on intergroup dynamics, which, in turn, influence individual clinical issues. For example, a recent study indicated that minority youth, in comparison with white adolescents, are more influenced by their peers and less by their parents in the area of academic achievement (Steinberg et al., 1992). It is also important to recognize not only the high degree of ethnic segregation that characterizes the social structure of most ethnically mixed high schools (Youth News, 1983; Gordon, 1990) but also the stratification within ethnic groups according to place of birth (American-born or foreign-born, Vietnamese vs. Chinese, etc.) social class, residence, and so on. One cannot assume that shared ethnicity guarantees a supportive relationship. Separate peer groups, support networks, social clubs, and the like are developed with little interaction among the different groups.

INTERVENTION

Two cases, representing composites of adolescents I have treated, are presented to illustrate possible approaches to clinical intervention with Asian American adolescents and their families. These cases represent the extremes of presenting problems. The first case addresses the frequently observed intergenerational acculturation conflicts; the second addresses the cultural developmental issues for a severely disturbed adolescent.

Case Example 1

Lily was a 16-year-old Korean adolescent attending a highly academic, selective public high school. Born in Korea, she had immigrated with her parents as a young child. She was referred by her English teacher to the guidance counselor who subsequently referred her to the psychologist because of concerns regarding suicidal ideation.

Reason for Referral

Lily was falling asleep in class, turning in assignments late, and sometimes failing to attend class. This occurred in several classes and represented a marked deterioration in her school performance; previously, she had been a straight-A student. On one of her recent test papers and on several of her homework assignments, she had drawn knives and hangings. She denied any suicidal ideation and said she was "just fooling around."

Family History

Lily was the oldest of three children. Both parents worked as laboratory technicians. They were extremely strict and held high expectations for the children. They expected Lily to excel academically and set an example for her younger siblings. They were demanding and restrictive about her social behavior, forbidding her to socialize with peers after school. Her parents felt that socializing would cut into study time, was wasteful, and would lead to trouble. Both parents were bilingual and had immigrated to the United States more than 10 years earlier.

Family Resistance

Initially, the family was unwilling to come to the school for a meeting. Her parents felt Lily was just being difficult and further restrictions would make her improve. The parents said they would talk to her.

Psychologist's Impressions

After meeting with Lily, the psychologist was concerned that Lily was depressed and experiencing severe anxiety. Lily was not suicidal but had many somatic complaints. She was in a very demanding academic situation with competitive, high-achieving peers in a school environment often described as a "pressure cooker." During the meeting, Lily was tearful and angry toward her parents, feeling unloved and unappreciated for her accomplishments.

The presenting issue in this case is not uncommon. The unrelenting parental pressure for academic excellence combined with unreasonable restrictions on life beyond school placed this adolescent in triple jeopardy: (1) the culture, community, and family placed a high value on education and scholarly achievement at any cost; (2) the culture devalued autonomy in adolescence; and (3) the adolescent was dealing with the concept of "face" and bringing pride or shame to the family. Simply by calling attention to her problems, she had brought shame and embarrassment to her family. She was also caught between saving face with her family and with her peers. Finally, she was also protective of the psychologist's "face," which would diminish if the parents refused to cooperate.

In order for the parents to engage in the intervention process, they must acknowledge a problem or an issue that is personally and culturally valid to them. Presenting Lily's problems in conceptually unfamiliar terms, such as "depression and psychological adjustment," or value-laden terms such as "unhappiness," may do little to enlist the support of the parents. The therapist needs to reframe the problem in a manner that draws on the parents' values and what they view as important or urgent. In this case, the therapist knew, from Lily, that her parents highly valued educational achievement. This issue became the *common ground*. The therapist phrased her goal as helping Lily to achieve the educational objectives that she, the therapist, also shared with the parents and to remove obstacles impeding Lily's progress. Reference to educational and college planning were also briefly mentioned. Reframing the problem in this manner succeeded in getting the parents to meet with the psychologist.

Careful structuring of the family meetings should reflect cultural patterns of role relationships and communication within the family. The family's level of acculturation and their language proficiency are essential factors in determining what combination of family members to meet with and in what order. In this case, the therapist met with the parents separately from the daughter. In this initial meeting, the therapist attempted to *convey respect for the parents' values and perspective*. Empathy is enriched by knowledge of the parents' subjective cultural experience.

Although the therapist may feel objectively that the parents are too academically rigid and demanding, awareness of the personal sacrifices made by many Asian immigrant/refugee families for the primary purpose of education for their children, may enable the therapist to more deeply understand the parents' perspective. *Conveying concern* for their frustrations regarding their daughter is the affective complement to the more cognitively oriented values focus.

Educating the parents in terms of the operations and expectations of the school system and the therapist is fundamental to developing any form of collaborative relationships (Huang & Gibbs, 1992). This information may be considered "a gift" (Sue & Zane, 1987) or the compensation the parents receive for engaging in an unknown process toward which they had much initial resistance (Huang, 1989). Examples in this case included discussing the objectives of the school in creating well-rounded, academically successful students who are attractive to colleges and presenting the range of student problems seen by the therapist.

Normalizing the problem diminishes the parents' alarm and feelings of incompetence, shame, and embarrassment. A simple phrase, such as "I see this often with some of my other Korean students," enables parents to feel less isolated. Normalizing within the ethnic group is more valuable than generalizing across all groups as, for some Asian parents, the standard to which they aspire is not the "typical American student." The critical referent group for comparison is often their own ethnic group.

An important intervention used in this case was *cultural brokering* (Spiegel, 1983). This is done in the presence of the parents and the daughter. Culture brokering involves the presentation of the parents' cultural viewpoint and the daughter's cultural viewpoint. This may involve information regarding perceptions and values about the parents' roles, the daughter's role, the daughter's behavior and experiences in the school, the parents' experiences, concerns and anxieties in a new society, the patterns of role relationships in the family, the pressures of outside demands on the daughter and the parents, and so on. Brokering should enable the parents and the daughter to remove themselves from a cycle of blame and inadequacy and allow them instead to "scapegoat" the acculturation process. The source of the current problems are not attributed to the child or parents but to the process of acculturation. Alternative explanations for the problem are generated, and brokering increases the repertoire of responses for both daughter and parents. This approach "plants the seeds" for consideration of new approaches and explanations rather than imposing or dictating a particular course of action.

A concluding aspect of intervention is *follow-up*. The therapist suggested a follow-up meeting or at least phone contact in several weeks "to see how things are going." The therapist used a crisis intervention approach in this case. A follow-up contact usually forces parents to consider the content of the meeting and to experience some account-ability. For some Asian American families, the response to a therapist is acquiescence and agreement, but upon returning home, they make few changes in existing patterns. A follow-up meeting may add incentive for change or at least consideration of the compromises or plans discussed in the initial meeting. The concept of "face" comes into play here. Oftentimes the family will not want to lose face vis-à-vis the therapist and may also be protective of the therapist's "face." A follow-up meeting in conjunction with the motivation to avoid losing face may ensure at least some consideration of the issues discussed.

Case Example 2

Wei was a 19-year-old, Chinese American male, born in Hong Kong. He came to the United States at 6 months of age and was the second and youngest son of Chinese immigrant parents. His father was an office worker with the city government and his mother an office clerk. Both parents and son were bilingual.

Reason for Referral

Wei was referred to outpatient treatment from the community mental health center inpatient crisis unit. This had been his second psychiatric hospitalization in 2 years. He was diagnosed as having paranoid schizo-phrenia. Each hospitalization was precipitated by a flagrant thought disorder—tangential speech, looseness of associations, prominent thought blocking, ideas of self-reference, angry affect, and threatening behavior. He also had a history of interpersonal difficulties. According to each hospital discharge report, Wei's relationship with his parents was charac-terized as "enmeshed, hostile dependent with conflicts around issues of goals, expectations, and judgment."

Due to space limitations, this case cannot be presented in full detail. However, three issues are briefly discussed: (1) the adolescent's recogni-tion and management of symptoms and symptom precipitants, (2) social-contextual issues, and (3) cultural and developmental issues.

Symptoms and Symptom Management

Wei was taught to recognize the events that signaled an impending decompensation: overpersonalizing all events, a heightened fearfulness and vigilance of people around him, and a color delusional system (where certain colors would take on symbolic meanings and send mes-sages to him). For example, Wei might see a person on the street wearing red; red was associated with Chinese and red in their faces meant they were angry at him. Blue meant they were not interested in him. People and objects would take on a color halo. The therapist worked with Wei to devise ways of coping with these signs. Some of the coping behavior involved removing himself from the public situation and returning to designated "safe" places. These are not atypical behaviors for individuals suffering from some forms of schizophrenia. However, in conjunction with the sociocultural context, the focus of intervention becomes more complex.

Social–Contextual Issues

Wei felt that racism and exclusion contributed to his problems. He often talked of "not belonging; not fitting in." When he was the only Chinese boy in his Catholic school class, no one wanted to play with him. He often struggled with issues of "feeling split between worlds—the white world and the Asian world." He often idealized Asia as the place where he would "be with my brothers, away from the racism and oppression here." Yet this also generated conflict because he felt he "knows how to get along with white people better."

These contextual factors, the reality of racism and social exclusion, contributed to the impaired development of an already fragile ego. Wei's subjective cultural experience included feelings of oppression, self-devaluation, split cultural identifications, and related identity confusion. Differentiating between race-based rejection and behavior-based rejection is difficult for both the adolescent and the therapist. This is akin to the dilemma of distinguishing between true, pathological paranoia and cultural paranoia. In this case, the therapeutic task was first to help Wei learn how his verbal and nonverbal behaviors may engender rejection. For example, Wei would glare at an individual and then annoyingly feel, "Why is he staring at me?" A second task was to teach Wei to identify situations within his control and situations beyond his control. For example, when racial slurs were directed at him, Wei needed to understand that in most of these situations, he did not control the cause or the effect. He needed to remove himself from the stressful situation because he lacked "recovery skills" in racially antagonistic situations. He also needed to know that some rejecting behavior would in fact be based on his race regardless of his character or behavior.

These sociocultural variables at times merged with Wei's color delusional system. If Wei experienced some social rejection or racial slur, sometimes his color delusional system would be stimulated, he would feel bombarded by color, and he would decompensate into a "me versus them" position drawn along color lines.

The Interplay of Cultural and Developmental Issues

For the Asian American individual straddling two distinct cultures, it is not always clear what comprises the "normal developmental tasks." Wei was 19. According to Western developmental stages, Wei should be going through emancipation from the family and the home. According to Asian cultural patterns, Wei should be assuming more responsibility in the family kinship network, not necessarily leaving home, however, which would be taken as an abandonment of home and family responsibilities. Clearly, the cultural demands were in conflict.

Wei's relationship with his parents had been characterized as "enmeshed, hostile dependent." The agenda for the mental health inpatient services was to remove him from a perceived psychopathogenic family system and assist him in the normal developmental task of autonomy from the family. However, each time Wei was removed from the home, he eventually decompensated, was hospitalized, and then returned to his parents' home. Clinically, could Wei and his parents individuate? Culturally, could they individuate? Was this a culturally appropriate objective? Developmentally and culturally, Wei and his parents still needed contact with each other. An arrangement was made where Wei would work part-time, live independently in a rooming house, and have several dinners a week with his parents. This plan bridged the different cultural expectations and developmental needs. It addressed mainstream expectations of separation and autonomy from parents by enabling him to live outside his parents' household. In terms of culturally based issues, Wei was able to fulfill the role of dutiful son and "check on" his parents, making sure they were "okay." Psychologically, this enabled Wei to "check in" with his parents and satisfy his needs for contact, "emotional refueling," and reassurance from them. For the parents, this arrangement fulfilled their need to have Wei remain as part of their family and their routine. It kept their family intact and enabled them to "maintain face." That is, they were still serving the role of parents and Wei was still the filial son. Total disengagement from the family, as proposed and attempted by the inpatient disposition team, would have been culturally incongruent, unacceptable, and difficult for the family to sustain.

CONCLUSION

Clinical work with Asian American adolescents is a nascent field still struggling with concepts, models, and parameters. New paradigms for assessment and intervention which incorporate cultural dynamics and contextual factors need further discussion and development. In some ways, the field recapitulates the challenges encountered by these youth.

These youth synthesize strategies for being Asian American. Similarly, the mental health field must build bridges—conceptually and operationally—between mainstream and ethnic psychology in order to more effectively serve this population.

REFERENCES

Ahearn, F., & Athey, J. (1992). *Refugee children.* Baltimore: Johns Hopkins University Press.

Asian immigrants say schoolmates harass them. (1987, March 28). *San Francisco Chronicle.*

Atkinson, D., Morten, G., & Sue, D. (1983). *Counseling American minorities.* Dubuque, IA: William C. Brown.

Bauman, K., & Wilson, R. (1974). Sexual behavior of unmarried university students in 1968 and 1972. *Journal of Sex Research,* 10, 327–333.

Berry J., & Kim, U. (1988). Acculturation and mental health. In P. Dasen, J. Berry, & N. Sartorius (Eds.), *Health and cross-cultural psychology.* Newbury Park, CA: Sage.

Berry, J., Kim, U., Minde, T., & Mok, D. (1987). Comparative studies of acculturative stress. *International Migration Review, 21,* 491–511.

Cross, W. (1991). *Shades of black: Diversity in African-American identity.* Philadelphia: Temple University Press.

Cummins, J. (1986). Empowering minority students: A framework for intervention. *Harvard Educational Review, 56*(1), 18–36.

Erikson, E. (1968). *Identity: Youth and crisis.* New York: Norton.

Fry, C. L. (1995). Kinship and individualtion: Cross-cultural perspectives on inter-generational relations. In V. L. Bengtson, K. W. Schaie, & L. M. Burton (Eds.), *Adult intergenerational relations: Effects of societal change* (pp. 126–168). New York: Springer.

Gordon, E. (1990). *Minority student achievement.* Report to Montgomery County Public Schools, Rockville, MD.

Guisinger, S., & Blatt, S. (1994). Individuality and relatedness. *American Psychologist, 49,* 104–111.

Harrison, A., Wilson, M., Pine, C., Chan, S., & Buriel, R. (1990). Family ecologies of ethnic minority children. *Child Development, 61,* 347–362.

Hsu, F. (1981). *Americans and Chinese: Passage to differences.* Honolulu: University of Hawaii Press.

Huang, K., Leong, F., & Wagner, N. (1994). Coping with peer stressors and associated dysphoria: Acculturation differences among Chinese-American children. *Counseling Psychology Quarterly, 7*(1), 53–68.

Huang, K., & Uba, L. (1992). Premarital sexual behavior among Chinese college students in the United States. *Archives of Sexual Behavior, 21*(3), 227–240.

Huang, L. N. (1989). Southeast Asian refugee children and adolescents. In J. Gibbs & L. N. Huang, *Children of color: Psychological interventions for minority youth.* San Francisco: Jossey-Bass.

Huang, L. N., & Gibbs, J. (1992). Partners or adversaries? Home–school collaboration across culture, race, and ethnicity. In S. Christenson & J. Conoley (Eds.), *Home–school collaboration: Enhancing children's academic and social competence.* Silver Spring, MD: National Association of School Psychologists.

Huang, L. N., & Ying, Y. (1989). Chinese American children and adolescents. In J. Gibbs & L. N. Huang, *Children of color: Psychological interventions with minority youth.* San Francisco: Jossey-Bass.

Lang, J., Munoz, R., Bernal, G., & Sorenson, J. (1982). Quality of life and psychological well-being in a bicultural Latino community. *Hispanic Journal of Behavioral Sciences, 4,* 433–450.

Le, D. (1983). Mental health and Vietnamese children. In G. J. Powell (Ed.), *The psychosocial development of minority group children* (pp. 373–384). New York: Brunner/Mazel.

Liu, W., Yu, E., Chang, D., & Fernandez, M. (1990). The mental health of Asian American teenagers: A research challenge. In A. Stiffman & L. Davis (Eds.), *Ethnic issues in adolescent mental health.* Newbury Park, CA: Sage.

Lucas, T., Henze, R., & Donato, R. (1990). Promoting the success of Latino language-minority students: An exploratory study of six high schools. *Harvard Educational Review, 60*(3), 315–340.

Murstein, B., & Holden, C. (1979). Sexual behavior and correlates among college students. *Adolescence, 14,* 625–639.

Nidorf, J. (1985). Mental health and refugee youths: A model for diagnostic training. In T. Owan (Ed.), *Southeast Asian mental health: Treatment, prevention, services, training, and research* (pp. 391–429). Washington, DC: U.S. Department of Health and Human Services.

Okie, S. (1988, October 31). Children reach for new heights in study of growth hormones. *The Washington Post,* pp. A1, A4.

Ou, U. S., & McAdoo, H. (1980). *Ethnic identity and self-esteem in Chinese children.* Report submitted to National Institute of Mental Health Center for Minority Group Mental Health Programs. Columbia, MD: Columbia Research Systems.

Parham, T., & Helms, J. (1985). Relation of racial identity attitudes to self-actualization and affective states of black students. *Journal of Counseling Psychology, 32,* 431–440.

Phinney, J. (1989). Stages of ethnic identity in minority group adolescents. *Journal of Early Adolescence, 9,* 34–49.

Phinney, J., & Alipuria, L., (1990). Ethnic identity in older adolescents from four ethnic groups. *Journal of Adolescence, 13,* 171–183.

Phinney, J., Lochner, B., & Murphy, R. (1990). Ethnic identity development and psychological adjustment in adolescence. In A. Stiffman & L. Davis (Eds.), *Ethnic issues in adolescent mental health* (pp. 53–72). Newbury Park, CA: Sage.

Pothier, P. (1976). *Mental health counseling with children.* Boston: Little, Brown.

Reisman, J. (1973). *Principles of psychotherapy with children.* New York: Wiley.

Shon, S., & Ja, D. (1982). Asian families. In M. McGoldrick, J. K. Pearce, & J. Giordano (Eds.), *Ethnicity and family therapy* (pp. 208–228). New York: Guilford Press.

Slaughter, D., Nakagawa, K., Takanishi, R., & Johnson, D. (1990). Toward cultural/ecological perspectives on schooling and achievement in African- and Asian-American children. *Child Development, 61,* 363–383.

Sluzki, C. (1979). Migration and family conflict. *Family Process, 18*(4), 379–390.

Spiegel, J. (1983). An ecological model of ethnic families. In M. McGoldrick, J. K. Pearce, & J. Giordano (Eds.), *Ethnicity and family therapy* (pp. 31–54). New York: Guilford Press.

Steinberg, L., Dornbusch, S., & Brown, B. (1992). Ethnic differences in adolescent achievement: An ecological perspective. *American Psychologist, 47*(6), 723–729.

Sue, S., & Zane, N. (1987). The role of culture and cultural techniques in psychotherapy: A critique and reformulation. *American Psychologist, 42*(1), 37–45.

Sung, B. (1987). *The adjustment experience of Chinese immigrant children in New York City.* New York: Center for Migration Studies.

Szapocznik, J., & Kurtines, W. (1980). Acculturation, biculturalism, and adjustment among Cuban Americans. In A. Padilla (Ed.), *Acculturation: Theory, models, and some new findings.* Boulder, CO: Westview.

Tajfel, H. (1978). *The social psychology of minorities.* New York: Minority Rights Group.

Uba, L. (1994). *Asian Americans: Personality patterns, identity, and mental health.* New York: Guilford Press.

Youth News. (1983). *Unfinished business: Racial isolation in desegregated schools.* A special report by Youth News, Oakland, CA.

12

Asian American Young Adults

LORENA WONG
MATTHEW R. MOCK

A CONCEPTUALIZATION OF ASIAN
AMERICAN YOUNG ADULTHOOD

Unlike Western cultures, in which young adulthood may be synonymous with separation and individuation, Asians tend to remain closely tied to their families. Although young adults may demonstrate the beginnings of physical separateness, as when they move away from home to attend college, remaining an integral part of the family is reinforced through frequent phone contacts, monetary ties, working in the family business, or returning to the home on weekends. The physical "launching" of Asian children may not occur until they are in their 30s (Tseng & Hsu, 1991). This reinforced contact, rather than seen as pathological, has often been essential to the survival of the family. Rather than independence, which is the Western norm, Asian families continue to value familial interdependence (Shon & Ja, 1982). Southeast Asian refugee families, for example, rely on older children who, often through acculturation, become more adept in the use of the English language. These older children serve not only as family interpreters but also as negotiators and bridges between Eastern and Western cultures. Often they may also be one of the potential primary wage earners on whom the family relies. Highly patriarchical in nature, eldest Asian sons are generally still expected to carry on as the head of the family in the absence of his father. Thus, young Asian men often face increased pressure to succeed academically and to major in those areas considered to be most respectable and financially rewarding by the family. In contrast, Asian parents often convey to their daughters that marrying into a good family and having children are the primary tasks of young adulthood. Therefore, Asian parents may not emphasize higher education and establishing a professional identity for their daughters.

For many Asians, young adulthood means achieving for the family by earning a degree in higher education. Issues around specific majors, grades, and ability to compete are therefore often stressed. However, with increased exposure to or immersion in Western cultures and values, and conflict between peer pressure and family expectations, young adult Asian Americans may begin to question Asian values.

Like all young adults, they may begin to see young adulthood as a means to achieve physical and psychological distance from the family.

Similar to other cultures, interpersonal relationships become more of a challenge. The beginnings of potential intimate relationships can stimulate conflicts in cultural identity and values. Some students who have been sheltered by the family or taught to focus primarily on educational goals rather than interpersonal relationships may experience social problems or a lack in effective communication skills. This may lead to heightened stress and anxiety and questioning of family relationship norms.

Interracial relationships may give rise to conflict between family messages highlighting the importance of Asian cultural identity and continuation of the family lineage and the possibilities of cultural diffusion through biracial offspring. Asian men, who will carry on the family name, may feel pressure to date women only within their specific Asian group.

Many adult Asians have been taught to value the continuity of relationships and to place the feelings of others above their own. They may misunderstand, experience self-doubt, or feel personally devalued when personal encounters are brief and transient, which is often the case in urban, Western settings.

Like most young adults, Asians experience a consolidation of their identity and values during this period. Some may question their own adherence to familial values. Some may stay closely allied to family values, socializing mostly with their Asian subgroup or affiliating only with Asian organizations. At the other extreme, some may not associate primarily with other Asians, unconsciously rejecting their family. Some Asians report having a "dual identity" defined by specific context. When they are at home, they are Asian ethnic identified (Chinese, Japanese, Vietnamese, etc.), as per parental expectations. When they are away, this identity may be suppressed, and they may represent themselves as more Americanized.

The identification and resolution of this "split" and its conflicts may be one of the primary tasks in working with a counselor or psychotherapist.

INDIVIDUAL LIFE CYCLE STRESSES AND THE IMPACT OF MIGRATION

Not withstanding the usual young adult developmental tasks of individuation, identity formation, and progression into adult life, the Asian American young adult's development is couched in cultural edicts. Frequently, these cultural influences intensify stress in young adulthood as the individual struggles between familial and cultural expectations and his or her growing need for autonomy and identity consolidation.

Two areas most notably affected by parental values are (1) career choice and (2) social life.

Career Choice

Given the fact that an Asian young adult's educational opportunity is viewed as a vehicle for familial economic and status enhancement, as well as a means for increased future generational security, the individual is sometimes subject to conflict in motivation. Often, the obligation to parents supersedes the individual's preferred choice of career pursuit. For example, the student pursues culturally sanctioned fields of science or business versus the arts or social sciences, which are not viewed as economically or socially sound. A career choice outside that which is approved by one's parents could effect some loss of emotional and financial support, thereby increasing stress.

Social Life

Nowhere is the stress of individual versus parental values more obvious than in the individual's choice of friends and partnerships. Socializing itself is viewed by some Asian parents as an unnecessary aspect of the young adult's life, a distraction to the main task of studying hard to eventually get a good job. Dating is often to be deferred until after one's education is completed. This message is generally conveyed more strongly to male young adults, who are to carry the family name, while female young adults are given the message to study hard but keep their eyes open for good prospective partners. Socializing is further inhibited if a young adult lives at home, which is commonly encouraged during the college years.

Because relationships are seen as important for preserving and carrying forth values, it stands to reason that interracial relationships are

perceived as a threat to ethnocentric culture. Depending on the generation of the parents, pressure to conform to social expectations can be so
intense as to lead to the young adult's estrangement from the family.
There may be guilt-inducing messages of disapproval or even disownment
in extreme cases.

Another common stressor for the Asian young adult is being placed
in the role of the negotiator between parents and the host culture. This
situations occurs when parents are monolingual or have great discomfort
in dealing with Western ways of interacting. These parents may depend
on their bilingual or English-speaking child to be interpreter, translator,
and negotiator of tasks requiring English language skills. The young adult
becomes the means to access societal resources for the family. In such
situations, the young adult's separation from the parents is ever more
difficult and complicated, as he or she takes on the caretaker role while
trying to increase his or her independence.

Other stresses on the Asian young adults include the following.

1. Peer pressure requires conformity in social behavior, particularly
in regard to drinking and sex. Also, because sex is rarely mentioned, let
alone discussed in Asian families, the Asian young adult often has a late
start in learning how to deal with relationships and sex or sexuality issues.
This can add to stress about social awkwardness.

2. Bicultural values often lead an individual to feel marginal within
a college or work environment. Not conforming to the majority culture
can affect gaining respect and recognition. For example, an individual
who is assertive in a more Western way, such as speaking out in class,
may possibly be given more respect, recognition, and perhaps a higher
grade than one who is not. In addition, common Asian modes of
communication, such as indirectness, avoidance of direct conflict, respect
for authority through verbal and nonverbal behavior, and deference to
others, are frequently not appreciated or understood by the majority
culture.

3. Adjustment to young adulthood becomes a greater challenge
when the young adult has recently migrated. Relocation from one home
and culture to another leads to multiple stresses of loss and redefining of
values. The manner in which one leaves one's homeland has major
implications for subsequent adjustment (Mock, in press). For example, a
family leaving a country as refugees to escape political and social strife
will likely have less preparedness and resources to deal with the new
environment. Multiple traumas, including splintering of the family, may
occur on the trip over. There are likely to be unresolved issues, and the
inability to return home, unlike an immigrant, can have a resounding
impact (Lee, 1990b; Mock, 1993). The young adult refugee in these cases,
along with the rest of the family, may be focused on survival and trying

to keep the family together. The usual pull for autonomy and separation in young adulthood would be superseded by a posttrauma need for family cohesiveness.

For young adults who leave their homeland under planned and secure circumstances frequently the impetus is to get a college education or achieve job status in the United States. In these cases, there is great pressure on the young adult to succeed and be instrumental in facilitating the remainder of the family immigration to the United States. There may be pressure to earn and send money back home.

Asian foreign students who have temporary status may feel conflicted about staying in the United States versus returning to their homeland. For some of these students, the pressure to excel in an unfamiliar culture, which offers little appropriate support, becomes so great that depression is a common consequence. Unfortunately, self-criticism to the point of suicidal ideation is not uncommon among the young adults pursuing foreign education. Most institutions are not adequately responsive to foreign students' needs (Thomas & Althen, 1989).

For the young adult who is unsure of majority cultural norms and has little guidance or support, the stress of adjustment can be overwhelming and the feeling of isolation and alienation pervasive. In order to restore some feeling of power and identity, some young adults who are having a difficult time with migration and implantation into a new culture may be susceptible to gangs or other groupings. Being a member of these groups, with their own set of rules, may restore some feelings of belonging.

4. Although experiences of racism or discrimination may not be new, to some young adult Asians, this may be the first time that they have to deal with such difficulties directly. With identity issues at the forefront, young Asians may become active against anti-Asian sentiment.

DEMOGRAPHICS

Asian Pacific Americans are one of the fastest growing ethnic minority groups in this nation, particularly in states like California, where there is a high concentration from primary and secondary migration. Asian immigrants and refugee families are responsible for much of this growth. Young adult Asians have accounted for a significant portion of the increasing numbers of Asians in higher education since the mid-1970s. Between 1976 and 1986, the Asian population in America doubled, and at the same time their numbers in postsecondary education nearly tripled, from 2O0,000 to more than 50,000 (Hsia, 1989). Since 1980, Asians have been the largest minority student group in the California State University system, and as of 1989 accounted for over 15% of the total student population (Asian Pacific American Education Advisory Committee, 1990). Since 1991, the entering freshman class at the University of California at Berkeley for each year has been 37% Asian, a majority over any other group. The total enrollment of Asian Americans in Bay Area colleges were as follows in 1992: City College, 36%; San Francisco State University, 28%; and Stanford University, 21.9% (Office of the President, Stanford University, 1991). At the University of California at Berkeley, the percentage of new entering freshmen who were Asian was 40.0% in 1993, 41.7% in 1994, 38.4% in 1995, and 39.6% in 1996. The consistent impact of Asian American students in the overall eight-campus University system is clear, with Asian undergraduate enrollment increasing from 20.7% of total enrollment in 1989 to 29.8% in 1994 (L. Wong, personal communication, June 11, 1997). Following the recent challenges to affirmative action, Asian enrollment will most likely increase but not without its backlash. With more than 50 ethnic/cultural groups defined as being Asian Pacific American whether native born, foreign born, or in transition, as in the case of immigrants, refugees, or foreign students—there will be continued challenges in meeting diverse needs.

EPIDEMIOLOGICAL STUDIES

Epidemiological studies on Asian American young adults, as well as on Asian Americans in general, are limited. Those studies that are available tend to be limited in sample size. Utilization rates of mental health services may be skewed by underreporting. Use of services may only occur in extreme crises that go beyond familial coping strategies.

However, it is clear that Asian American young adults are far from being a "model minority." In our experience in Asian focused community mental health and several university settings, young adult Asian Americans are often in need of both primary intervention and secondary prevention mental health counseling. Issues that are commonly seen include conflict with family, low self-esteem, relationship stress, conflicts in dealing with dual American and specific Asian subgroup cultural identity, and uncertainty of one's future. These problems are commonly manifested in psychosomatic stress (students may often be referred by health centers), academic or work stress, feelings of depression and even suicidality, general confusion, or substance abuse. In the San Francisco Bay Area there are specific programs dealing with substance abuse and domestic violence among Asians.

Asian young adult men and women often struggle with the conflict between traditional and societal sex-role messages. For young adult Asian women, conveying their needs, asserting themselves in relationships, and sorting out future goals may often become a concern. Asian men often question their core identity as it is expressed in relationships. Both young men and women struggle to overcome stereotypes that they have internalized (Sue & Morishima, 1982; Hatamiya, 1991). Also past teachings and internalized messages from primary same-sex role models, particularly mother and father, are often questioned during this period.

SOCIOCULTURAL ISSUES IN ASSESSMENT AND TREATMENT

Assessment of the Asian American young adult needs to be a process of sensitive engagement, data collection, and some education as needed. It is a multidimensional process which goes beyond traditional first evaluations (Lee, 1990a; Tseng & Hsu, 1991). Framing the assessment as a way of familiarizing oneself with important events, concerns, developments and influences to better understand of the young adult can facilitate getting the individual to experience the psychotherapist as helpful.

The period of young adulthood is very dynamic in its response to emotional, social, and physical changes. Young adults experience great external stimulation, with forces pulling in many directions, including safety of home and familiarity versus exploration and adventure, dependence versus autonomy, more serious pairing in relationships, responsibilities to family versus serious responsibility to self (demonstrated particularly in academic and career pursuits), greater emotional and sexual intimacy, and physical and social maturation.

With all the complexities of young adulthood, it is important to assess the many factors that influence on the individual's life and adjustment. Among the factors that need to be considered in assessing the Asian young adult are the following.

1. Generation, gender, and birth order. These often prescribe certain role behaviors and carry specific expectations from the individual's family and community.

2. Level of English language comprehension and articulation. This clearly affects an individual's ability to access various resources and negotiate a more comfortable adjustment in the United States.

3. Socioeconomic status and status change in the case of those who migrated. This will help the psychotherapist to understand what resources the young adult has and what other resources would be helpful to access.

4. Traumatic experiences. An understanding and appreciation of the individual or family's distant or recent experience with trauma provides the sensitivity needed in working with young adults. Also, it could cue in the therapist to identifying triggers for intense emotional response. Internal or repetitious conflicts may be manifestations of previous losses by the individual or family.

5. Coping strategies. Often, a family has experienced war, oppression, or family separation during migration. Many of these Asian families demonstrate survival in the face of adversity. Highlighting this cultural coping mechanism may help to change the common perception that psychotherapy focuses solely on problems and psychopathology (Lee, 1990b). Reinforcing the concepts of resilience and hardiness in coping amid multiple, prolonged stressors can prove to be very therapeutic (Mock, 1991).

6. Substance abuse. Substance and alcohol abuse are not uncommon among Asian young adults. This is particularly true during the freshman year in college, when the young adult, spending more time away from home, is experimenting relatively freely and experiencing peer pressure. Young adulthood is a period in which many substance and alcohol users become abusers. In fact, early adulthood is the period of highest alcohol-related injuries. Early intervention can make tremendous differences in the individual's future use.

7. Sexual, physical, and emotional abuse. Often it is during the period of young adulthood when the individual begins to examine past abuse, he or she is exploring relationships with partners. With too much frequency, the issues of past sexual, physical, and emotional abuse present themselves in the therapy situation in college campuses. Empowerment, assertiveness, and self-esteem building are necessary goals in the treatment of the abused young adult. Education, information, and referral to various treatment and support modalities are useful in these situations.

8. Sexual activity and sexuality. Many aspects of identity are burgeoning at this time, and sexuality is one of the most notable and permeates many levels of social interaction. Education and support can help the young adult clarify his or her needs, especially if the individual's experiences are limited. Assessing sexual activity and practices is also important in learning how well young adults are taking care of themselves. Though often embarrassing, communicating or reinforcing safe sex practices in an educational manner is very important.

9. Suicidality. Depression and suicidality are not uncommon to Asians. Asians are generally raised with a deep sense of obligation and an expectation to achieve. Real and perceived pressure can be very intense for such individuals. Suicidal ideation is not uncommon when the individual does not achieve expected success. Foreign students, for example, who have to deal not only with regular student stress but also with cultural adjustment and feelings of isolation and homesickness, are at high risk for spiraling self-doubt and depression.

10. Support system. It is critical to have knowledge of the Asian young adult's support system because it not only gives some indication of the individual's functioning and resourcefulness but also fills in gaps. Extending the individual's support network (via referral to social groups,

churches, community or family association groups, etc.) can make a significant difference in the individual's social adjustment and well-being.

SPECIAL BARRIERS AND EFFECTIVE INTERVENTIONS IN WORKING WITH ASIAN AMERICAN YOUNG ADULTS

College may be the first major step away from home for many Asian American young adults, but they are still very much tied to their family. The feelings of obligation and commitment to serving the family remain omnipresent. When Asian American young adults encounter difficulties that might cause them to seek professional intervention, they still hesitate to do so for fear of betraying or shaming their family. They are unaccustomed to seeking help, preferring to resolve issues on their own without burdening others. This is further compounded by the role of shame which makes it difficult for the young adult to express need. These barriers, based in Asian culture, as well as the stigma and lack of definition attached to the notion of counseling or psychotherapy, lead young adult Asians in need to choose not to seek therapy, or to do so only when their problems have become quite serious (Mock, 1994). They may do so only at the recommendation of other authority figures (e.g., doctors or professors), and even then with hesitation, uncertainty, or trepidation.

Institutional barriers often exacerbate the accessibility issue of mental health services. Although multicultural training of mental health professionals is strongly endorsed in California, relatively few Asians are going into the counseling field. Without consistent, visible Asian staff and with lack of bilingual capability, many clients perceive that they will not be understood or properly served.

Oftentimes Asian young adults need first to be educated about the counseling process. Problems may initially manifest themselves in the form of academic or physical issues. Because this is culturally syntonic, problem solving in these areas may be very useful in demonstrating credibility and beginning a therapeutic alliance. Once they form such an alliance, client and therapist can begin to address other core issues related to family, interpersonal relationships, or other adjustment problems. An astute awareness of differing world views and cross-cultural expressions of diagnoses such as depression are critical for effective interventions (Mock, 1995).

Because psychotherapy is a more Western form of healing, more acculturated Asian young adults tend to seek out psychotherapists. Young Asian women tend to seek psychotherapy more than Asian men do. When more recent newcomers or Asian foreign students come for psychotherapy, they often seek someone who not only understands their specific culture but speaks their language. Recent Asian immigrants or foreign students may seek out counseling for a variety of reasons relating to adjusting to the American culture (meeting people, feeling isolated or alienated, feeling a clash in values), problem solving, or needing social services assistance (continuation of status, financial support issues, etc.). While treating Asians in psychotherapy, Asian therapists in particular need to stay attuned to thoughts and reactions in this face-to-face encounter. Clients are likely to have underlying fears of exposure or vulnerability since the Asian community is perceived as being quite small and close.

The therapist should clearly convey and reinforce the notions of confidentiality. In a college campus setting, in addition to being perceived as a source of assistance, psychotherapists are perceived as authorities and community figures. It is important for therapists to clarify their role and sensitively address perceived hesitations to disclose. Also, when appropriate, normalizing some of the client's problems may be reassuring and may help to form a positive working alliance.

In treating Asian young adults, financial considerations must often be quickly addressed. Many young adults are not yet financially independent. They work to support school, and additional monies are often used to help support the family. It is not unusual for many Chinese students to live close to campus during the weekdays and return to the home on the weekends and work in the family business. Therefore, payment for services may become an impediment as the issue of financial independence is raised.

Asian young adults, as part of the continual maintenance of a therapeutic alliance, may ask personal questions of the therapist, including earned degrees, the therapist's experience in dealing with their particular problem, and his or her success in past treatment of others. Rather than viewing this curiosity in a negative manner, it may be more useful to treat this as an attempt to assess the credibility and expertise of the therapist. As we discussed earlier, credibility is an important therapeutic tool among Asians. Also, clients who experience some type of giving will remain engaged and motivated at an optimal level (Sue & Zane, 1987).

College and university counseling centers can be ideal settings in which to work with young adult Asians. Asian counselors often work closely with on-campus student health centers. A psychoeducational approach may also prove to be an effective outreach tool that is not only culturally syntonic but quite fitting in the setting.

In college or university settings, counselors should also work closely with faculty and staff who refer. To avoid false or unrealistic expectations about the outcome of personal, psychological counseling, those referring should be educated about conveying ways in which counseling may be helpful.

CONCLUSIONS AND RECOMMENDATIONS

Young adulthood is a challenging, often difficult time of adjustments. Young adults experience greater distance from their family and new relationships, core questions about academic and career interests and identity issues arise. For young adult Asians, this is often a period during which they realign themselves with their parents and become exposed to a wider range of social relationships. At a minimum, they may encounter a split in values and may feel challenged to resolve these conflicts, for example, by dating or socializing, carrying forth family values, and choosing areas in which to concentrate in work or college. Their own feelings of what it means to be Asian may come sharply into focus.

The psychotherapeutic process can be extremely useful helping them to voice some of these difficult issues. Culturally relevant and sensitive services to Asian young adults can establish a healthy forum to address core issues and thus prevent more difficult problems.

REFERENCES

Asian Pacific American Education Advisory Committee. (1990). *Enriching California's future: Asian Pacific Americans in the CSU.* 1–45.

Hatamiya, L. (1991). *Walk with pride: Taking steps to address anti-Asian violence.* Japanese American Citizen's League.

Hsia, J. (1989). The demographics of diversity: Asian Americans and higher education. *Change, 9,* 20–27.

Lee, E. (1990a). Assessment and treatment of Chinese-American immigrant families. In G. Saba, B. Karrer, & K. Hardy (Eds.), *Minorities and family therapy* (pp. 99–122). New York: Haworth Press.

Lee, E. (1990b). Family therapy with Southeast Asian families. In M. P. Mirkin (Ed.), *The social and political contexts of family therapy* (pp. 331–354). Needham Heights, MA: Allyn & Bacon.

Mock, M. (1991). *Life trauma, social support, and personality characteristics: Their impact on the psychological adjustment of Southeast Asians.* Doctoral dissertation, California School of Professional Psychology, Berkeley/Alameda.

Mock, M. (1993, July/August). Hardiness and resilience of Southeast Asian refugees. *Family Therapy News,* p. 15.

Mock, M. (1994, March). Asian-Pacific mental health: The importance of sociocultural factors in framing effective interventions. *Access Silent Asia Conference Proceedings.*

Mock, M. (1995, October). Multicultural expressions of clinical depression. *Family Therapy News,* pp. 21–22.

Mock, M. (in press). Clinical reflections of refugee families. In M. McGoldrick (Ed.), *Families in cultural context: Culture, class, and gender.*

Office of the President, Stanford University. (1991). *Stanford statistics* (Vol. 9). Palo Alto, CA: Stanford University Press.

Shon, S., & Ja, D. (1982). Asian families. In M. McGoldrick, J. K. Pearce, & J. Giordano (Eds.), *Ethnicity and family therapy* (pp. 208–228). New York: Guilford Press.

Sue, S., & Morishima, J. (1982). *The mental health of Asian Americans.* San Francisco: Jossey-Bass.

Sue, S., & Zane, N. (1987). The role of culture and cultural techniques in psychotherapy: A critique and reformulation. *American Psychologist, 42,* 37–45.

Thomas, K., & Althen, G. (1989). Counseling foreign students. In P. Pedersen, J. Draguns, W. Lonner, & J. Trimble (Eds.), *Counseling across cultures* (pp. 205–241). Honolulu: University of Hawaii Press.

Tseng, W., & Hsu, J. (1991). *Culture and family: Problems and therapy.* New York: Haworth Press.

13

Asian American Elderly

RUDOLF SING-KEE KAO

MARY LEONG LAM

Aging is a lifelong process—challenging individuals to constantly adapt to the reality of their changing capabilities and environment (Ikels, 1983). Aging persons are increasingly called on to adapt to loss, to change in identity, and to decreasing ability to be active (Jackson, 1980). Cumulative losses experienced in later life make older adults more vulnerable and dependent on others to maintain their independent functioning (Wan, 1985). Incidences of mental illness increase as people age. Mental disorders in the aged are of two kinds: the organic disorders, which have a physical cause, and the functional disorders, for which no physical cause has been found and whose origin appears to be emotional—related to the personality and life experiences of the individual (Butler & Lewis, 1977). Functional disorders may be prevalent among first- and second-generation ethnic aged people who have learned to rely on relatives or friends to help them negotiate the environment that surrounds them. With the loss of these helpers, as a result of geographic moves or death, such individuals may experience such symptoms of emotional trouble as depression, hypochondria, insomnia, or even paranoia (Gelfand, 1982).

Like all older persons, the Asian elderly are confronted by declining strength, increased leisure time, and the imminence of death. As immigrants, the Asian elderly are also confronted by the trauma of migration, the erosion of cultural and family values, and the harsh disruption of their life cycle. Described as a high-risk population with increased mental health needs and few resources, Asian elderly immigrants draw on limited resources to confront major life stresses (Sue & Morishima, 1982). Unfortunately, a growing number of Asian elderly are unable to cope or have difficulty maintaining their ability to care for themselves or to function safely in their community. It is at such times that the Asian elderly may become the consumer of mental health services.

This chapter looks at existing studies, the impact of migration and individual life cycle stress on the Asian elderly, sociocultural issues and barriers, and treatment. The information provided in this chapter is based on characteristics commonly found in Asian elderly immigrants who reside in San Francisco's Chinatown area.

DEMOGRAPHIC DATA

According to the 1990 Census, of the total Asian Pacific Islander population, 12.6% (919,800) are over 55 years of age. The dramatic increase of Asian Pacific Islanders have produced an "at risk" population of Asian elderly immigrants whose life cycle has been severely disrupted. As the influences of cultural norms and traditional structures diminishes, the problems of the Asian elderly have multiplied. Inadequate income, reduced physical capabilities, and social isolation combine to make the Asian immigrant's "golden years" a period of degeneration and suffering.

EPIDEMIOLOGICAL STUDIES

In a study of mental illness among older people, Lowenthal (1964) examined 530 elderly patients who had appeared in the psychiatric ward at San Francisco General Hospital. Their presenting problems fell into five broad categories: (1) disturbances of thought or feeling, including abnormal fears, confusion, hallucinations and delusions, and depression; (2) potentially harmful behavior, including subcategories as unmanageable, running away or getting lost, threats of violence, and "senility"; (3) harmful behavior, including safety hazards, violence, refusal of food or medical care, and suicide attempts; (4) physical factors, falls, malnutrition, and a generally enfeebled condition; and (5) environmental factors referring to reasons not directly connected with the condition of the patient, including inability or unwillingness of another person to care for the patient. The significant fact regarding the presenting problems is that two-thirds of the presenting problems had prevailed for a year or more—thus demonstrating the capacity of the family or community to tolerate or to manage these symptoms for long periods.

In the Resthaven study comparing a sample of inpatient Chinese patients with a matched sample of Caucasian inpatients in Los Angeles (Sue & Wagner, 1973), the two major findings were (1) the severe mental health problems in the Chinatown area tend to occur in immigrants and (2) the Chinese inpatients are, typically, more psychiatrically disturbed when admitted than Caucasian inpatients.

In a survey of Chinese patients admitted to San Francisco Psychiatric unit in 1964, Dr. Stanley Wang (Report of the SF Chinese Community Citizens' Survey & Fact Finding Committee, 1969), showed that there was a high utilization of police vehicles for transportation—suggesting that it took a crisis, requiring intervention of the police, to finally bring many of the mentally ill into the hospital.

Koranyi's (1981) investigation of psychiatric illness among recent elderly immigrants in Canada revealed that the frequent emergence of severe psychological and even organic pathologies can be observed in elderly immigrants' inability to find or retain participation with their respective ethnic enclaves. (Ethnic enclaves might include a well-established social–cultural organization, church group, or any place where the elderly immigrant is provided an opportunity to recreate a fragment of the "old country.") Adverse family relations was also noted as a significant contributing factor. The role of ethnic enclave was most prominently demonstrated in the comparison of a group of elderly immigrants who had made a good adaptation subsequent to their arrival but were later uprooted again when they followed their children to a new location. This group was unable to rejoin or locate an ethnic enclave in their new locale and within weeks to months developed depression and/or other mild organic symptoms.

In her study of adaptation in old age among Japanese and Vietnamese elderly women, Yee (1987) found that older women may be afforded a more functional role in the family than is the older male. Whereas older males suffered a significant downward shift in status, older women were able to maintain a useful function within the family, such as taking care of grandchildren or performing household chores. Yee's study noted Rumbaut's (1985, cited in Yee, 1987) conclusion that "immigrants who are most at risk for psychological distress are the least educated and the least proficient in English, the most dependent upon welfare, the poorest, the most unemployed, the oldest with health problems and those with the most traumatic migration history."

Peralta and Horikawa (1978) studied the Asian American elderly in the greater Philadelphia area and concluded that elderly Asian Americans are economically disadvantaged and underutilized available public financial assistance and social services. Specifically, the elderly Asian lack adequate English-speaking ability, find it difficult to negotiate the confusing bureaucratic system, and avoid social services because of the social services agency's lack of response to Asian American's needs. Confronted by major cultural differences, the Asian American elderly face great difficulty adjusting satisfactorily to the stresses of life within American society and are forced to accept the harsh revision of their life cycle.

LIFE CYCLE

Asian elderly immigrants are aging in a society very different from the one in which they spent their formative years. To grow old in a society in which the older members are valued as well as given deference and respect is a relatively easy task. To age gracefully in a society in which the contributions of the elderly are restricted and devalued and in which the old are regarded collectively as helpless dependents is a much more demanding task. Asian elderly immigrants are confronted with a cultural conflict fueled by the difference between how Asians view the elderly and how Americans view the elderly.

For instance, China has often been described as a "gerontocracy" because of the position of the elderly in the family and the general veneration of the aged in the Chinese world view (Chen, 1979). In Chinese tradition, the elderly have a revered position in the family and in society. Growing up in China, the majority of Chinese elderly immigrants lived in a society in which (until 1949) the government officially endorsed the practice of ancestor worship. Dictated by Confucian values of filial piety, public and private relationships treated the elderly with deference and respect (Davis-Friedmann, 1983).

Anthropologist Francis Hsu discusses American and Chinese differences in aging. American elders emphasize independence as a means to maintain their self-esteem. The Chinese elder, however, encourages a mutual dependence framework whereby parents care for their children with the expectation that when they become elderly, their grown children will care for them. Thus, although Asian elders look forward to retiring to bear the fruits of their children's labor, their American counterparts struggle to avoid becoming a burden to their children, often becoming recipients of social programs (i.e., social security or pension plans). This minimizes the responsibility of the children in the financial support of elderly parents. The American elder also live in a culture that encourages young couples to live in separate residences. Regardless of whether they are married or single, many children move away from their elder parents. Traditional Chinese elders tend to have full control over family and financial decisions, regardless of whether they live apart from or with their children. Thus, the Chinese elder's authoritative position is modified but not surrendered (Hsu, 1981).

IMPACT OF MIGRATION AND INDIVIDUAL LIFE CYCLE STRESSES

Immigration strips the Asian elder of his or her rites of passage and disrupts the elder's life cycle. The pattern of immigration for Asians to migrate to the United States has contributed to the breakdown of family traditions as families have had to suffer through long years of separation. During the separation, younger generations have adopted Western values, traditions, and customs. Emphasis on material success, individualism, and nuclear family autonomy often creates pressures on the children of Asian elderly immigrants that lead to a disregard for their elderly parents (Lum et al., 1980). The absence of societal and community pressure on the adult children to take responsibility for their aged parents contributes to the gradual loosening of family ties and the erosion of the old value of filial piety. The generation gap grows as the Chinese elderly immigrant resists acculturation and makes little or no effort toward assimilation (Chen, 1979).

The Early Asian Elderly Immigrants

For Asian elderly immigrants who have been settled in the United States since the 1920s, the life cycle was disrupted when they discovered that they would be unable to return to their homeland to enjoy the fruits of their labor. Blatant racism and hostility from American society forced Asian elderly immigrants to find refuge in an ethnic enclave (Chinatown) where they learned to keep a low profile and to become suspicious of government officials. Immigration restrictions deprived Asian immigrants from returning to their homeland at crucial points of the life cycle's rite of passage (when a parent passed away, a parent's birthday, children's birth, etc.). It is ironic that the sojourners who provided cheap labor for the railroads and mining camps now lived off savings, refusing welfare and suffering from bad health, malnutrition, and mental illness (Chen, 1979).

Early-wave immigrants who were able to bring their family to the United States fared better as the passage of time and participation in rites of passage within the American society helped them to adapt to new roles within the life cycle. There is no clear analytical system for predicting which individual will adapt well or will function without serious psychological disturbance in American society. Most of the people in Ikels's (1983) study of Chinese aged in Boston were convinced that adapting to American culture was a function of level of education, time spent in the United States, and the community in which one lived.

The Early Asian Immigrant Women

The Asian immigrant women's lives were especially changed by immigration to America. The traditional role of Asian women underwent drastic changes as they sought to adapt to their new environment. Confucian theology defines a woman's role as follows: When young, she must serve her father; when married, she must serve her husband; and when old, she must serve her son. Once married, she had to live with her husband's family serving as a dutiful daughter for her mother-in-law. Migration uprooted the early Asian immigrant women from their traditional roles and planted them in a foreign culture where they had to develop new roles of identity. They could no longer rely on the traditional values and tasks taught to them by their mother and grandmothers. Instead, they were faced with the overwhelming task of redefining their role as wife and mother. Although grateful to be in the United States, many found adaptation to a new way of life difficult—especially older women and those who had been separated from their husbands for many years. Without an adequate support system, the early Asian immigrant women struggled to become self-sufficient and to raise their children in a vastly different culture.

Asians Who Immigrate as Elders

In a stable society, by early adulthood most people have acquired a reasonably clear idea of what they should be able to expect of themselves and others as they move into or out of their productive years (Ikels, 1983). Changes in the life cycle may be more difficult for the Asian elderly who immigrates in the elderly years. Revisions in their perception of their roles in relation to the family and society need to be considered.

> The elderly newcomer may be surprised that there are no servants in the children's homes and that they have to perform household tasks they did not have to do before. Just when they thought they could relax and be attended to—they find that they are saddled with child care and no other adults are in the house during the day ... no servants, no paid companion, no dutiful daughter-in-law. Major sources of intergenerational tension in Chinese families in the United States lie in role definitions, child rearing and goals of marriage. Families in which generations have acculturated at different paces or in different ways frequently operate with conflicting assumptions about family goals. (Ikels, 1983, pp. 179, 181)

Many monolingual Chinese elderly end up revising their views on intergenerational living when they arrive in the United States and find their children living too far away for easy access to Chinatown. For many who could not speak English, settling in an area with other Chinese was the only possible way to retain a sense of control over their lives. For other elderly, immigrating to the United States provides the opportunity to become financially independent of their children as they learn they are eligible for public assistance. Most Chinese elderly immigrants prefer the children to move in with them rather than vice versa. Moving into the child's home confuses the lines of authority—particularly when the older person is still healthy and active. Although the Chinese elderly immigrant may choose to live independently, the value placed on independence is still not attractive to most older Chinese. They have chosen a separate residence more for survival purposes (near Chinatown) or to avoid potential conflict over family roles than because of a genuine preference for independent living (Ikels, 1983).

SOCIOCULTURAL ISSUES IN ASSESSMENT

Due to the breakdown of a close-knit family unit and traditional family values, many Asian elderly suffer different kinds of mental impairments. Complicated even further by the change of environment and the language barrier, many do not or cannot seek help voluntarily. Unfortunately, by the time the troubled Asian elderly is brought to the attention of a third party (i.e., relatives, friends, neighbors, social agency, hospital, or building manager) for help—his or her mental condition has deteriorated to the point that he or she requires psychiatric hospitalization.

After 1965, the large influx of Asian immigrants coming to the United States introduced a new "transitional extended family situation" phase that is especially difficult for the Asian elderly. Because immigration legislation utilizes a preference system, individual family members must immigrate to the United States at different times. For instance, a parent petition for a child is the most expedient means of immigration. In Hong Kong, brothers and sisters of U.S. citizens (the fifth preference) have a $9\frac{1}{2}$-year wait for immigration (cited in Ikels, 1983). Although some Asian elderly immigrate to America for family reunions and retirement, others are burdened with the responsibility of sponsoring children. Thus the stability of the family is broken as the Asian elderly is left with an extended family that is in transition, waiting for the immigration process to be completed. Unfortunately, this new transitional extended family situation fosters a growing estrangement between children and parents or grandparents and often leads to role confusion, identity crisis, and loss of self-value. It is not unusual for the Asian elderly to experience anger, depression, and a sense of alienation resulting in severe mental breakdown. Thus, in assessing the Asian elderly client, clinicians should try to understand the individual's transitional extended family situation (immigration history of the client and the client's family, client's relationship with children, etc.).

Another sociocultural issue to consider in the assessment of the Asian elderly has to do with the "language" the elderly use to describe their problems at the initial interview. For instance, many of the Asian elderly clients seen at an outpatient clinic in San Francisco's Chinatown are referred by medical practitioners. In the initial visit, the elderly client almost always complain of physical problems (headaches, insomnia, heart palpitations, forgetfulness, poor concentration, loss of physical energy, etc.). One reason may be that many Asian elderly believe seeking help for physical problems is socially acceptable. In fact, seldom will an elderly client use terms that are directly related to psychotic problems, as mental illness continues to be a subject that could cast shame on the entire family. Some Asian elderly clients also believe that being mentally ill is retribution for a wrongful deed committed in the past. They share the Buddhist belief that what they are suffering from in this life is most likely related to some wrong they committed in a past life. In addition, they believe that the life cycle consists of one's previous life, one's present life and one's future life. Thus, an Asian elderly client may deny the seriousness of his problems for fear that if something bad is happening to him now, it will also affect him badly in the next life. Finally, some Asian elderly also believe that mental illness is caused by evil spirits. Some clinicians may attempt to have "reality-based" discussions on evil spirits and try to correct their client's perception. This is a grave mistake as it indicates the clinician's lack of understanding for the client's culture. The client may also feel rejected by the clinician. During an assessment, the clinician's goal should be to provide the Asian elderly client a safe atmosphere to reveal his belief systems. To help the client overcome his fear of mental illness, the clinician should work with the client to accept that the illness is not because of what the client did wrong in the past. Focusing clients on specific causes surrounding their symptoms may also help (anxiety due to separation from loved ones, depression due to their needs not being met, disorientation because they are unfamiliar with the language or customs of their new environment, etc.). When the elderly believe that their illness is caused by evil spirits, clinicians should not argue about the reality of evil spirits. One approach the clinician may use with such a client is to acknowledge his or her belief and then offer the client the possibility that the illness may be related to causes other than evil spirits. This approach permits the elderly client to consider discussing real life stresses in therapy.

When assessing the Asian elderly female immigrant, the clinician needs to consider the traditional role of women in the Asian culture. Today, many of the early Asian immigrant women who are now elderly face bitter disappointments, as the traditions and values that had so clearly defined their roles in society over the decades are no longer respected by their children or their children's spouses. Some common complaints expressed by Asian elderly women at the outpatient clinic in San Francisco's Chinatown include feeling abandoned by children who move away from home and the lack of respect (and obedience) from daughters-in-law. For instance, in China, mothers can dictate what food their sons should be served by their wives, but in America, many daughters-in-law simply ignore the mother's wishes.

Finally, it is important for the clinician to recognize that the Asian elderly immigrant's view of the world is different. In the first interview, most clinicians inquire about the client's work history or education. However, many elderly Asian immigrants come from rural villages where there was minimal opportunity for formal employment or education. Thus, the elderly client may awkwardly respond that he did not "work" when, in actuality, he may have spent 10 to 12 hours a day tending the fields or fishing for food. Or, if a client reports she worked "selling things," clinicians may make the erroneous assumption that the client worked in a store when, in fact, the client had to carry her heavy wares several miles into town to sell at a street corner. "Who was the first President of the United States?" is the type of question a clinician might use to assess whether a client is oriented. Such a questions posed to an Asian elderly immigrant may go unanswered—not because the client is disoriented but because the client is unfamiliar with this country's political system. It is essential for the clinician to attempt to understand the client's responses within the context of how that client views the world. For example, the elderly client who is afraid of going to sea may be remembering attempts to escape wars by sea and the many losses he or she suffered during the escapes.

SPECIAL BARRIERS

Because most Asian elderly do not voluntarily seek out mental health services, the first step in assessment usually takes place in the elder's home. Mental health professionals representing either a government or private agency can expect the Asian elder to meet them with resistance and fear. To be helpful, clinicians must be ready to "enter their world" to empathize with the Asian elderly in their fear and pain. Because most Asian elderly seldom discuss their personal or family problems with outsiders, the clinician will have to be accepted as part of their family before meaningful communication can take place. Clinicians who treat their clients with detached emotions will have difficulty gaining their trust. Elderly clients are concerned with whether the clinician is someone who understands them and can be depended on to help them in their time of need. Within the boundaries of a therapeutic relationship, the clinician is called on to become a positive transference figure.

The desire to see the therapist as an "expert" is mentioned often as a factor in working with Asian Americans. Although this may be true in some situations, the emphasis on the clinician as an "expert" may not be effective in other cases with Asian elderly clients. On the first visit, clinicians should be aware that the use of an official title to identify themselves would not only create an emotional distance from the elderly client, but would also emphasize the clinician's status as an outsider. Instead, the clinician should address the elderly in a respectful manner and let them see his or her willingness to become a family member surrogate in order to gain acceptance. To establish rapport with Asian elderly, the clinician's first objective should be to introduce a climate of emotional safety. The clinician should address the client by his or her respectful title. The opening dialogue should allow clients to have a sense of personal control and to talk of things about which they are knowledgeable. When assessing the Asian elderly, it is extremely helpful to encourage the client to talk about their birthplace or native land and skills they feel proud of. Forging an emotional connection with clients opens the way to engage them in treatment. (Most Asian elderly feel a much closer emotional connection if the therapist can let them know that he or she is from the same village and is familiar with their native land and customs. The therapist can also just simply acknowledge that he or she has heard about their native land.)

By developing a strong emotional connection with the client, the clinician is also providing the Asian elderly an outlet where they can discuss topics freely and eventually become less defensive. In the beginning stage of treatment, some Asian elderly immigrants may present their therapists with simple tasks (e.g., interpreting a letter). They are indirectly questioning the clinician's willingness and ability to help. Clinicians are challenged to interpret the client's requests and respond in a way that will build a therapeutic relationship. After creating a nonthreatening, friendly, and casual environment of understanding, respect, and trust for the elderly, the clinician can move into the next phase. This phase focuses on assisting the elderly client to be able to present their issues and then engaging the client to accept therapy in a culturally relevant way.

One of the most common barriers in working with this special group is the issue of time-limited therapy. Usually it takes longer for the Asian elderly to become engaged in therapy. For many of the Chinese elderly immigrants who utilize services at an outpatient clinic in San Francisco's Chinatown, brief therapy does not work well because many of the elderly clients already feel abandoned by their family. The goal of treatment for such clients is to help them link up with a support system before termination (in-home support service, case management, family association or social club, etc.). For instance, a clinician may accompany the elderly client to a nutrition meal site to link that client up with a social service. Without a well-planned support system, the Asian elderly may suffer further emotional damage.

The offering of gifts by Asian elderly clients may be another barrier clinicians face in working with this special population. Most elderly offer gifts as a token of appreciation when they feel that they have received help from you. However, agency policies usually prohibit clinicians from accepting monetary gifts in exchange for treatment. Explain to the elderly that perhaps a small handmade craft or homemade cookies would be appreciated if they truly insist on giving a gift. This not only provides an opportunity for them to value their cultural skills but also serves as a therapeutic tool to provide them with a sense of pride and a feeling of reciprocation.

Another barrier is the cultural belief of what some Chinese elderly call *yeet hay* (Cantonese pronunciation). The literal translation for *yeet hay* is "hot air." In the Taoist theory of *yin–yang*, there is always a balance of nature relevant to every living thing and good health depends on a proper balance of nature within the individual. For instance, there needs to be a balance of hot with cold or sadness with happiness. Often, elderly Chinese clients may have a trusting relationship with their therapist but will refuse to take medication for fear of *yeet hay*. This is most likely because they believe that the medicine will unbalance their system and will give them too much "hot air," thus causing them to become irritable or agitated. It seems that every nuance in the client's environment affects the individual negatively or positively; thus, it is not surprising that the client presents with multiple physical complaints as immigration means that their bodies must adapt to new environments, new food, and a new climate.

Some Asian elderly immigrants are hesitant to utilize services because they may be unfamiliar with how mental illness affects their immigrant status in the United States. They are afraid that any indication of mental illness would prohibit them from being able to petition their family to America. Elderly immigrants may also refuse to seek treatment for fear of becoming a burden to their sponsors. The first 3 years for Asian elderly immigrants are especially stressful as their age and lack of work experience make it difficult for them to find employment and, yet, they cannot qualify for public assistance. Faced with financial hardship, many elderly immigrants not only avoid seeking mental health services but also put off seeking medical services until their illness becomes more severe. Clinicians might find it helpful to educate such clients by explaining that receiving mental health services will not necessarily be burdensome to their sponsor or prohibit them from eventually becoming sponsors for other family members.

It is helpful to involve family members in treatment with the Asian elderly client, but it is not advisable to use family members as translators. This is because the elderly client's problems may be related to family members, and so clients might find it especially difficult to discuss their issues aloud. Also, when family members make a referral, it is important to look at the motivation behind it. Some children of elderly immigrants may exaggerate symptoms as an excuse to have the troublesome elder removed from their home. However, it is important to remember that family members do play a key role in providing detailed information about the elderly client's background and history.

Finally, another barrier that clinicians may face is that many Asian elderly expect that if the doctor is good, they should be able to see some positive result immediately. There is a Chinese saying that translates, "If you stand a bamboo in the ground, you should be able to see the shadow of the bamboo." Thus, some Asian elderly clients may wonder whether their doctor is an ineffectual bamboo if they do not see any direct benefit from their treatment. So, if an elderly client presents her complaints and is not given anything to help, she may end up shopping around for a doctor who will give her medicine. Unfortunately, such clients usually end up dissatisfied with the medicine (because there are no immediate results) and then see several other doctors and receive even more medicine. (During initial assessments, clinicians will find it helpful to ask Asian elderly clients to bring in all their medications so that the client's medical history and medication intake become clear.) To address this barrier, a clinician might focus the initial phase of treatment on addressing somatic complaints and providing some immediate results (i.e., medication to improve the client's sleep or ease his or her headaches). After building trust with the elderly client, the therapist can introduce breathing and other relaxation exercises.

INTERVENTION AND TREATMENT

To effectively work with the Asian elderly, clinicians should practice "mental reservation" in all phases of treatment. Mental reservation is client-based communication where the clinician avoids explaining specific details to the elderly, reserving the right to bring up the details again at a more critical moment when the client is safely engaged in treatment. For instance, many elderly Asian immigrants have never been exposed to the concept of mental health services. In fact, their only association with mental illness may be an extremely negative one where emotionally unstable individuals are "caught and locked away." Thus, if a mental health professional introduces himself as a "mental health worker," the elderly client may conjure up an image of being caught and locked away. By reserving the specific details of his job title and simply introducing himself as an employee of the social services agency for which he works, the mental health worker will be able to make contact with the client.

The clinician can also use mental reservation when elderly clients invite the clinician to lunch or ask for the clinician's home address. Rather than responding with a detailed explanation of why such requests may be inappropriate, the clinician may respond with "I've already eaten," "If there is an opportunity, we'll do it," or "This is not a good time to give you my address." Such responses acknowledge the elderly client's gesture of goodwill and allow the clinician to maintain his or her professional boundaries. The following case example demonstrates how mental reservation works.

CASE EXAMPLE

Mrs. W is a 74-year-old married Chinese woman who has been repeatedly referred to several different social services agencies by her husband. The referrals reported that Mrs. W was exhibiting increasing "bizarre" behavior, such as talking to herself, offering "ashed" tea to her husband, and waiting for her "deceased" son in the middle of the night. The husband stated that his wife always refused to open the door to the various outreach workers who had attempted to visit her in the past. She would insist that she was not "sick" or "crazy" and refuse to talk to anyone from mental health agencies.

When the mental health clinician made the first home visit, he simply introduced himself as Mr. K from a city agency (without mentioning mental health—reserving the disclosure of this information for a later time when the client is more receptive) and said that he would like to discuss recent changes in programs providing benefits to the elderly (renter's credit, assistance with electric or phone bill, social security adjustments if her home had no kitchen, etc.). (Because Mrs. W was not ready for therapy, the clinician introduced a specific topic that would be of interest to most elderly persons.) Upon hearing this, Mrs. W immediately opened the door and let the clinician in. After a few exchanges of general conversation, the clinician pointed out that it sounded as if she was from the village of Ningpo. The clinician then commented that Ningpo was very nice and began communicating with Mrs. W in her native dialect. (The communication is based on something that is familiar and safe for her.) To Mrs. W's surprise, she was happy to talk about herself! She described herself as illiterate, unable to read or write Chinese. She had married her husband when she was 18, when he returned to China in 1945. Mrs. W talked about being a firm believer of Buddha and how much she enjoyed cooking and embroidery. (The client is communicating about things about which she is knowledgeable, and that provides her with a sense of control.)

A year ago, Mrs. W's only son had died in an automobile accident. Mrs. W became very depressed, blaming herself for not having made her son marry before he died. She also blamed her husband's Americanized way of raising their son and stated that "if they were living in China, things would be different and her son would probably still be alive." (The clinician allows the client to ventilate and is empathic with the client's feelings.) The worker patiently listened and promised to look into the possibility of low-income rental rebate benefits for which Mrs. W might be eligible. (This provides an opportunity for future visits as well as bridges the communication from ventilation about the past to present issues.)

At the fourth session, Mrs. W was able to share her feelings more openly and explained why she had to put ashes into her husband's tea. She emphasized that she did it because she "wanted to have her husband back." Since her son's death, Mrs. W's husband had been spending more time at the night club with his friends. Mrs. W further explained that the ashes were burnt from the sutra she had chanted. She firmly believed that if her husband drank the tea with the ashes in it, he would spend time at home with her. Mrs. W also admitted talking to her son's soul the previous month because it was the anniversary of his death. The clinician discussed other possible ways to help change her husband's behavior and suggested that it might be more effective if Mrs. W could pray for change in her husband's behavior at the temple instead of burning ashes at home. And in response to Mrs. W's wish to comfort her son's soul, the clinician suggested offering a shrine inside the temple. Mrs. W gladly agreed to the clinician's suggestions. (Culturally relevant interventions are often overlooked by social services professionals and family members.)

When Mrs. W's behavior changed, Mr. W spent less time away from home. He was able to understand Mrs. W's behavior as cultural rather than "crazy." A few sessions later, both Mr. and Mrs. W focused more on how to communicate without flinging verbal accusations at one another. Another goal was for the elderly couple to learn to accept each other's behavior as sometimes functional and necessary.

As their behavior changed, Mr. and Mrs. W's relationship continued to improve. It became evident that Mrs. W could now openly discuss health issues and was willing to come into the clinic for medication to help her sleep better. At the same time, Mrs. W was introduced to a ladies group at a community senior center. She began attending the senior center 3 hours a day to complete her embroidery work. When the senior center had its art festival, Mrs. W won first prize for her embroidery. Proud of her achievement and talent, Mrs. W decided to devote 1 day a week as an instructor of the embroidery class at the senior center. To show her appreciation, Mrs. W and her husband insisted on presenting the clinician with an original, delicate hand-embroidered pillow case.

RECOMMENDATIONS

- Reeducation should occur both in the home and at school so that Asian families can begin to address their attitudes toward mental health and learn how to avoid the negative psychic makeup of "ageism."

- Communication between health professionals and patients need to improve. Practitioners who work with the Asian elderly's physical problems should develop a cooperative and consultant relationship with mental health providers, thus becoming allies in persuading patients to seek and accept needed mental health services.

- A growing number of Asian elderly immigrants reside in smaller cities throughout the United States. Unfortunately, only larger cities with a high concentration of Asians provide bilingual services. In smaller communities throughout the country, there is a need to increase the availability and accessibility of services from personnel who understand the culture and customs of Asian elderly.

- The general public tends to minimize mental health problems among the Asian elderly population. This may be due to the stereotype that the elderly is well cared for within the Asian community and a lack of understanding regarding the mental health needs of the Asian elderly. However, regardless of their ethnic background, all elderly individuals should have equal access to services and be able to receive mental health services with respect and dignity.

- Some social services agencies also tend to minimize problems faced by Asian elderly immigrants and may refer them to community service organizations that do not provide mental health services. Mental health agencies should establish liaisons with local social services (protective services, legal services, in-home support services, etc.) so that they may be readily contacted in specific situations.

- The traditional extended family system may be encouraged if all members can benefit from living positively together.

CONCLUSION

Fear and shame have always inhibited the Asian elderly from reaching out for required mental health care. Many Asian elderly immigrants hold lifelong beliefs that "outsiders" cannot be trusted and that "you should never have anything to do with government agencies as long as you live." To avoid hassles, they intentionally avoid seeking services. It is indeed a challenge for mental health practitioners to engage the Asian elderly in treatment.

Creating an environment of understanding, respect, trust, and safety sets the foundation for the acceptance of services by the Asian elderly. Clinicians will find it helpful to look at how the individual Asian elderly's life cycle has been disrupted by immigration as well as the cultural conflict caused by differences in how the aged are viewed. Most important, empathy continues to be the therapeutic tool most effective in working with this special population.

REFERENCES

Butler, R., & Lewis, M. (1977). *Aging and mental health.* St. Louis: C. V. Mosby.

Chen, P. N. (1979). A study of Chinese American elderly residing in hotel rooms. *Social Casework, 60*(2), 89–95.

Davis-Friedmann, D. (1983). *Long lives: Chinese elderly and the communist revolution.* Cambridge, MA: Harvard University Press.

Gelfand, D. (1982). *Aging: The ethnic factor.* Boston: Little, Brown.

Hsu, F. (1981). *American and Chinese: Passage to differences.* Honolulu: University of Hawaii Press.

Ikels, C. (1983). *Aging and adaptation: Chinese in Hong Kong and the United States.* Hamden, CT: Archon Books.

Jackson, J. J. (1980). *Minorities and aging.* Belmont, CA: Wadsworth.

Koranyi, E. (1981). Immigrant's adaptation in aged population. In L. Etinger & D. Schwartz (Eds.), *Strangers in the worlds* (pp. 220–231). Bern, Switzerland: Hans Huber.

Lowenthal, M. (1964). *Lives in distress: The path of the elderly to the psychiatric ward.* New York: Basic Books.

Lum, D., Cheung, L. Y. S., Cho, E. R., Tang, T. Y., & Yau, H. B. (1980). The psychosocial needs of the Chinese elderly. *Social Casework, 61*(2), 100–106.

Report of the SF Chinese Community Citizens' Survey & Fact Finding Committee. (1969). San Francisco: H. J. Carle.

Sue, S., & Morishima, J. (1982). *The mental health of Asian Americans.* San Francisco: Jossey-Bass.

Sue, S., & Wagner, N. (1973). Asian Americans: Social and psychological perspectives. In R. Kalish & S. Yuen (Eds.), *Americans of East Asian ancestry: Aging and the aged* (pp. 236–349). Ben Lomond, CA: Science and Behavior Books.

Wan, T. (1985). *Well being for the elderly.* New York: Lexington Press.

Yee, B. (1987). Adaptation in old age: Japanese and Vietnamese elderly woman. *Asian American Psychological Journal, 12*(1) 38–50.

Part III

Therapeutic Issues in Working with Asian Americans with DSM-IV Diagnoses

14

Assessment and Treatment of Schizophrenia among Asian Americans

KENNETH K. GEE

MUTSUMI M. ISHII

Schizophrenia, more so than other mental illnesses in Asian Americans, presents special difficulties in assessment and treatment by mental health professionals. The stigma of mental illness that many Asian families feel is heightened when the family is forced to cope with schizophrenia in a family member. Stigma disables help seeking and encourages assessment and treatment noncompliance via denial and minimization. By examining epidemiological prevalence, understanding cultural and familial views of schizophrenia, and identifying unique assessment and treatment issues of schizophrenia in Asian Americans, treatment alliances with both Asian patients and their families can be better established.

Asian Americans in the United States are a heterogeneous group. Not only intergroup differences but also intragroup differences exist as a result of differing levels of acculturation, histories of migration, education, religion, socioeconomic class, and age. Furthermore, the dearth of research on schizophrenia in Asian American populations forces us to rely on studies conducted in other Asian countries that often have very different social environments. Conclusions drawn for one Asian group should not be blindly applied to all others. This is a reality we acknowledge. Nevertheless, some similarities do exist and can be useful as guides to clinical assessment and treatment.

EPIDEMIOLOGY

United States

The National Institute of Mental Health Epidemiologic Catchment Area Program (NIMH-ECA) was hailed as the landmark endeavor in psychiatric epidemiology (Regier et al., 1984; Freedman, 1984). The study sampled nearly 20,000 community respondents at five study sites in the United States from 1978 to 1986. The study design utilized the Diagnostic Interview Schedule/Diagnostic and Statistical Manual III (DIS/DSM-III) (Robins et al., 1981) and found that over a 6-month period, nearly 20% of Americans had previously or currently met criteria for a DIS disorder. The most frequent disorders involved anxiety and depression. The 6-month prevalence for schizophrenia ranged from 0.6% in the rural areas to 1.1% in the urban areas (see Table 14.1).

Unfortunately, Asian American groups were not included in the study because of the inadequate numbers of Asian Americans interviewed. It is unclear why an Asian sample could not have been selectively chosen at the Los Angeles site, as was done for the Hispanic sample. Because of the absence of epidemiological data in the United States on schizophrenia prevalence for Asian American groups, we are forced to look at studies of other countries: mainland China, Taiwan, Japan, and Korea. Outside of these four developed or rapidly developing countries, there is a disturbing paucity of data.

TABLE 14.1. Lifetime Prevalence (%) of Schizophrenia in Five Countries

Country	Overall	Urban	Rural	Small towns
United States[a] (DIS)	—	1.1%	0.6%	—
Taiwan (DIS)	0.27%	0.3%	0.23%	0.23%
Korea (DIS)	0.47%	0.34%	0.65%	—
China (5 studies) (PSE/ICD-9)	0.19%–0.47%	—	—	—
Japan (17 studies) (key informant)	0.19–1.79% (M = 0.55%)	—	—	—

[a]Six-month prevalence.

Taiwan

The Taiwan Psychiatric Epidemiological Project took place between 1982 and 1986 (Hwu, Yeh, & Chang, 1989). The study utilized a multistage random sampling method to identify 11,004 community respondents—5,005 from metropolitan Taipei, 3,004 from two small towns, and 2,995 from six rural villages. The instrument used was the Chinese Mandarin Version of the DIS (DIS-CM) which was translated from English to Mandarin and back-translated to English by a second clinician (Hwu, Yeh, & Chang, 1986a, 1986b). This version was reviewed by Professor Lee Robins (Compton et al., 1991), one of the original authors of the DIS, and then assessed for interrater reliability and validity. The lifetime prevalence rates for schizophrenia are shown in Table 14.1. The combined rates for the three settings was 0.27% (0.3% for Taipei; 0.23% for the small towns and rural villages).

Korea

The DIS was also utilized for this major study undertaken in the mid-1980s (Lee et al., 1990). The instrument was translated and back-translated by a team of psychiatrists and psychologists from Seoul National University and the Pacific American Mental Health Research Center at the University of Illinois in Chicago. The instrument was then validated using psychiatric inpatients and controls and then evaluated for its test—retest reliability.

A two-stage cluster sampling method selected a total of 5,100 community respondents: 3,134 from urban Seoul and 1,966 from the rural countryside. Table 14.1 shows the lifetime prevalence rates for schizophrenia. The overall prevalence was 0.47% (0.34% for urban and 0.65% for rural).

China

There were a total of 61 psychiatric epidemiological studies conducted between 1958 and 1981 (Liu, 1987). By 1981, only 6 of the 61 surveys had been published. In these 6 surveys, local health personnel and neighborhood cadres undertook case identification of all persons suspected of having a psychiatric problem. These "key informant" identified cases were then assessed individually to establish a diagnosis. The prevalence of schizophrenia ranged from 0.77 to 4.80% (Lin & Kleinman, 1981).

Since 1981, five community surveys have looked at schizophrenia prevalence (Cheung, 1991). Three of these surveyed Han Chinese, who comprise the largest ethnic group in China. The others looked at psychiatric disorders among two Chinese ethnic minorities—Baima Tibetans in Sichuan Province and Uygurs in Xinjiang Province.

These later studies used the two-stage method rather than the older "key informant" method. A large number of individuals were initially screened with questionnaires to identify probable cases during the first stage. The Chinese version of the Present State Exam/International Classification of Diseases–9 (PSE/ICD-9) was then administered by a psychiatrist or trained physician to confirm or rule out the diagnosis.

The rates for schizophrenia ranged from 0.193–0.475% which is similar to rates in Taiwan (see Table 14.1). Rates were similar between the Han Chinese and ethnic Uygurs. There were no cases identified for the Baima Tibetans.

Japan

There are approximately 17 prevalence studies of schizophrenia in Japan dating back to 1940 (Nakane, Ohta, & Radford, 1992). Lifetime prevalence rates from these studies ranged from 0.19–1.79% with a mean prevalence rate of 0.55% (see Table 14.1). Sample sizes ranged from 540 to 12,027.

Nakane et al. (1992) felt that many of these studies suffered methodological problems which limit the interpretation and generalization of their results. Most of these studies focused on island or rural populations where the communities are particularly isolated and remote. These communities tended to have higher rates of consanguineous marriages. Researchers were usually outsiders to the community and may have been viewed with suspicion by the local people. Key informant case finding was used. Finally, standard definitions and criteria were not used, so comparisons between these studies and studies in other countries must be made with caution.

In summary, the best designed epidemiological studies that we reviewed were those done in Taiwan and Korea, which used the DIS instrument for assessment on large-scale, carefully sampled community populations. The similarity in study design allows comparisons with the NIMH-ECA study done in the United States. The data indicate a slightly lower lifetime prevalence of schizophrenia in both Taiwan and Korea compared to the United States.

Comparisons with China and Japan are more difficult to make in light of differences in study designs. The prevalences in the China studies show a general agreement with those prevalences reported in the United States, Taiwan, and Korea. The Japanese studies show a much wider range of prevalences. However, if two of the cited studies are excluded, the data show some conformity with other Asian countries and the United States. Currently, there are no studies looking at prevalence rates for schizophrenia among Asian Americans. Until these are done, we will be forced to infer from other country sources.

CULTURAL AND FAMILIAL VIEWS OF SCHIZOPHRENIA

To successfully assess and treat Asians with schizophrenia, the clinician must first view patients in the context of their relationships with their family and society. Treatment of an Asian with schizophrenia must inherently involve consideration of the family's attitudes toward mental illness and its concern for its reputation in Asian society, as an Asian's identity is always closely integrated with the family's identity. In working with Asian schizophrenic patients and their families, it is important to understand how schizophrenia is viewed by the patient, family, and Asian society. By understanding these views, a therapeutic alliance with the patient and family will be established. Viewing the patient's identity as part of a greater whole with family and Asian society is often difficult to do with Western perspectives, which emphasize the importance of the individual. Acknowledging what the family identifies as problems, what causes these problems, and how the family addresses and seeks help for these problems are all important issues in forming a therapeutic alliance to facilitate a culturally sensitive psychiatric assessment and treatment.

Symptoms and Problems of Schizophrenia as Perceived by Asian American Families

The symptoms and problems of schizophrenia as viewed by Asian families are different than those viewed from a Western psychiatric perspective. The hallucinations, delusions, agitation, and disruptions in social function that are the hallmark target symptoms of the Western approach to schizophrenia are not necessarily what Asian families view as being most important. As viewed by Asian families, the most important problem caused by schizophrenia is stigmatization. In Filipinos (Araneta, 1993), mental illness such as schizophrenia is caused by a weak will, which can be inherited by other family members. Denial of and secrecy surrounding mental illness are important to protect the family reputation as well as to protect family members from the stress of shame. For the Japanese, family honor is a primary concern. Mental illness is seen as deviating from conformity to society and is a family dishonor. Mental illness is stigmatized because the symptoms expressed are individualistic and do not increase belonging to family or society (Fuji, Fukushima, & Yamamoto, 1993). For the Japanese, schizophrenia is even more strongly stigmatized than other mental illnesses (McDonald-Scott et al., Machizawa, & Hiroyuki, 1992). For Chinese families, having a family member with mental illness brings shame upon the entire family and makes marriage difficult not only for the patient but for the rest of the family's progeny. The importance of family reputation in marriage may result in families keeping the mental illness of a son secret in order to carry on the family name, or of a daughter in order to rid the family of embarrassment (Lin & Lin, 1980).

Even specific target symptoms, such as auditory hallucinations and delusions, are understood in a different manner by Asian patients and their families. Rather than focusing on the unreality of auditory hallucinations, Chinese families may initially validate and endorse them as possession by ancestors speaking for the family and reflect the reality of spirits and ghosts, especially if the hallucinations occur around the time or anniversary of a family member's death. Lin and Lin (1980) described a culture-bound syndrome called *hsieh-ping*, where a family member experiences visual and auditory hallucinations, identifies with a dead ancestor for up to several hours, and imitates the manner of a deceased family member. A first-break schizophrenic episode may be initially misinterpreted as *hsieh-ping*, where important family directives and fortunes may be foretold. In addition, delusions may be accepted by families when expressed as a concern over contagion. Westermeyer, Lyfoung, Wahmenholm, and Westermeyer (1989) described several case reports in which Hmong families endorsed a family member's delusions of contagion from parasites or venereal disease. Although this was seen as a *folie à famille*, in which several family members had major depression with psychotic features, it is important to note that many Asian families may endorse rather than challenge psychotic symptoms. On the other hand, the Khmer are likely as a community to isolate a person with schizophrenia, fearing possession by spirits. Khmer spirits are appeased by regular offerings; lapses may cause accidents and mental illness (Rangaraj, 1980). To the Filipino, spirit possession may be the actions of *anitos*, agents of God which act to punish family misdeeds (Araneta, 1993).

Causes of Problems in Schizophrenia as Seen by Asian American Families

Asian families may view mental illness, particularly schizophrenia, as being caused by agents alien to the Western perspective. Clinicians must acknowledge these causes if assessment and treatment are to succeed. These views are strongest in both immigrant and unacculturated/monolingual families, and they may even have faint echoes in highly acculturated families. For example, Southeast Asians and Filipinos commonly believe that spirit possession underlies what a Western psychiatrist would call schizophrenia. The Khmer, according to Rangaraj (1980), believe that psychosis is caused by possession by dead ancestors or those dying suddenly or traumatically. Spirits of ancestors, the guardian spirit of the village, guardian angels, black magic, and spirits of geographic features may all possess the schizophrenic. Family discord raises angry ancestral spirits, which may possess the person with schizophrenia. The guardian spirit of the village, *Neak Tha,* living nearby a venerable tree, protects the village but will punish those who violate village norms. Birth events may foretell later psychotic breaks. For example, a Khmer born with both a caul (placental membranes which drape the head upon birth) and a nuchal cord will be protected by this double sign if a Buddhist ritual is performed placing a *Sla Thor* (representing the body and placenta) near a Buddha. If done, the Khmer will have skin resistant to wounds; if not done properly, the Khmer will be prone to madness and headaches. Black magic may result in possession if a Khmer seeking vengeance calls on a black magician (*Krou Thmop*) to evoke spirits of dead people (usually those dying of sudden causes) to harm the victim. The Filipinos believe that psychosis is caused by possession by agents of God (*anitos*), souls of the dead (*multo* and *tomawo*), spirits of life (e.g., *dwendes, enkantos, kapres, haan tao,* and *santermos*), or curses placed by shamans (e.g., *mankukulam, tomay,* and *hiwit*) (Araneta, 1993).

Lin and Lin (1980) described a six-dimensional model of understanding the Chinese perspective on mental illness which can be applied specifically to schizophrenia. These six dimensions are moral, religious, physiological, psychological, social, and genetic. In the moral dimension, schizophrenia can be seen as being a volitional deviation from conformity to family and society. The importance of honoring the family and contributing to society is paramount in Asian cultures. The expression of agitation, hallucinations, delusions, and disorganization is seen by the family as dishonoring its reputation and by society as disrupting smooth social functioning. The patient's inability to control psychotic and social symptoms as well as the family's inability to control the patient can raise individual and familial shame that disables help seeking. In the religious dimension, schizophrenia can be seen as retribution by the wrath of gods and ancestors for indiscretions in past or current lives. To understand this belief, one must understand the concepts of both Buddhist reincarnation based on conduct and Taoist beliefs in the supernatural intervening in daily life.

The physiological dimension formulates schizophrenia as disharmony or imbalance of opposing forces. The importance of balancing opposing forces such as *yin* and *yang* can explain patient and family concerns over various physiological functions. For example, a Chinese family's concern about a patient's overactive or underactive functioning, either sexual or somatic, must be respected and heeded in order to develop a therapeutic alliance. Asians also pay attention to the social dimension, where much weight is given to not disrupting important social responsibilities to the family, such as filial piety and enhancing the reputation of the family via marriage and work. Schizophrenia, which often disrupts such social functions, can devastate an Asian patient, who may be shunned by the family. Finally, there is a genetic dimension to the Asian view of schizophrenia. Asians view schizophrenia as Western psychiatry views schizophrenia in that there is an inherited biological component to schizophrenia. In addition, Asians believe in the genetic inheritance of punishment for ancestral misconduct. Thus, for families considering the marriage of an offspring to a another family, the genetic transmission of schizophrenia would not only affect the marriage and future offspring but would involve the entire family's progeny.

Not only patients and families but also Asian mental health care providers pay attention to the physiological dimension. Yang (1988) proposed a Chinese Five-Pattern Character Inventory which measures disruptions in balancing five important character forces. In Chinese schizophrenic patients, the Inventory shows elevations in both *taiyin* (excessive cowardice, conservatism, obsessiveness, selfishness, and lethargy) and *shaoyin* (excessive timidity, prudence, coldness, jealousy, and delicacy). These elevations, which roughly correspond to negative symptoms as seen by Western psychiatry, demonstrate Asian concern with the imbalance of forces as well as with complying with societal demand for conformity. In addition, according to the physiological perspective, schizophrenic patients have excessive *yin*, which exhibits itself through inhibition and weak *yang*, which demonstrates itself via excitatory behavior. Bipolar affective disorder, on the other hand, has imbalance in *yin* and *yang* in the opposite direction. According to Gaw (1993), possible causes of mental illness are thought to include disturbances in *yin* and *yang* (a duality that is at the same time oppositional and complementary), imbalances in the five elements (i.e., wood, fire, earth, metal, water), and inadequate *ch'i* (the life force).

Help-Seeking Behavior of Families with Schizophrenic Patients

Because mental illness, particularly schizophrenia, carries a stigma, the help-seeking behavior of Asian Americans (specifically the Chinese) generally can be described as a process: initial denial, attempts at containment of illness within the family, attempts at containment within the extended family or community, use of traditional healing methods, referral to a general practitioner, reluctant attempts to use psychiatric treatment and hospitalization, and eventual scapegoating and rejection of the affected family member (Lin & Lin, 1980). Once a problem is acknowledged, according to Cheung (1987), Chinese families demonstrate three different patterns for coping with mental illness. If the patient and family view psychosis as being purely psychological (e.g., volitional disobedience resulting in psychosis), the family is likely to delay seeking help outside the family. On the other hand, those families that view psychosis as being purely somatic, such as deficiencies in hormones or vitamins, or those with mixed psychological/somatic views, are likely to approach medical professionals, usually general practitioners. Families with purely somatic views of psychosis are more likely to consult practitioners of traditional medicine. Mental health consultation can be delayed by months or even years, depending on the pattern of coping.

Acculturation can modify the pattern of help seeking. For example, in Japan people consult folk healers, but Japanese Americans do not usually do so (Fujii et al., 1993). Even Japanese nationals raised near urban centers in Japan may be increasingly westernized around help seeking, although in the rural areas they first seek priests and herbal medicines and only later are referred to general practitioners. Seeking a psychiatrist and psychiatric hospitalization is still seen as a last resort. Japanese patients and their families are likely to be extremely deferential to the physician or psychiatrist, leaving all decisions to the doctor. Questioning the physician's authority is not likely (McDonald-Scott et al., 1992).

Help seeking by Asians can have unforeseen consequences. According to Lin, Tardiff, Donetz, and Goresky (1978), Chinese immigrant families in Vancouver exhibited help-seeking behavior characterized by early, prolonged efforts to address mental illness within the family setting. The family sought medical intervention only if the family setting proved unsuccessful; family members rarely utilized legal and social services. Only in the end did Chinese immigrants seek psychiatric intervention. Compared to Caucasians and Native Canadian Indians seen in the same catchment area, Chinese immigrant patients tended to have more florid psychosis. This may have been the result of delays in seeking help from psychiatrists. Families may successfully hide psychosis for a prolonged period, with tolerance of even florid symptoms if they are not too disruptive. Compared to the beneficent tolerance of psychosis when kept within the family, once the family seeks help outside, the same psychotic behavior is less accepted and the family member may be shunned. Similarly, if family, social agencies, or general practitioners recognized psychosis as a mental illness early in help seeking, psychosis was seen in more strongly negative terms by the family than if later recognized as mental illness by a mental health professional, who could explain the symptoms in the contexts of biological, social, and cultural factors.

Treatment of Schizophrenia in Countries of Origin

Treatments sought and accepted by Asian Americans can be colored by popular treatment choices in their countries of origin. A common pattern of treatment of mental illness is to contain the illness within the family. For example, in the Philippines, psychosis is initially denied. The symptoms may be explained by exhaustion, frustration, or external stressors. The family may encourage rest, avoidance of stress, and buildup of energy reserves by going to church, praying, making offerings, and indulging the patient's wishes. If these initial measures fail, the family may avoid familial shame by isolating and secluding the patient. Seeking help outside the family from priests, healers, general practitioners, and then psychiatrists occurs only if measures within the family fail (Araneta, 1993).

Traditional healers and priests are usually the first outside agents the family seeks in dealing with psychosis. In Khmer society, there are four types of healers, called *Krou Khmer*: (1) the *Krou Thanam Sangkao*, who treat patients in a somatic way akin to traditional Chinese doctors (the liver, for example, is seen as the center of emotions); (2) the *Krou Banebat*, who work principally through meditation; (3) the *Krou Robien*, who work through the manufacture of talismans; and (4) the *Krou Thmop*, who work via black magic. Khmer healers may use traditional herbal medicines, apply physical treatments such as burning incense with a metal cup over the affected organ (cupping), rub coins, or pinch the skin over the affected organ. Magic treatments such as ritualistic showering of patients with holy water or rice may also be employed (Rangaraj, 1980). The Khmer healer classifies psychosis in terms of *ckuet*, a social term which understands mental illness in the context of poor behavior and community misfortune. Diagnosis is made not by clustering symptoms in the traditional Western manner but by empathically understanding the patient and his or her world (Eisenbruch, 1992). Healers sought by Filipinos for psychosis may include psychic surgeons, *bulo-bulo* (magicians), *arbolarios* (herb doctors), shamans, or masseurs. Physicians are generally sought only when death is imminent (Araneta, 1993). For Koreans, a *mudang*, or shaman may perform *goot*, a ceremony which harmonizes relationships with spirits by dancing. While this ceremony may decompensate schizophrenics, goot is still thought to be cathartic and a stabilizer of family relationships (Kim, 1993).

Many Asian countries of origin also use herbal medicines in the treatment of mental illness. These medicines are usually natural products of plants and often not concentrated by sophisticated processing. As a result, Asians often perceive herbal medicines as being less harmful than Western medication. Some herbal medicines may contain atropine-like substances which may cause or exacerbate such anticholinergic effects as dry mucosa, constipation, or delirium. Herbal medicines are often mixtures of plant herbs made by the healer to create harmonious or balanced effects, which may increase the acceptance of polypharmacy. Asian physicians may mimic the healer in prescribing multiple medications without necessarily telling the patient the rationale behind their medications. Like the healer who mixes plant herbs without telling the patient what or how much of herbs is in the herbal medicine, the Asian physician may mix medications unknown in purpose to the patient; this unknown knowledge may increase the subjective potency of the medications and may be more appealing to patients (Chien, 1993).

The value of work as therapy in many countries of origin assumes that productivity for the greater good of family and society is therapeutic. This may not seem so alien when one considers the value of occupational therapy and rehabilitation training in Western day treatment programs for persons with schizophrenia. For the Chinese, long-term treatment consists of educating the patient about schizophrenia and the value of work. Successful long-term treatment of schizophrenia consists of measuring productivity in factory work and adherence to work discipline (Guo, 1988). Lin and Lin (1980) reported that during the earlier years of the People's Republic of China, treatment could include exhorting political reattunement, with belief in Mao replacing belief in Confucious in mandates for good industrious behavior.

When Asian persons with schizophrenia are treated by physicians and hospitals in their countries of origin, treatment within the family and through traditional means of healing has generally failed. For Chinese physicians, psychiatry was not a specialized field until introduced well after the end of the 19th century; physicians still tend to see mental illness as having strong physiological components. Schizophrenic symptoms are likely to be viewed in the cultural context of violating familial or societal respect (e.g., delusions rejecting membership within the family, rejecting family leadership, disavowing marriages, disavowing pregnancies, and devaluing patronage by elders or delusions of false arrest or slander by others). Such a cultural display of delusions may have as much to do with the schizophrenic patient's disruption of the social fabric of the family as the Asian physician's sensitivity to the shame raised by observing these delusions.

Psychiatric hospitalization is usually seen as a dire last resort. For Indochinese Asians, hospitals are seen as places where people die. Psychiatrists are rare, and treatment may frequently involve extreme measures such as electroconvulsive therapy. Psychiatric hospitals may be seen by the Indochinese as places of punishment and harm. In addition, according to Fujii et al. (1993), the Japanese are extremely reluctant to hospitalize family members even for medical reasons because they perceive the care at home as better. When families are forced to hospitalize a family member for medical reasons, they bring many gifts and personal items and home-cooked food into the hospital. Asians think raising morale is extremely important in recovery from medical illness, and discussing a medical diagnosis with a patient in Japan is considered detrimental, for fear of weakening a patient's stamina. On the other hand, psychiatric hospitalization in Japan is treated differently. To avoid stigmatization, the psychiatric hospitalization is kept a secret, known only to a few family members. Visitation is kept to a minimum, usually to avoid chance discovery and therefore family shame. For Asian immigrants, psychiatric hospitalization may represent an extreme measure; asking for a family meeting may be met with polite but firm resistance.

Treatment Expectations of Asian American Families with Schizophrenic Patients

Treatment expectations for Asian American schizophrenic patients focus on the restoration of social conformity and function within the family. Lin and Lin (1980) discussed the expectation that Chinese families will be able to have the affected family member married to enhance the family's reputation. If such an event occurs, the family may expect post hoc that the mental illness will never recur, now that the patient is married and functioning appropriately. The expectation for a transient course in schizophrenia may also be seen in Asian families in their beliefs about medications.

Medications, even for schizophrenia, may be used by Asian patients and their families for only a short time during the acute phase of active psychosis. Asian patients may not comply with neuroleptic medication because they fear addiction or bodily harm. In obtaining informed consent, doctors must alert patients to such possible permanent or transient side effects as neuroleptic malignant syndrome, anticholinergic constipation, sedation, blurry vision, tardive dyskinesia, and extrapyramidal syndrome, which, unfortunately, may dovetail with cultural fears of medications and cause noncompliance. Experience with these side effects, however mild, may confirm fears of bodily harm and permanently affect the future help- seeking behavior of patients and family. For example, an Asian patient who experiences cogwheeling rigidity from neuroleptic medication may never use the medication again. Once doctors mention neuroleptic side effects, patients may complain of drug side effects even though they have been completely noncompliant with medication (Chien, 1993). Asian families often view Western medication as being too strong; families and patients often self-reduce doses without informing the physician to cater to a commonly held belief that schizophrenia, like other mental illnesses, arises from weak will (Araneta, 1993).

SPECIAL DIAGNOSTIC AND ASSESSMENT ISSUES OF ASIAN AMERICANS WITH SCHIZOPHRENIA

Accurate diagnosis and assessment of schizophrenia in Asians require careful evaluation of symptoms in the context of cultural and spiritual norms. In the initial assessment of an Asian patient with psychosis, more time and attention to contextual cues are required. As Lin (1990) noted, the interviewer must carefully cultivate the initial rapport. For example, a Caucasian mental health worker must carefully address the possible war trauma or immigration harassment experiences of an Indochinese patient's family before attempting to form a treatment alliance. Assessing of a monolingual Asian patient with traditional cultural beliefs will require more than double the time needed for other patients without cultural issues because more time is needed to effectively translate the statements of the examiner, patient, and the family. In addition, time is needed to distinguish between patient/family issues and any coloring of those issues from the interpreter, who is usually more acculturated and may carry minimization or elaborative bias. Time is also needed to obtain a longitudinal understanding of immigration and acculturation. For example, it is important to understand prerefugee, refugee, and postrefugee histories in Indochinese refugees. Lin (1990) described a developmental path of refugee immigration that influences the course of mental illness: life in the homeland, life escaping the homeland, life as a transient refugee, and life as an immigrant in resettlement. Involving and validating the family's concerns in assessment of the patient with schizophrenia also require time and attention; if this is not carefully done, the patient and family become alienated.

Assessment of the psychotic Asian patient may require revision in psychometric testing. Western tests, which are based on Western norms and concepts, may lose validity and reliability when used for Asian patients. A Chinese Scales for Assessment of Positive and Negative Symptoms has been positively correlated with a Chinese version of the Brief Psychiatric Rating Scale (Phillips et al., 1991). Completely Asian scales based on Asian concepts may be more useful in rating psychosis symptoms; the Chinese Five-Pattern Character Inventory may be useful in discriminating between psychotic manic patients and those with schizophrenia (Yang et al., 1988).

From a phenomenological perspective, symptoms must be evaluated in the context of normal Asian cultural beliefs. Beliefs in spirits, influence of deceased elders on family, and power of past misdeeds done by the family to punish the individual are all powerful realities for Asians. In discerning psychosis from culturally validated phenomena, several discriminators are useful. Information on lack of community validation for the patient's experiences can be obtained from the translator. Knowledge of lack of family validation for the patient's experiences is also useful in an evaluation of psychotic symptoms. This lack of validation by community and family usually results in experiences of shame for the patient and family, with rejection by family and community. Concern with unusual experiences that are culturally determined is usually time-limited. Asians who experience culturally determined symptoms adapt normally both before and after symptomatology and are without other pathological symptoms such as social withdrawal or disorganization. The content of psychosis usually is in part or totally in conflict with normal Asian beliefs (Westermeyer et al., 1989).

Discrimination of psychosis from culturally validated experiences also requires understanding culture-bound syndromes. Culture-bound syndromes are accepted folk illnesses that may have analogues among other cultures. These culture- bound syndromes, which are pathological and deviate from social norms, do not have exact correlates in *Diagnostic and Statistical Manual* (DSM) classification, and may represent in different patients different DSM diagnoses. Examples of culture-bound syndromes that may be related to schizophrenia include (1) *hsieh-ping*, which involves prodromal dysphoria, agitation, possession by spirits, glossolalia, and hallucinations; (2) *pa-leng*, which involves paranoia about cold temperatures; and (3) *pa-feng*, which is paranoia about wind. *Phii pob* is a Thai example of a culture-bound syndrome that involves spirit possession. *Shin-byung* is a Korean syndrome that involves initial somatization followed by a trance state and possession by family spirits.

A proposal for DSM-IV recommended considering culture (Mezzich et al., 1993). Symptoms may be expressed differently in Asians. Visual hallucinations, which would likely indicate organic factors if viewed purely from a Western perspective, are more common in Asian cultural contexts. Flat or blunted affect, which would indicate undifferentiated rather than paranoid schizophrenia, must be assessed in context of cultural norms in expressing affect; otherwise, an affective component can be missed. The time course and function of Asian patients with psychosis can also be misleading if the mental health worker gathers a psychiatric history without paying attention to cultural context of episodes. An individual who has psychotic episodes while living in a developing country may recover more rapidly, with better treatment course and social function outcome, than an individual who experiences such episodes while living in a developed country. DSM diagnostic categories may ignore the context of culture in Indochinese refugees (Eisenbruch, 1992). Asian Americans may be more likely to be diagnosed as schizophrenics than Caucasians, may be more likely to be seen as having major affective disorders than African Americans and Latinos, and may have a lower rate of substance abuse than Caucasians, blacks, or Latinos. This difference may be based on stereotyping and misassumptions about ethnic identity (Flaskerud & Hu, 1992). Symptom expression may be different among different Asian ethnicities. For example, Filipino Americans with schizophrenia may express paranoid symptoms with supernatural content, and Korean Americans may express such symptoms with persecutory delusions (Araneta, 1993; Kim, 1993).

Clinicians must take care when formulating differential diagnoses. The DSM-IV Outline for Cultural Formulation (Lu, Lim, & Mezzich, 1995) provides an outstanding clinical tool for using the fourth edition of the *Diagnostic and Statistical Manual of Mental Disorders* (American Psychiatric Association, 1994) with Asian Americans. As noted earlier, schizophrenia may be diagnosed more frequently in Asians than Caucasians, reflecting errors based on a misreading of symptoms as a result of cultural differences. One important differential diagnosis in Asian immigrants is brief reactive psychosis. Extreme stresses as a result of trauma experienced during escape may cause a higher prevalence of reactive psychoses in refugees than in the nonimmigrant population. Psychopathology can appear to be more severe because of experiential and cultural differences between Asian patients and their diagnosticians, who may have a propensity to overdiagnose schizophrenia. Paranoia may be a maladaptive response to overstimulation by unfamiliar cultural cues, inability to resolve communication problems with understanding and speaking a foreign language, and inability to resolve alien ambiguous social interactions. These problems may also lead to the formation of delusions and illusions/hallucinations (Lin, 1990).

EFFECTIVE TREATMENT STRATEGIES FOR SCHIZOPHRENIA IN ASIAN AMERICANS

Effective treatment for schizophrenia in Asians involves rapport building, careful cultural attunement, effective use of translators, engagement of family, and judicious discussion of diagnosis and treatment with family. It is important to establish rapport during interviewing. Mental health providers can do so by avoiding identification with any likely prejudicial agency. For example, it is important to clearly communicate that the mental health provider and clinic are not affiliated with immigration services, entitlement agencies, or other services with which the family or patient may have experienced bias or judgmental attitudes. Clinicians may facilitate initial rapport by beginning with somatic symptoms, then moving to personal, family, and social problems. Interest and investment in understanding culture and personal/family experience as immigrants can greatly enhance initial rapport. Clinicians must take care to avoid heightening stigmatization or shame.

A bilingual staff can help to achieve cultural attunement. Bilingual staff includes interpreters, who are usually limited to bidirectional language competency and layman's understanding of cultural context; bilingual peer counselors, who may have a better understanding of culture and symptomatology; cultural brokers, who can help determine the congruency of symptoms with culture; and bilingual cotherapists, who can help integrate Western supportive therapy and medication management strategies with traditional approaches. Careful collaboration with a bicultural, bilingual translator can potentiate assessment and diagnosis (Westermeyer, 1989). Asking for literal translations, using simple sentences, avoiding technical terms, and emotionally charged issues, and allowing extra time can help facilitate treatment with a translator (Lin &

Lin, 1980). Creative integration and validation of traditional healing methods with therapeutic and pharmacotherapeutic strategies can enhance compliance and treatment success. The psychiatrist's acceptance of herbal medication "augmentation" to ameliorate concerns about the strength of Western medication may increase a patient's acceptance of neuroleptic medication. However, the psychiatrist must take care when concomitant use of medication occurs. Managing medication with brief, frequent visits may increase effectiveness of treatment. Tangible benefits of treatment, such as medication and referrals to social services and legal aid, can increase compliance. The respectful pursuit of family approval of treatment also increases compliance (Jaranson, 1990).

Lin and Lin (1980) underscored the importance of the therapist's leadership; quick and decisive action is valuable when the family is in crisis. They advised using a medical approach with many medical cues (e.g., taking blood pressure, measuring body weight, ordering blood tests, and conducting diagnostic screens/scales). They also promoted giving advice on physiological matters with which the family may be concerned, such as balancing the hotness and coldness of foods. McDonald-Scott et al. (1992) reported that Japanese psychiatrists commonly practice benevolent diagnostic deception, which may be of value in working with some Asian persons with schizophrenia; they offer vague diagnoses, such as neurasthenia, neurosis, or psychogenic fugue, to avoid giving the patient the stigma of schizophrenia. However, discussions with family involve more open diagnostic disclosure to prepare the family for mobilizing parental caretaking and to help the family to cope with effects of schizophrenia on marriage potential and employability of siblings.

There may be limits to optimizing treatment of Asians with mental illness. In Indochinese Asians, matching language and ethnicity increases compliance with treatment but does not affect Global Assessment of Functioning Scale (GAF) scores. However, the best outcomes in GAF scores come from combined supportive therapy and medication rather than no medication (Flaskerud & Liu, 1990). Because of the cultural stigmatization of mental illness by Asians, schizophrenia is likely to be hidden or masked by the family until symptoms are severe. Even so, when the family seeks acute services after delayed help seeking, Asians are still less likely to be admitted to the hospital than Caucasians, possibly because of a culturally related compliance with authority in the emergency-room setting or inaccurate assessments resulting from cultural and language factors. However, once admitted, a longer untreated course of psychosis prior to presentation is more likely to cause Asians to have a longer length of stay (Snowden & Cheung, 1990). In addition, working with Asians may be sporadic and may necessitate the acceptance of patient and family involvement in other systems of health care (e.g., herbal healers, priests, and family caretaking). This may be the reason why Asians are underrepresented in community mental health systems (Flaskerud & Hu, 1992).

ETHNOPSYCHOPHARMACOLOGY

Prior to the mid-1980s, only a limited number of studies compared the efficacy of psychotropic medication in patients from different cultures. This dearth stems from the lack of diagnostic instruments validated across cultures to provide consistency in diagnosis and measures of functional improvement. The majority of studies from the mid-1970s to the early 1980s conducted in India, Pakistan, China, Japan, Malaysia, and Indonesia indicated that patients from the Asia region had clinical response to lower doses of neuroleptic medication, as compared to Americans and Europeans (Lin, Poland, & Lesser, 1986; Yamamoto, Fung, Lo, & Reese, 1979).

Lin and Finder (1983) conducted a retrospective chart review comparing the neuroleptic dosage of 13 hospitalized Asian or Asian American patients with 13 Caucasian patients matched for age, sex, diagnosis, and chronicity. When body weight differences were standardized, they found that the Asian patients required a lower dose of neuroleptics for symptom remission. Furthermore, extrapyramidal symptoms (EPS) occurred at a lower dose of neuroleptic in the Asian patients. Sramek, Sayles, and Simpson (1986) attempted to replicate Lin and Finder's (1983) results using a similar retrospective chart review of 30 Asian patients and 30 matched Caucasian patients at Metropolitan State Hospital. They found no differences in the dosages required or the degree of EPS between the two groups.

Binder and Levy (1981) compared the frequency of EPS (e.g., acute dystonia, rigidity, and akathisia) in a sample of 20 Asian, 20 black, and 40 Caucasian schizophrenic patients treated with similar doses of haloperidol (Haldol). They found that EPS was most frequent in the Asian group (95%) versus the Caucasian group (75%) and Black group (60%).

Potkin et al. (1984) conducted a prospective pharmacokinetic study comparing plasma haloperidol levels in a sample of 18 Chinese schizophrenics in Beijing and 18 U.S. non-Asian schizophrenic patients matched for sex and body weight. Patients were diagnosed by ICD-9 and DSM-III criteria. Oral haloperidol doses were fixed at 0.4 mg haloperidol per day per kilogram of body weight for 6 weeks. The Chinese schizophrenic sample had plasma haloperidol levels that were 52% higher than the U.S. non-Asian schizophrenic sample.

Lin, Poland, Lau, and Rubin (1988) compared serum haloperidol levels after giving a small test dose of haloperidol (0.5 mg given intramuscularly or 1.0 mg given orally) to 34 normal (nonschizophrenic) male volunteers (12 Caucasians, 11 American-born Asians, and 11 foreign-born

Asians). Both Asian groups had significantly higher serum haloperidol levels than the Caucasian group.

Lin et al. (1989) prospectively studied 16 Asian and 13 Caucasian schizophrenic patients treated sequentially with weight adjusted fixed doses (0.15 mg per kg) and clinically determined (variable) doses of haloperidol. Diagnoses were established using the Structured Clinical Interview for DSM-III (SCID). During the fixed dose phase (initial 2 weeks of the study), the Asian group had slightly higher serum haloperidol concentrations and significantly higher incidence of EPS.

During the subsequent clinically determined (variable) dose phase, Asian patients required significantly lower doses (6.5 mg vs. 11.5 mg per day) to reach neuroleptic threshold (the highest haloperidol dose at which the patient did not require anticholinergic medication and manifested minimal EPS (McEvoy, Stiller, & Farr, 1986). The Asian patients also required a significantly smaller dose (5.1 vs. 14.3 mg per day) for optional clinical response as determined by the dose at the point of the lowest Brich Psychiatric Rating Scale score. Significantly lower serum haloperidol levels for Asians at the neuroleptic threshold (4.3 vs. 7.8 mg per ml) and the optimal response point (3.6 vs. 7.6 mg per ml) further suggest that brain receptor differences may play a factor in these culturally variable responses.

In conclusion, whether Asians require lower dosages of neuroleptic medication than their Caucasian counterparts remains controversial. The majority of the prospective studies cited here indicate that Asians may indeed respond to lower neuroleptic dosages or may achieve higher neuroleptic serum levels at the same neuroleptic dose. Also, Asians may have a greater susceptibility to EPS. Future prospective, well-controlled ethnopsychopharmacological studies with larger samples of patient subjects need to be done. In the meantime, judicious individualized dosing must be used to minimize the incidence of EPS and the future risks of tardive dyskinesia.

TARDIVE DYSKINESIA

Tardive dyskinesia (TD) is a disorder of abnormal involuntary movements associated with prolonged use of antipsychotic drugs. Studies have reported a wide range in TD prevalence in patients receiving antipsychotic drugs, varying from 0.5 to 70% (Fleischhauer, Kocher, Hobi, & Gilsdorf, 1985; Crane & Smith, 1980). Kane and Smith (1982) reviewed 56 studies involving 34,555 patients and found an average prevalence of 20%.

The etiology of TD remains obscure; however, age has been consistently found as a risk factor. Several studies (Crane & Smeets, 1974; Toenniessen, Casey, & McFarland, 1985; Chacko, Marmion, Molinari, &

Adams, 1985) have shown a higher prevalence of TD in elderly psychiatric patients in the range of 40–67%. A prospective study of TD by Saltz et al. (1989) showed an incidence rate of 49% after cumulative neuroleptic exposure of 40 weeks. They concluded that those over the age of 55 may be especially susceptible to TD with neuroleptic use.

All of the aformentioned studies were conducted primarily in North America or Europe. The studies on Asian samples are far fewer (there is no data on Asian Americans) and summarized by Chiu, Shum, Lau, Lam, and Lee (1992). They reported approximately 11 Asian studies published up to 1992 involving 8,647 patients with an average prevalence of 11.6% with a range from 2.5% to 27.6%. In the same article, Chiu et al. (1992) evaluated 917 Chinese psychiatric patients in Hong Kong for prevalence of TD. All inpatients of a Hong Kong mental hospital were surveyed with the Abnormal Involuntary Movement Scale, and standard research criteria (Schooler & Kane, 1982) were used to make the diagnosis of TD. They found a 9.3% prevalence rate for TD with mean chlorpromazine equivalent doses of 876 mg per day at the time of assessment. The majority of the patients ($N = 602$) were schizophrenic (by ICD-9 criteria), among whom the prevalence of TD was 8.5%.

Tan and Tay (1991) looked at the prevalence of tardive dyskinesia in a sample of 514 elderly (60 years or older) psychiatric patients in Singapore. Ethnicities represented include 461 Chinese, 20 Indian, 19 Malay, 13 Eurasian, and 1 Jew. There were 384 (75%) patients with schizophrenia. The prevalence of TD was 27.3% for the overall sample and 28.4% for the schizophrenia sample. These figures were significantly lower than those found in North America and Europe. Furthermore, the prevalence of TD in the Eurasian group (54%) was higher than for the three Asian groups (21–27%).

Binder, Kazamatsuri, Nishimura, and McNeil (1987) looked at neuroleptic drug response in a sample of 126 patients in Japan. They found a 20.6% prevalence of TD. Though doses for individual neuroleptics were low, the practice of polypharmacy (concurrent use of more than one neuroleptic) resulted in as high or higher mean daily doses of neuroleptic drugs (in chlorpromazine equivalents) than Western standards. Koshino et al. (1992) examined all 647 inpatients of four hospitals in the Hokuriku district in central Japan for TD prevalence. TD was diagnosed using the criteria of Schooler and Kane (1982) with the Abnormal Involuntary Movement Scale. The mean age of their sample was 49.8 years and the mean dose of antipsychotic drugs was 277 mg of chlorpromazine equivalents. There were 508 (77%) patients with schizophrenia. They found an overall prevalence of 22.3% for TD and a prevalence of 22.8% for the schizophrenia sample.

Chiu, Wing, Kwong, Leung, and Lam (1993) examined the prevalence of TD in four samples of elderly Chinese in Hong Kong. They were drawn from all outpatients attending a psychogeriatric clinic, all inpatients over 60 years of age from a mental hospital, elderly patients attending a geriatric day hospital, and healthy elderly from a local senior citizen center. Median age for each of the groups was 73, 71, 75, and 74 years, respectively. Only the outpatient clinic and mental hospital samples had a history of neuroleptic exposure and showed a 25.9% prevalence of TD.

In summary, though relatively few studies look at the prevalence of TD in Asians, the majority of them seem to indicate a lower prevalence of TD for Asians. Furthermore, this lower prevalence appears to hold for elderly Asian populations as well. The specific reasons for this are unclear. Possible explanations may involve lower antipsychotic dosages used in Asian countries or genetic differences in antipsychotic sensitivity.

CASE EXAMPLE

The following case illustrates the importance of involving the family in the assessment and treatment of an Asian with schizophrenia. In this case, the inadequate development of a therapeutic alliance with the family and insufficient attention to the problems as perceived by the family served to create a prolonged and severe course of illness.

AN is a 30-year-old bilingual bicultural Vietnamese male who was brought to the psychiatric emergency room by police on an involuntary psychiatric hold for psychotic disorganization in the context of treatment noncompliance and a family mistrustful of mental health providers. His family's neighbors called police after hearing screaming and smelling urine and feces in the backyard. Upon investigation, police found AN locked in a home-built shed in the yard of the family home. He was wearing dirty clothes and was living in urine and feces spread over a concrete floor.

His past psychiatric history was remarkable for a first psychotic break at age 20, with a total of seven hospitalizations. His last hospitalization at age 25 was precipitated by assaultiveness and poor eating while committed to a long-term psychiatric facility. He was stabilized on a lower dose of thiothixene than he was given while at the long-term psychiatric facility and was discharged to his family with community mental health follow-up. During this hospital stay, the family strongly protested his involuntary commitment and verbalized a strong mistrust of involuntary care. As an outpatient, AN was only seen sporadically due to family noncompliance and his case was closed a year later with no further contact for 5 years. AN had no serious suicidal history except for self-mutilative behavior (slapping himself). He had a history of breaking objects and pushing/slapping people but no assaultive history with weapons. He had no significant medical or drug/alcohol history.

His family history was remarkable for a mother who had an intermittent history of treatment with antipsychotics and a questionable history of depression. His father also had an intermittent history of treatment with antipsychotics and was reportedly emotionally abusive to the family. During the patient's hospital course, his brother decompensated and may have had a psychotic break. He had a maternal uncle in Vietnam who was chronically mentally ill and was on medications. The family could not clarify the uncle's diagnosis or treatment.

AN's social history was remarkable for immigration at age 12 with the intact family. Although his primary language and culture was Vietnamese, he was fluently bilingual and bicultural. He was the oldest of five children, all of whom had some college education and were living at home at the time of his hospitalization. AN suffered his first break while he was a senior in college, after stressors of a broken relationship with a Caucasian female and a move off-campus with Caucasian roommates. His family disapproved of both his girlfriend and his roommates; his family believed that his first break occurred because his roommates reportedly placed "poison" drugs in his food.

His family was intensely mistrustful of mental health providers and had a poor understanding of schizophrenia. They believed his psychotic disorganization was due to weakness and poor tolerance to the recent heat. Due to parental and patient exposure to antipsychotics, the family believed that antipsychotics always begat severe side effects and were of minimal use in obtaining school success. They believed that they themselves could make the patient better with their own food and by returning the patient to school. The family was convinced that the patient's minor facial injury from a fall while in the locked facility was a sign of beatings by mental health providers, and they did not want the patient to be hospitalized again. His family had prior contacts with police. His parents had been incarcerated in the past for resisting forced eviction and, at that time, the children were placed in a foster home. During this hospitalization, the police arrested all family members on charges of neglect to an adult. He was stabilized on a relatively low dose of Navane with Cogentin and discharged to a board and care home with case management.

This case illustrates the problems in treating schizophrenia in an Asian American due to different cultural and family views of schizophrenia. The stigma of a family member with schizophrenia likely disabled help-seeking behavior and prolonged attempts by the family to contain the patient's symptoms (taking the extreme measure of building essentially a seclusion room in the family yard). The family had a poor understanding of schizophrenia, even among the more acculturated siblings. Viewing psychotic disorganization as a matter of weak will arises from a moral view of mental illness. Similarly, the notion that hot weather could account for psychosis and that food can cure psychosis can be understood from the physiological view of mental illness.

The family was mistrustful of mental health providers and did not maintain a therapeutic alliance. The clinician could have better addressed the family's concern about possible physical abuse of the patient while at a long-term psychiatric facility by discussing the differences between American and Vietnamese psychiatric hospitals. Also, the clinician did not address the   possible misidentification of mental health care providers with the police and the past breakup of the family. In addition, the family's mistrust of Caucasians, as seen in bias against the patient's girlfriend and roommates, illustrated the need to clarify the role of a Caucasian mental health provider, who might have been viewed as being part of the police or part of a culture the family mistrusted. The clinician could have better addressed the family's concern about the potency of antipsychotics and dreaded side effects. Indeed, their concern may have been warranted given that the patient was stabilized on lower doses of Navane than was given at the long-term psychiatric facility.

REFERENCES

American Psychiatric Association. (1994). *Diagnostic and statistical manual of mental disorders* (4th ed.). Washington, DC: Author.

Araneta, E. G., Jr. (1993). Psychiatric care of Pilipino Americans. In A. C. Gaw (Ed.), *Culture, ethnicity, and mental illness* (pp. 377–411). Washington, DC: American Psychiatric Press.

Binder, R. L., & Levy, R. (1981). Extrapyramidal reactions in Asians. *American Journal of Psychiatry, 138*(9), 1243–1244.

Binder, R. L., Kazamatsuri, H., Nishimura, T., & McNeil, D. (1987). Tardive dyskinesia and neuroleptic-induced Parkinsonism in Japan. *American Journal of Psychiatry, 144*(11), 1494–1496.

Chacko, R. C., Marmion, J., Molinari, V., & Adams, G. (1985). The prevalence of tardive dyskinesia in geropsychiatric outpatients. *Journal of Clinical Psychiatry, 46*(2), 55–57.

Cheung, F. M. (1987). Conceptualization of psychiatric illness and help-seeking behavior among Chinese. *Culture, Medicine and Psychiatry, 11,* 97–106.

Cheung, P. (1991). Adult psychiatric epidemiology in China in the 80's. *Culture, Medicine and Psychiatry, 15,* 479–496.

Chien, C. (1993). Ethnopsychopharmacology. In A. C. Gaw (Ed.), *Culture, ethnicity, and mental illness* (pp. 413–430). Washington, DC: American Psychiatric Press.

Chiu, H., Shum, P., Lau, J., Lam, L., & Lee, S. (1992). Prevalence of tardive dyskinesia, tardive dystonia, and respiratory dyskinesia among Chinese psychiatric patients in Hong Kong. *American Journal of Psychiatry, 149*(8), 1081–1085.

Chiu, H. F. K., Wing, Y. K., Kwong, P. K., Leung, C. M., & Lam, L. C. W. (1993).

Prevalence of tardive dyskinesia in samples of elderly people in Hong Kong. *Acta Psychiatrica Scandinavica, 87,* 266–268.

Compton III, W. M., Helzer, J. E., Hwu, H. G., Yeh, E. K., Mcevoy, L., Tipp, J. E., & Spitznagel, E. L. (1991). New methods in cross-cultural psychiatry: Psychiatric illness in Taiwan and the United States. *American Journal of Psychiatry, 148*(12), 1697–1704.

Crane, G. E., & Smeets, R. A. (1974). Tardive dyskinesia and drug therapy in geriatric patients. *Archives of General Psychiatry, 30,* 341–343.

Crane, G. E., & Smith, R. C. (1980). The prevalence of tardive dyskinesia. In W. E. Fann, R. C. Smith, J. M. Davis, & E. F. Domino (Eds.), *Tardive dyskinesia: Research and treatment* (pp. 269–79). New York: Spectrum.

Eisenbruch, M. (1992). Toward a culturally sensitive DSM: Cultural bereavement in Cambodian refugees and the traditional healer as taxonomist. *Journal of Nervous and Mental Disease, 180*(1), 8–10.

Flaskerud, J. H., & Hu, L. T. (1992). Relationship of ethnicity to psychiatric diagnosis. *Journal of Nervous and Mental Disease, 180*(5), 296–303.

Flaskerud, J. H., & Liu, P. Y. (1990). Influence of therapist ethnicity and language on therapy outcomes of Southeast Asian clients. *International Journal of Social Psychiatry, 36*(1), 18–29.

Fleischhauer, J., Kocher, R., Hobi, V., & Gilsdorf, U. (1985). Prevalence of tardive dyskinesia in a clinic population. In D. E. Casey, T. N. Chase, A. V. Christensen, & J. Gerlach (Eds.), *Dyskinesia: Research and treatment* (pp. 162–72). Berlin: Springer-Verlag.

Freedman, D. X. (1984). Psychiatry epidemiology counts. *Archives of General Psychiatry, 41,* 931–933.

Fujii, J. S., Fukushima, S. N., & Yamamoto, J. (1993). Psychiatric care of Japanese Americans. In A. C. Gaw (Ed.), *Culture, ethnicity, and mental illness* (pp. 305–345). Washington, DC: American Psychiatric Press.

Gaw, A. C. (1993). Psychiatric care of Chinese Americans. In A. C. Gaw (Ed.), *Culture, ethnicity, and mental illness* (pp. 245–279). Washington, DC: American Psychiatric Press.

Guo, E. Y. (1988, August 14–18). *Recovery treatment of schizophrenic patients.* Paper presented at Joint Meeting of the APA and the Chinese Medical Association Advances in Psychiatry: Chinese and American (Chinese Part), Beijing, China.

Hwu, H. G., Yeh, E. K., & Chang, L. Y. (1986a). Chinese diagnostic interview schedule. I. Agreement with psychiatrist's diagnosis. *Acta Psychiatrica Scandinavica, 73,* 225–233.

Hwu, H. G., Yeh, E. K., & Chang, L. Y. (1986b). Chinese diagnostic interview schedule. II. A validity study on estimation of lifetime prevalence. *Acta Psychiatrica Scandinavica, 73,* 348–357.

Hwu, H. G., Yeh, E. K., & Chang, L. Y. (1989). Prevalence of psychiatric disorders in Taiwan defined by the Chinese diagnostic Interview Schedule. *Acta Psychiatrica Scandinavica, 79,* 136–147.

Jaranson, J. M. (1990). Mental health treatment of refugees and immigrants. In W. H. Holtzman & T. H. Bornemann (Eds.), *Mental health of immigrants and refugees: Proceedings of a conference sponsored by Hogg Foundation for Mental Health and World Federation for Mental Health* (pp. 207–215). Austin, TX: Hogg Foundation.

Kane, J., & Smith, J. (1982). Tardive dyskinesia: Prevalence and risk factors. *Archives of General Psychiatry, 39,* 473–481.

Kim, L. I. C. (1993). Psychiatric care of Korean Americans. In A. C. Gaw (Ed.), *Culture, ethnicity, and mental illness* (pp. 347–375). Washington, DC: American Psychiatric Press.

Koshino, Y., Madokoro, S., Ito, T., Horie, T., Mukai, M., & Isaki, K. (1992). A survey of tardive dyskinesia in psychiatric inpatients in Japan. *Clinical Neuropharmacology, 15*(1), 34–43.

Lee, C. K., Kwak, Y. S., Yamamoto, J., Rhee, H., Kim, Y. S., Han, J. H., Choi, J. O., & Lee, Y. H. (1990). Psychiatric epidemiology in Korea: Part II—Urban and rural differences. *Journal of Nervous and Mental Disease, 178*(4), 247–252.

Lin, K. M. (1990). Assessment and diagnostic issues in the psychiatric care of refugee patients. In W. H. Holtzman & T. H. Bornemann (Eds.), *Mental health of immigrants and refugees: Proceedings of a conference sponsored by Hogg Foundation for Mental Health and World Federation for Mental Health* (pp. 198–206). Austin, TX: Hogg Foundation.

Lin, K. M., & Finder, E. (1983). Neuroleptic dosage for Asians. *American Journal of Psychiatry, 140*(4), 490–491.

Lin, K. M., & Kleinman, A. (1981). Recent development of psychiatric epidemiology in China. *Culture, Medicine and Psychiatry, 5,* 135–143.

Lin, K. M., Poland, R. E., & Lesser, I. M. (1986). Ethnicity and psychopharmacology. *Culture, Medicine and Psychiatry, 10,* 151–165.

Lin, K. M., Poland, R. E., Lau, J. K., & Rubin, R. T. (1988). Haloperidol and prolactin concentrations in Asians and Caucasians. *Journal of Clinical Psychopharmacology, 8*(3), 195–201.

Lin, K. M., Poland, R. E., Nuccio, I., Matsuda, K., Hathuc, N., Su, T. P., & Fu, P. (1989). A longitudinal assessment of haloperidol doses and serum concentrations in Asian and Caucasian schizophrenic patients. *American Journal of Psychiatry, 146*(10), 1307–1311.

Lin, T. Y., & Lin, M. C. (1980). Love, denial and rejection: Responses of Chinese families to mental illness. In A. Kleinman & T. Y. Lin (Eds.), *Normal and abnormal behavior in Chinese culture* (pp. 387–401). Dordrecht, Netherlands: D. Riedel.

Lin, T. Y., Tardiff, K., Donetz, G., & Goresky, W. (1978). Ethnicity and patterns of help-seeking. *Culture, Medicine and Psychiatry, 2,* 3–13.

Liu, W. T. (1987). The Shanghai Psychiatric Epidemiological Survey. In W. T. Liu (Ed.), *The Pacific/Asian American Mental Health Research Centre: A decade review of mental health research, training and services.* Chicago: University of Illinois.

Lu, F., Lim, R., & Mezzich, J. (1995). In J. Oldham & M. Riba (Eds.), *Review of psychiatry* (Vol. 14, pp. 477–510). Washington, DC: American Psychiatric Press.

McDonald-Scott, P., Machizawa, S., & Hiroyuki, S. (1992). Diagnostic disclosure: A tale in two cultures. *Psychological Medicine, 22,* 147–157.

McEvoy, J. P., Stiller, R. L., & Farr, R. (1986). Plasma haloperidol levels drawn at neuroleptic threshold doses: A Pilot Study. *Journal of Clinical Psychopharmacology, 6,* 133–138.

Mezzich, J. E., Kleinman, A., Fabrega, H., Good B., Johnson-Powell, G., Lin, K. H., Manson, S., & Parron, D. (1993). *Cultural proposals and supporting papers for*

DSM-IV (3rd rev. ed.). Paper submitted to the DSM-IV Task Force by the Steering Committee NIMH-Sponsored Group on Culture and Diagnosis.

Nakane, Y., Ohta, Y., & Radford, M. H. B. (1992). Epidemiological studies of schizophrenia in Japan. *Schizophrenia Bulletin, 18*(1), 75–84.

Phillips, M. R., Xiong, W., Wang, R. W., Gao, Y. H., Wang, X. Q., & Zhang, N. P. (1991). Reliability and validity of the Chinese versions of the scales for assessment of positive and negative symptoms. *Acta Psychiatrica Scandinavica, 84*(4), 364–370.

Potkin, S. G., Shen, Y., Pardes, H., Phelps, B. H., Zhou, D., Shu, L., Korpi, E., & Wyatt, R. J. (1984). Haloperidol concentrations elevated in Chinese patients. *Psychiatry Research, 12,* 167–172.

Rangaraj, A. G. (1980, April 14). *The role of traditional medicine in relief operations–Introduction to Khmer traditional medicine based on experience in the refugee camps in Thailand.* Memorandum by United Nations High Commissioner for Refugees, UNHCR Regional Office, Bangkok, Thailand.

Regier, D. A., Myers, J. K., Kramer, M., Robins, L. N., Blazer, D. G., Hough, R. L., Eaton, W. W., & Locke, B. Z. (1984). The NIMH epidemiologic catchment area program. *Archives of General Psychiatry, 41,* 934–941.

Robins, L., Helzer, J., & Croughan, J. (1981). National Institute of Mental Health Diagnostic Interview Schedule: Its history, characteristics, and validity. *Archives of General Psychiatry, 38,* 381–389.

Saltz, B., Kane, J., Woerner, M., Lieberman, J., Alvir, J., Blank, D., Kahaner, K., & Foley, C. (1989). Prospective study of tardive dyskinesia in the elderly. *Psychopharmacology Bulletin, 25*(1), 52–56.

Schooler, N. R., & Kane, J. M. (1982). Research diagnoses for tardive dyskinesia. *Archives of General Psychiatry, 39,* 486–487.

Snowden, L. R., & Cheung, F. K. (1990). Use of inpatient mental health services by members of ethnic minority groups. *American Psychologist, 45*(3), 347–355.

Sramek, J. J., Sayles, M. A., & Simpson, G. M. (1986). Neuroleptic dosage for Asians: A failure to replicate. *American Journal of Psychiatry, 143*(4), 535–536.

Tan, C. H., & Tay, L. K. (1991). Tardive dyskinesia in elderly psychiatric patients in Singapore. *Australian and New Zealand Journal of Psychiatry, 25,* 119–122.

Toenniessen, L. M., Casey, D. E., & McFarland, B. H. (1985). Tardive dyskinesia in the aged. *Archives of General Psychiatry, 42,* 278–284.

Westermeyer, J. (1989). Clinical assessment. In J. Westermeyer (Ed.), *Psychiatric care of migrants: A clinical guide* (pp. 63–110). Washington, DC: American Psychiatric Press.

Westermeyer, J., Lyfoung, T., Wahmenholm, K., & Westermeyer, M. (1989). Delusions of fatal contagion among refugee patients. *Psychosomatics, 30*(4), 374–382.

Yamamoto, J., Fung, D., Lo, S., & Reese, S. (1979). Psychopharmacology for Asian American and Pacific Islanders. *Psychopharmacology Bulletin, 15,* 29–31.

Yang, Q. (1988, April 18). *The test of schizophrenics and maniacs with five-pattern character inventory of traditional Chinese medicine.* Paper presented at Joint Meeting of the APA and the Chinese Medical Association Advances in Psychiatry: Chinese and American (Chinese Part), Beijing, China.

15

Psychotherapy for East Asian Americans with Major Depression

YU-WEN YING

This chapter discusses psychotherapeutic treatment methods for depressed East Asian Americans. As the next chapter addresses treatment with Southeast Asians, the focus here is limited to Chinese, Japanese, and Korean Americans. East Asians do not represent a homogeneous group, and clinicians must assess each individual client's experiences and values when undertaking treatment. Most important, the client's acculturation level often influences how the client views his or her problems and what kinds of treatment methods are likely to be well received and prove to be effective. The chapter focuses on the less acculturated East Asians, who pose the greatest challenge to the Western-trained clinician.

CULTURAL CONTEXT

Because of their physical proximity and cross-cultural fertilization, there are great many similarities among Chinese, Japanese, and Korean cultures. Although differences may be found (see, e.g., Hsu, 1985), this chapter emphasizes their similarities. East Asian cultures are most concerned with harmony of the parts of a whole (Kaptchuk, 1983). This may be applied to the relationship between man and nature, between individuals, and within a person. When harmony is present, a person's (physical and psychological) well-being is ensured.

Confucianism has had the most pervasive impact on the lives of East Asians by prescribing rules for correct interpersonal behavior that ensure harmonious relationships (Huang & Ying, 1989; Tomie, 1991; Lee & Cynn, 1991). In fact, traditionally, East Asians are defined by their relations and family. Thus, Hsu (1985) has suggested that in contrast to the West, where the sense of self is derived from how one is different from others, in the East it comes from interaction with others. In contrast to the West, the family of origin retains a central position in a person's life, which is traditionally not replaced by friendships or marriage. Usually, the oldest male is the head of household and commands respect and obedience. In turn, he is responsible for the welfare of the family. Women play a supportive and primarily subservient role to fathers, husbands, and grown sons. Clear distinctions are made between insiders and outsiders, that is, family members and nonfamily members. Close friends are usually viewed as adopted family members and insiders. Family members are highly interdependent and obliged to place the family's welfare above their own.

This focus on relationship permeates every aspect of life and East Asians' *weltanschauung*. As Kaptchuk (1983) writes, "In the West, the final concern is always the creator or cause . . . for the Chinese, the web has no weaver, . . . the desire [is] to understand the interrelationships" (p. 15). In addition to social relationship, another important interrelationship is that between *yin* and *yang*, the female and male, cold and hot forces. The balance of *yin* and *yang* in an individual's body results in physical harmony, just as the balance of male and female forces in a family ensures social harmony. In addition, *chi* (or energy) allows for the smooth function of the body. If *chi* is depleted and fails to flow smoothly, dysfunction results (Kaptchuk, 1983). Harmony is synonymous with health and well-being. When imbalances occur (either between people or between the internal *yin* and *yang* forces or due to disrupted or depleted *chi*), disharmony results and symptoms emerge (Tseng, 1975). Harmony may be attained by adhering to Confucian teachings and behaving properly and by eating foods that balance the *yin* and *yang* elements. Popularly practiced *chi*-exercises (or *chi-gong*) also aim at increasing the amount of *chi* and its smooth flow in the body.

ACCULTURATION

Because East Asian Americans have differential acculturation levels, their adherence to the cultural beliefs vary greatly. First-generation immigrants tend to espouse more traditional values. However, this also varies by their age at arrival and socioeconomic status; those who came at a younger age and who have a middle-class background are more likely to be exposed to and embrace more Western values and thus are more acculturated. Second-generation Asian Americans are more likely to be bicultural, retaining both Asian and European American values. In the case of Japanese Americans, because of the high outmarriage rate among second-generation Niseis, the Sanseis (third-generation Japanese Americans) are likely to be from ethnically mixed households (Nagata, 1989). Thus, their beliefs are likely to be a blend of Japanese culture, their non-Japanese parent's culture, and the predominant European American culture.

Disharmony may occur within a family because more acculturated children adhere to a different set of norms (e.g., European American) than that of their parents, who may subscribe to more traditional East Asian norms (Huang & Ying, 1989; Nagata, 1989; Lee & Cynn, 1991; Sluzki, 1979). In addition, differential acculturation levels may be observed between the spouses due to differential exposure to mainstream American values. Because family relationships are central to the well-being of most East Asian Americans, assessing the presence of differential acculturation levels in a family may be essential.

DEPRESSION IN EAST ASIAN AMERICANS

The prevalence of major depression in East Asians is currently unknown. However, a study including Chinese, Japanese, and Korean Americans showed they experienced levels of depression symptoms comparable to those of European Americans (Kuo, 1984). A more recent study suggested that, at least for the Chinese, the presence of depression symptoms may have been underestimated in the earlier study and was in fact significantly higher than that of European Americans, especially for those who were immigrants and from a lower socioeconomic background (i.e., the less acculturated) (Ying, 1988). In light of these findings, the development of effective treatment methods for depression in East Asian Americans is especially important.

PROBLEM CONCEPTUALIZATION

In the West, major depression is a commonly used diagnosis. Although East Asians have been found to experience depression levels comparable to or higher than those of European Americans (Kuo, 1984; Ying, 1988), depression is not necessarily experienced or understood the same way across these two groups. It has been repeatedly suggested that depression is primarily experienced as egocentric in the West (guilt is a prominent symptom) but involves primarily interpersonal and/somatic difficulties in the East (Chan, 1990; Kleinman & Lin, 1981; Marsella, Kinzie, & Gordon, 1973; Tseng, 1975; Ying, 1990). In addition, Kleinman (1986; Kleinman & Kleinman, 1985) has conducted extensive studies in Chinese societies that show major depression to be greatly underdiagnosed. However, neurasthenia, suggesting a physical component to the illness, is a frequently used diagnosis. Again, as previously discussed, this diagnosis suggests disharmony in the body.

In a study of Chinese immigrant women, major depression was believed to involve both psychological and somatic processes, without specifying which came first (Ying, 1990). The somatic process may involve an imbalance of the *yin* and *yang* forces and blocked or diminished *chi* (Kaptchuk, 1983). Although this has been commonly referred to as somatization, the East Asian conception of it is different in an important way. The Western conception suggests that a psychological illness is being expressed through somatic means (often with the implication that this is less sophisticated than a psychological expression). Consequently, the Western-trained clinician may be more interested in the psychological processes underlying the somatic expression. However, the East Asian American client may feel both the soma and psyche deserve attention, and neither is necessarily the cause of the other. This discrepancy may severely interfere with effective treatment unless the clinician recognizes and incorporates the client's perspective in the intervention.

PSYCHOTHERAPEUTIC METHODS

Sue and Zane (1987) have suggested that in the treatment of ethnic minority clients, clinicians must demonstrate credibility by sharing the client's problem conceptualization and treatment goal and utilize methods acceptable to the client. In addition, the therapist needs to present a gift to the client early on (i.e., intervene in a manner that is experienced by the client as helpful). Previous discussion has focused on the importance of harmony in the world view of less acculturated East Asian Americans and how this affects their problem conceptualization. This section identifies effective treatment methods and illustrates them using a case vignette.

Mrs. Lee was a 40-year-old Chinese woman who immigrated to the United States at the age of 13. She spoke fluent but accented English. She lived with her husband and 17-year-old son who was about to leave home for college.Mrs. Lee had worked as an administrative assistant for 18 years at a local company but had been on disability for the last 6 months because she had persistent and severe headaches. The persistent pain led to her inability to sleep and loss of appetite.

Mrs. Lee came to the first session with a detailed history of her headaches and named the numerous neurologists she had seen who could not identify any organic causes and thus suggested that she seek psychotherapy. She did consult an experienced European American therapist. He diagnosed her as being depressed due to empty-nest syndrome and saw her headaches as an expression of sadness and need for attention. Mrs. Lee disagreed with the clinician and insisted that she was depressed because of the headaches and not vice versa. One time when she was in severe pain and could hardly breathe, she called to cancel her appointment. Her therapist advised her to come in to discuss the pain. Mrs. Lee felt angry about his lack of consideration and refused further treatment. She saw him for a total of three sessions. Subsequently, she decided to seek help from an Asian therapist. At their first meeting, Mrs. Lee reported feeling depressed and having no interest in any activity. She had no appetite and could hardly sleep. She could not concentrate, and worried constantly about her illness.

Mrs. Lee ended her presentation by expressing the desire to seek further medical assistance. Currently, her primary physician was prescribing medication to help her sleep, but it had no significant effect on her headaches. The therapist expressed empathy for her sense of frustration and supported her wish to consult other medical specialists. She inquired whether Mrs. Lee had tried other methods of help. She reported that she had been seeing a *chi-gong* teacher for a few weeks and practiced it regularly, which eased her pain. The therapist encouraged her to continue her practice. She also informed Mrs. Lee that she would teach her other exercises that might have a similar effect in helping her regain harmony in her body. The client expressed interest in learning these exercises.

The therapist also briefly discussed the nature of psychotherapy and related that she would not prescribe any medication but supported Mrs. Lee's use of the sleeping pills. The therapist expressed interest in hearing whatever was troubling Mrs. Lee and would endeavor to assist her with these problems. She asked Mrs. Lee if she had any questions. Mrs. Lee did not. On her way out, she commented that she was glad she had come to see a Chinese woman therapist.

The first therapist made several errors which resulted in premature termination. He demanded that Mrs. Lee surrender her view of the problem and embrace his explanation of somatization (i.e., her physical symptoms were merely expressions of psychological distress and in and of themselves not important). He insisted that she come in when her pain was acute to explore and understand its roots without having persuaded her of the usefulness of doing this. No "gift" was rendered (see Sue & Zane, 1987), as the clinician failed to provide relief or promise of relief within three sessions. Consequently, credibility was never established and the client decided to terminate. In reporting this experience, Mrs. Lee was also warning the new therapist not to repeat the mistakes of the former therapist. The new clinician did not. She did not challenge the client's problem conceptualization. She supported both the client's effort to restore harmony to her body through *chi-gong* and her desire to seek further medical assistance. The client was not asked to change any beliefs and was promised healing methods (breathing and relaxation) that were consistent with these beliefs.

Although the client had a brief encounter with a previous therapist, she did not understand or accept his methods. To diminish her anxiety about what therapy would be like with the second clinician, the therapist briefly explained what to expect in treatment. This is particularly helpful with East Asian American clients with limited or no prior knowledge of Western psychotherapy. However, in and of itself, it is not sufficient. The clinician also needs to intervene effectively. The therapist's intervention in the first session consisted of supporting and empathizing with the client and promising to teach other techniques similar to *chi-gong*, which might further reduce Mrs. Lee's symptoms. The client left the first session feeling heard and understood.

In the next session, the therapist introduced and demonstrated breathing and relaxation similar to *chi-gong*, which an individual may practice to restore physical and psychological harmony and comfort. Although the headaches did not disappear entirely, their severity decreased. The therapist and client practiced together in the office and the client agreed to practice regularly at home, along with *chi-gong*. She was still considering seeking another medical opinion. The following four sessions were devoted to continued practice and reinforcement of the practice of *chi-gong*, breathing, and relaxation. Mrs. Lee reported sleeping better and feeling more hopeful about recovery. She no longer mentioned wanting to seek additional medical assistance.

Although Mrs. Lee was resistant to the methods of the first clinician, she proved to be very cooperative with the interventions of the second therapist. In fact, Mrs. Lee was remarkably conscientious about practicing breathing and relaxation regularly along with *chi-gong*. At this point, the clinician was primarily concerned with symptom reduction—the gift she was giving the client. Only after the client experienced improvement and the therapist gained credibility could the therapist address other areas of the client's life.

In discussing her life with the therapist, Mrs. Lee mentioned that in addition to her husband and son, she was very close to her family of origin (including her parents and siblings). She lived on the same block as her in-laws, but had no significant nonfamily relationships. Of the various people in her life, Mrs. Lee was most disturbed by her mother-in-law's intrusiveness. Her mother-in-law was quite concerned about Mrs. Lee's headaches and would often drop by unannounced and bring her food.

Mrs. Lee complained that her mother-in-law's dishes were too greasy and she had no appetite for them. Also, she felt burdened by her mother-in-law's worries. This led to a discussion of past conflicts between mother- and daughter-in-law. Her mother-in-law had strongly opposed her son's marriage to Mrs. Lee because they had only just finished high school. However, Mrs. Lee was pregnant and the marriage could not be postponed. To show her displeasure, the mother-in-law refused to give them a banquet, the social acknowledgment of the union. Because of their limited financial resources, the young couple lived with their in-laws during the initial years of their marriage. These were difficult years for Mrs. Lee, as her mother-in-law often interfered with their lives.

The therapist supported Mrs. Lee's long-standing feeling of hurt. At the same time, she worked with Mrs. Lee to better appreciate her mother-in-law's good intentions. She reminded Mrs. Lee that, especially for older Chinese women, cooking was the primary means to express affection and nurturance. Perhaps, the therapist suggested, if she could acknowledge this and express gratitude to her mother-in-law and then suggest that she call before coming (in case Mrs. Lee was resting or out walking), she would not waste a trip. Also, the therapist suggested that Mrs. Lee tell her mother-in-law that because of her illness, she had little appetite and would enjoy her mother-in-law's cooking better if she used less oil. Mrs. Lee agreed to try and her mother-in-law began to modify her behavior.

Interestingly, Mrs. Lee now agreed that she had been indeed too young to marry. She had never dated anyone other than her husband. She was especially worried about her son, who often received telephone calls from girls. She warned him to focus on his studies and not to waste his time on girls. However, the therapist suspected he was already dating behind Mrs. Lee's back. The therapist suggested that in order not to repeat her own "mistake" (client's term), it might be better for her son to meet and date girls now so he would be able to choose the one with whom he was most compatible. Mrs. Lee also accepted this advice. Her son brought his girlfriend home whom Mrs. Lee liked a great deal.

When Mrs. Lee began to experience symptom reduction and was on her way to restoring her physical, bodily harmony, she initiated discussion of interpersonal disharmony. The first therapist had considered this the most important realm but failed to engage Mrs. Lee in discussion when he dismissed her physical symptoms. He had considered interpersonal disharmony the cause of Mrs. Lee's symptoms and had told her so. She had disagreed vehemently. In contrast, the current therapist recognized that interpersonal relationships were related to the client's physical pain but did not dwell on the question of cause and effect. Instead, she recommended methods that were consistent with Mrs. Lee's world view to restore harmony in her interpersonal relationships.

Given both her problem conceptualization and description of her social world, it was apparent that although Mrs. Lee worked in a large United States corporation, she lived a very traditional Chinese life and was not very acculturated. The therapist kept this in mind when she offered assistance to Mrs. Lee. In the case of the mother-in-law, the therapist did not question Mrs. Lee about her inability to express her annoyance with her mother-in-law because she understood that Mrs. Lee's mother-in-law occupied a superior position in her family and could not be confronted directly. Yet, Mrs. Lee did not need to suffer in silence, either. The therapist suggested that if Mrs. Lee could convey her appreciation, as a good daughter-in-law should, and use her current role as a patient (who deserved special care), it was likely that the mother-in-law would modify her ways to please Mrs. Lee.

With regard to her son's dating, Mrs. Lee was willing to change her stance from forbidding dating to allowing it if it did not interfere with his studies because the therapist had accumulated sufficient credibility subsequent to the client's gradual symptom relief. The therapist used the client's view that she ought to have dated more men before marrying her husband right out of high school to persuade Mrs. Lee that the only way her son would not do the same was to date more girls. As the therapist suspected, he was already dating (and Mrs. Lee agreed), and it was better to let him know that his mother accepted this as long as he was not neglecting his schoolwork. Mrs. Lee was persuaded without much difficulty.

Mrs. Lee continued to make progress, reporting less frequent and severe headaches, decreasing the use of sleeping pills, resuming more of her usual activities, and beginning to consider returning to work. She expressed some reservation about this as she felt overwhelmed by the demands of her boss. In fact, she wondered whether this was the cause of her pains. Mrs. Lee felt abused by how much work she was given but never complained, as she felt it was her duty to do whatever her superior demanded of her. When the therapist suggested that perhaps the boss would not be aware of the her distress unless she told him, Mrs. Lee acknowledged that she had assumed they already knew. Later she commented, "Maybe I should speak up, huh?" She was able to do so when she returned to work in 5 months' time. Her task was made significantly easier as, in her absence, her boss found it necessary to hire two people to cover for her.

The only major setting outside the family where Mrs. Lee traveled was her worksite. There, she also behaved in a traditional Chinese manner by being a subservient, loyal employee and did not express any discontent with the amount of work she was assigned. However, her employer did not understand that this silence did not indicate satisfaction. He continued to give Mrs. Lee more work as she seemed to be able to handle the assignments. Here again, rather than assuming that something was wrong with Mrs. Lee because she failed to assert herself appropriately, the therapist understood that her behavior would have indeed been appropriate in a Chinese cultural context. Instead, she educated Mrs. Lee on cross-cultural differences, and Mrs. Lee quickly recognized other more effective means of alerting her European American superiors of her distress. The fact that Mrs. Lee was able to implement this recommendation as soon as she understood that her superiors failed to realize her distress suggested that her previous lack of assertion was not likely to be due to a deeply rooted problem.

When Mrs. Lee had discussed all the major relationships that were conflictual for her (she had repeatedly reported having a harmonious and good relationship with her family of origin), the therapist inquired about Mr. Lee. Mrs. Lee reported he was very busy and often worked late into the night, and she rarely saw him. While Mrs. Lee did not appear troubled by this, the therapist noted Mr. Lee's absence to herself. But she did not press Mrs. Lee and continued to work with her on the other areas of her life. Mrs. Lee reported steady improvement of her symptoms, discontinued taking medication, and was prepared to return to work.

As Mrs. Lee had already discussed her other important relationships at length, it was striking that she said so little of her husband. However, to press Mrs. Lee before she felt a need or inclination to discuss her husband was likely to meet with resistance. Thus, the therapist chose to wait.

Two months into treatment, Mrs. Lee called the therapist between sessions. She sounded distraught. She had just received a telephone call from a woman who claimed to have been dating her husband for five years. When the woman's suspicions grew, as Mr. Lee would never spend the night with her, she followed him home one day to his house, thereby discovering that he was already married. Mrs. Lee was extremely upset and requested an emergency session. During this meeting, Mrs. Lee admitted that she had suspected Mr. Lee of having affairs all these years. He was rarely home, even on weekends. Yet she chose not to press him when he denied involvement with other women "for the sake of my son." Mrs. Lee also reported that her husband often complained she paid him no attention, but she felt this was childish. She took care of his physical needs and was raising his son to be a responsible young adult. This was what a good Chinese wife did. Her husband retorted that she was a good mother but a bad wife.

When Mrs. Lee confronted her husband with the telephone call, he denied knowing this woman. At this time, Mrs. Lee's headaches returned, but they were not of the same magnitude as they had been initially. Nonetheless, she postponed her return to work. The therapist encouraged her to practice breathing, relaxation. and *chi-gong* and expressed empathy for her distress.

Although Mrs. Lee was extremely angry and hurt, she maintained that she could not divorce her husband because a woman married for life, and she depended on Mr. Lee to support her. Upon further discussion, however, it became apparent that Mrs. Lee could and was supporting herself on her salary. In fact, she had saved enough money to put her son through college. In contrast, Mr. Lee had been spending money recklessly and was living off his credit cards.

The therapist wondered if the client had considered whether her husband was fulfilling his obligations as husband and father. Mrs. Lee realized that throughout the years she had been both mother and father to her son, and that her husband was mostly absent from her life as well. The therapist praised her achievements professionally and as a mother. Her son explicitly expressed support for Mrs. Lee and the divorce. He encouraged her to obtain a college education. In contrast, her in-laws begged her not to leave and complained of chest pains. Her parents also encouraged her to stay in the marriage. In the end, Mrs. Lee recognized she had a choice, and although she decided to give her husband another chance, she did not do so because she felt she could not survive without him.

Although Mrs. Lee wanted her husband to join her in treatment, he refused. He also continued to deny the affair. The therapist assisted Mrs. Lee in developing more effective interpersonal communication skills to strengthen her marriage. Mrs. Lee reported that her husband was coming home for dinner regularly now and spent the weekends at home. Mrs. Lee returned to work 3 months after she learned of the affairs, at first part-time and then full-time. Her work responsibilities were significantly reduced, as per her request. Her headaches had subsided to a large extent and treatment ended.

When Mrs. Lee contacted the therapist to share the news about her husband's affair, it was apparent that the therapist had been accepted as an insider. As the client had no close nonfamily relationships, it was essential that the clinician not assume an intimacy before the client indicated that such an intimacy indeed existed. The "discovery" of the husband's affair was at once surprising, but had also been clearly fore-shadowed by the husband's remarkable absence throughout his wife's illness. By not pursuing this until the client chose to do so, the therapist avoided the possibility of the client refusing to acknowledge it.

As members of her family with different acculturation levels began giving Mrs. Lee different advice (the older generation opposed divorce and her son supported it), the therapist's task was to explore Mrs. Lee's reasons for favoring or disfavoring one over the other. It became apparent that Mr. and Mrs. Lee were themselves at different acculturation levels.

Mrs. Lee held the traditional belief that a good wife cared for her husband's physical needs and raised his children properly. Mr. Lee's view of a good wife was a woman who kept herself attractive and kept the romance going. Mrs. Lee expected her husband to place his family first, as is the obligation of a Chinese head of household, but Mr. Lee was more interested in pursuing his personal pleasures. When the therapist raised the question of whether Mr. Lee fulfilled the obligations of a traditional Chinese husband, she was addressing the difference in their values. By recognizing this difference, Mrs. Lee could then consider whether she needed or wanted to be in a marriage where her expectations were not shared by her husband. When Mrs. Lee justified remaining in the marriage because she felt incompetent, the therapist helped Mrs. Lee's recognize her demonstrated competence, both at home and work. In the end, when Mrs. Lee remained in her marriage, she did not do so because she felt she had no alternative. Instead, she *chose* to stay, but not unconditionally; she would leave if her husband had another affair.

In addition to the comments already offered on the therapist's interventions throughout the case, two other points should be made. First, in responding quickly to the client's headaches, the therapist balanced the need for an assessment during the initial session and provided assistance with symptom reduction. If the therapist had insisted on conducting a lengthy assessment at the outset of treatment, the client might have perceived this as intrusive (inappropriate for a nonfamily member) and not relevant and might have refused further treatment.

Second, Western-trained clinicians, even when they are ethnically Asian, are likely to be more acculturated than their Asian American clients. This difference poses interesting challenges in the therapeutic encounter. In the case illustrated here, the therapist was sufficiently bicultural to empathize with Mrs. Lee. At the same time, although she felt pessimistic about Mr. Lee mending his ways, she did not advise Mrs. Lee to leave her husband. Instead, she invited Mrs. Lee to reflect on her reasons for remaining. The exploration began with Mrs. Lee feeling she had no choice but to stay and ended with her experiencing a choice in the matter.

Six months after termination, Mrs. Lee contacted the therapist to inform her that Mr. Lee had continued his relationship with his mistress. Mrs. Lee decided to go ahead with divorce proceedings. She thanked the therapist for helping her discover the possibility of this choice.

CONCLUSION

East Asian Americans are a heterogeneous group. The less acculturated East Asian Americans are likely to pose the greatest challenge to Western-trained clinicians. Thus, this chapter focused on treatment with this group. Unless the clinician can step into the *weltanschauung* of the client, it is unlikely that he or she can implement interventions that will be accepted and useful to the client. However, if the clinician is able to do so, even a relatively unacculturated East Asian American client is likely to benefit greatly from psychotherapy.

REFERENCES

Chan, D. (1990), The meaning of depression: The Chinese word associations. *Psychologia: An International Journal of Psychology in the Orient, 33*(3), 191–196.

Hsu, F. L. K. (1985). The self in cross-cultural perspective. In A. J. Marsella, G. DeVos, & F. L. K. Hsu (Eds.), *Culture and self* (pp. 24–55). London: Tavistock.

Huang, L. N., & Ying, Y. (1989). Chinese American children and adolescents. In J. T. Gibbs & L. N. Huang (Eds.), *Children of color: Psychological interventions with minority youth* (pp. 30–66). San Francisco: Jossey-Bass.

Kaptchuk, T. J. (1983). *The web that has no weaver: Understanding Chinese medicine.* Chicago: Congdon & Weed.

Kleinman, A. K. (1986). *Solid origins of distress and disease: Depression, neurasthenia, and pain in modern China.* New Haven, CT: Yale University Press.

Kleinman, A., & Kleinman, J. (1985). Somatization: The interconnectedness in Chinese society among culture, depressive experiences, and the meanings of pain. In A. Kleinman & B. Good (Eds.), *Culture and depression* (pp. 429–490). Berkeley: University of California Press.

Kleinman, A. M., & Lin, T. Y. (1981). Introduction. In A. M. Kleinman & T. Y. Lin (Eds.), *Normal and abnormal behavior in Chinese cultures* (pp. xiii–xxiii). Dordrecht, The Netherlands: Reidel.

Kuo, W. (1984). Prevalence of depression among Asian Americans. *Journal of Nervous and Mental Disease, 172,* 449–457.

Lee, J. C., & Cynn, V. E. H. (1991). Issues in counseling 1.5 generation Korean Americans. In C. C. Lee & B. L. Richardson (Eds.), *Multicultural issues in counseling: New approaches to diversity* (pp. 127–142). Alexandria, VA: American Association for Counseling and Development.

Marsella, A. J., Kinzie, J. D., & Gordon, P. (1973). Ethnocultural variations in the expression of depression. *Journal of Cross-Cultural Psychology, 4,* 435–458.

Nagata, D. (1989). Japanese American children and adolescents. In J. T. Gibbs & L. N. Huang (Eds.), *Children of color: Psychological interventions with minority youth* (pp. 67–113). San Francisco: Jossey-Bass.

Sluzki, C. E. (1979). Migration and family conflict. *Family Process, 18*(4), 379–390.

Sue, S., & Zane, N. (1987). The role of culture and cultural techniques in psychotherapy. *American Psychologist, 42*(1), 37–45.

Tomie, S. I. (1991). Counseling Japanese Americans: From internment to reparation. In C. C. Lee & B. L. Richardson (Eds.), *Multicultural issues in counseling: New approaches to diversity* (pp. 91–105). Alexandria, VA: American Association for Counseling and Development.

Tseng, W. S. (1975). The nature of somatic complaints among psychiatric patients: The Chinese case. *Comprehensive Psychiatry, 16,* 237-246.

Ying, Y. (1988). Depressive symptomatology among Chinese- Americans as measured by the CES-D. *Journal of Clinical Psychology, 44*(5), 739–746.

Ying, Y. (1990). Explanatory models of major depression and implications for help-seeking among immigrant Chinese-American women. *Culture, Medicine and Psychiatry, 14,* 393–408.

16

Treatment of Depressive Disorders in Refugees

J. DAVID KINZIE
PAUL K. LEUNG
JAMES K. BOEHNLEIN

Affective disorders, primarily depression, are some of the most common psychiatric disorders. According to a published community study (Regier et al., 1988), at any one time 3.5% of American men and 6.6% of American women would qualify as having an affective disorder. About 8.3% of people will suffer a major affective disorder at some time in their life. Depression is a complicated biopsychosocial phenomenon, and some depressive disorders clearly have strong biological factors in their development. However, studies have shown that there are strong social triggers to the development of many depressive disorders (Dohrenwend et al., 1992; Brown & Harris, 1978), often related to psychosocial stresses and losses.

As noted in other chapters, Indochinese refugees have suffered huge losses, including the loss of their country, social position, economic status, often their family and social network, as well as the support from their language and religion. Certainly, being forced to leave one's homeland is a major social and cultural disruption, and for many it results in depressive feelings and symptoms.

For the current Indochinese refugees, these losses are complicated by a history of frequently severe psychological and physical trauma.

Cambodians, who endured 4 years of concentration camp experience, severe forced labor, starvation, and beatings and saw family and friends executed or die without medical treatment under the Pol Pot regime epitomize those who have suffered. Many Vietnamese, Laotian, Mien, and Hmong have suffered tremendously, as well, from the effects of warfare and traumas endured while escaping (e.g., being shot at by rival militia or being attacked at sea by pirates). Refugee camps were quite unpredictable and dangerous.

As the refugees arrived in the United States they faced further disruption to their lives, experiencing local prejudice, poverty, living in poor neighborhoods with high rates of crime and violence, disintegrating family relationships resulting in broken marriages and homes, and increased use of alcohol and drugs. Refugees continue to have low to marginal economic status, and the repercussions of poverty contribute to their losses, sense of frustration, and, for many, clinical depression.

EPIDEMIOLOGY OF DEPRESSION AMONG REFUGEE GROUPS

The exact prevalence of depressive disorders among refugees is unknown. In our own clinic, 48% had a major depressive disorder (Kinzie & Manson, 1983). A clinical group studied by Mollica, Wyshak, and Lavelle (1987) also found 71% had an affective disorder, and both groups also reported very high rates of posttraumatic stress disorder. Using community samples, an early study (Lin, Tazuma, & Masuda, 1979) found widespread symptoms of depression, anxiety, and somatic preoccupation among Vietnamese refugees. These symptoms continued to increase even 3 years after resettlement (Masuda, Lin, & Tazuma, 1980). Beiser (1988) reported on a study of depressive symptoms among Southeast Asian refugees in Vancouver, British Columbia. The longer the refugees had been in Canada, the fewer the depressive symptoms. However, 10 to 12 months after they arrived, unattached Laotians and Vietnamese refugees experienced the highest degree of depression and incidence remained high even after 12 months. A study in California using the Psychological Well-Being Scale showed marked differences in depression among various ethnic groups (Rambaut, 1985). Here, Cambodians showed the highest level of depression, and along with the Hmong had much higher depressive scores than did the Vietnamese and the Chinese.

Because patients with depression often present to a medical clinic with somatic complaints, it is not surprising to find that high rates of depression are observed among Vietnamese seeking medical treatment. A study by Lin (1983) showed that most Vietnamese with physical complaints were suffering from depression. A recently completed project using the Vietnamese Depression Scale among 476 adult Vietnamese who presented to one of 10 public health clinics at least 2 months after arrival in the United States found that 20% met a criterion for depression (Buchwald, Manson, Dingas, Keane, & Kinzie, 1993). Being female, divorced, separated, widowed, older, or poorly educated was a significant risk factor for positive screening.

Although it is commonly stated that refugees and Asians frequently somatize, most of the patients in this study do express psychological symptoms, and this is consistent with our own clinical experience. In summary, depressive symptoms are very common among refugees. Depression and posttraumatic stress disorder (PTSD) represent the most common psychiatric disorders, affecting perhaps 20% of the refugees in the community, and perhaps 50 to 70% of refugees in a psychiatric clinic.

DIAGNOSIS

Diagnosing depression among refugees is not always a straightforward process. The majority of patients probably never present to a psychiatrist or mental health professional for treatment because of the stigma Asians attach to mental illness. It is very unusual for people to present the first time to a mental health clinic or to a psychiatrist for a self-made diagnosis of a mental disorder. In many ways, patients find it more acceptable and perhaps emotionally and financially easier to present to general practitioners, public health nurses, or medical facilities with multiple somatic complaints which they believe, or profess to believe, are organic in origin. Almost all our depressed patients, except those admitted to the hospital after a suicide attempt, have been referred by physicians in public health clinics after an extensive physical evaluation that was not productive.

Aside from the stigma and somatizing aspects, taking an appropriate history from a depressed refugee patient is particularly difficult. It requires a great deal of time to build up a treating relationship. Clinicians must be aware of nonverbal communication and be fluent in the patient's language or have assistance from a bilingual ethnic mental health worker, to establish rapport and communicate symptoms and treatment plans. Most important in establishing a relationship is not to be hurried and to pay attention to the physical symptoms the patient brings to the interview. Only after these are addressed and taken seriously can the therapist move to other areas of the patient's life, such as symptoms of depression, interpersonal and intrapsychic stresses, and previous symptoms, stresses, or coping strategies.

It is also essential to provide continuity of care (i.e., to be committed to treating the patient physically, psychologically, and socially). Patients must be able to trust the clinician and feel that they are cared for and understood before symptom relief can occur. Patient and clinician must explore the major symptoms of depression: sleep and appetite disturbances, problems with concentration and attention, feelings of hopelessness and worthlessness, anhedonia, and suicidal ideation. Clinicians must determine suicidal potential, although the rate of actual suicide in our experience has been less than the American average. Nonlethal suicide attempts are very common, reflecting both hopelessness and severe emotional pain.

Clinicians must also consider some specific aspects of depression. First, patients have tremendous concern for body function. Headaches, backaches, poor sleep, weakness, and digestive trouble tend to preoccupy Asians and often are the central focus of the interview.

Second, many ethnic groups have multiple terms for dysphoria that defy translation into English and must be recognized as representing strong general discomfort or distress. Some expressions of distress have been translated as "hot and bothered," or feeling "like I am going crazy," or I have a "heavy heart."

The affect of depression may be more subtle, with less obvious signs of distress exhibited. Even severely disturbed Asian patients can maintain a respectful decorum in the presence of a Western professional, downplay their own symptoms, and show a social grace that belies their despair. Subtle changes within their own reference group must be recognized, including increased psychomotor retardation and subtly sad faces.

The more we work with depression in Asians, the more we find that the clinical situation is often complicated by social or personal factors that go undiscovered until some time into treatment. For instance, until several years ago we did not recognize the reason that so many of our patients had not improved, we systematically reevaluated all of our patients and found a very significant number also had severe PTSD (Kinzie et al., 1990). The comorbidity of PTSD and depression have a much more guarded prognosis. Patients tend to improve less rapidly and to have their symptoms recur more frequently than do those with normal depression. A full evaluation for PTSD is mandatory when assessing refugees. Many of our patients originally diagnosed with depression underwent a more chaotic and bizarre course. Later, they were found to have a psychosis, usually schizophrenia, which was hidden because of their denial of major psychotic symptoms during the original evaluation. A number of patients also have comorbid psychosis and PTSD and tend to have a very chronic course.

Medical problems are also common, with the prevalence of hypertension and diabetes high among older refugees. Although hypertension does not produce many symptoms, antihypertensive drugs can exacerbate depression, and diabetes can mimic some symptoms of depression (such as fatigue and weakness). Alcohol and drug abuse problems are becoming increasingly common among Asians, a complication that can greatly affect both the clinical picture and the outcome of treatment. These must be considered when formulating the differential diagnosis.

TREATMENT OF DEPRESSIVE DISORDERS

Numerous studies reveal that Asians have difficulty accepting mental health treatment programs (Sue & McKinney, 1975). Most of our patients see numerous healers of various types and have been prescribed a large number of different medications which they usually do not take. A credible program treating a large number of refugees from each ethnic group in a setting in which each person feels comfortable will, over time, foster hope and motivation through treatment, recognition of peers' progress, and support and encouragement provided by fellow patients. This has been our program's goal and has given us substantial credibility as well as fostering confidence in new patients when they first seek treatment with us. A successful program and the presence of patients from all ethnic groups, sincerely committed to treatment and regularly participating, inspires confidence and provides a solid foundation for the uprooted individual. This may be the first time in a long while that patients feel they can count on anything or anyone or feel unity with others like them who are also experiencing adversity.

The first interview is crucial in establishing the impression that the examiner is a competent, well-trained professional who is patient, understanding, and respectful of patients and their culture and values, and who will provide patients with a safe haven to tell their stories. Often this is one of the few times in the patient's life that this has happened.

In taking a thorough history the clinician should explore family relationships, traumas, moves, and social and cultural stresses; by so doing, the clinician can evaluate the types of losses and difficulties experienced and their effects. The patient's expectations of the treatment need to be discussed. Complicated psychological themes may be operating, involving losses, jealousies, disrespect, and internal conflicts, or folk and cultural beliefs about displeasing the spirits of ancestors or not performing the correct rituals at death, feeling shame for breaking various social or cultural taboos, or harboring spirits who damage a person's body through maleficence. At this early point in treatment, clinician and patient should reach a joint agreement regarding the character of symptoms. Often a stress symptom model is useful; that is, the clinician recounts to the patient the severity of stresses and losses he or she has experienced over time and then explains that symptoms such as poor sleep, poor appetite, inability to concentrate, depression, and so on, are the manner in which the body and mind are trying to cope with all these losses. The therapist can add, often quite correctly, that the patient has coped very well, and that even the strongest persons may experience times when their body and mind cannot cope efficiently. This removes the problem from the stigmatic "crazy" category into one more acceptable and understandable to the patient. Learning that this is a normal reaction to difficult times can relieve a patient's guilt about these reactions.

The next most important aspect of treatment is to give the patient hope. Explaining his or her symptoms and how medicines and psychotherapy will work and describing how treatment will progress and what the patient can expect can go far to inspire hope and reduce demoralization. Then, symptom reduction with medication in particular can be quite rapid. The majority of patients in our program have experienced a substantial reduction in symptoms using this method.

It is also important for therapists to find ways to reduce the ongoing stress and pressure their patients suffer. Public assistance may be necessary to help with financial difficulties and to obtain health insurance coverage. A conference with the family early in the treatment course is helpful when there are interpersonal and family problems. Education aimed at reducing the patient's and family's stress can also be effective.

We require two things of our patients, and we have found these useful therapeutically. First, suicide and/or suicide attempts are prohibited. Second, patients are expected to keep their appointments. These rules are designed to convey to patients that we are involved in treatment together, and that we expect them to be committed both to being alive and to their treatment. This interactive alliance greatly increases compliance and lets patients know that we take their treatment, and their lives, quite seriously. We frequently employ Buddhist concepts prohibiting suicide: It is their faith, their karma, to live this life they have been given, and they must continue to live it, particularly for their children's sake and for the work that they have left to do. For suicidal Southeast Asian patients, emphasizing their role and responsibility as a family member, whether it be their importance as parent, spouse, or child, creates a compelling incentive to want to live.

ANTIDEPRESSANT MEDICATION

The effectiveness of antidepressant medicine among Asians has been a controversial topic in the literature. A great deal has been written indicating that medication is not effective or that lower doses are required. We have been able to determine that one of the primary problems in using antidepressant medicine for Asians is their noncompliance (Kinzie, Leung, Boehnlein, & Fleck, 1987). Others also have found this a problem (Kroll et al., 1990). It is very difficult to convince Asian patients with many somatic symptoms to tolerate some of the additional somatic side effects of medications. Fatigue, constipation, dry mouth, and blurred vision can increase the patient's discomfort and frustrations. One of our first studies on drug levels of antidepressant medicine among Asians revealed a high noncompliance rate, particularly among the Mien and the Vietnamese. Through education, projecting our expectations of patients, and monitoring their blood levels we produced a greatly improved compliance rate in all groups but one. The Mien have been unable to tolerate many antidepressant medicines (Moore & Boehnlein, 1991a, 1991b). Clinically it is important to test blood levels to determine compliance rates. Through experience we have found that Asians in general need the same dosages to achieve blood levels equivalent to those of Americans. The typical dose is 150–200 mg of imipramine or desipramine per day. Although Asians tend to have trouble tolerating this dose originally, continued use at this dose greatly reduces symptoms. Noncompliance or too low a dose of the antidepressant remain the two primary problems in treatment failure.

Selective serotonin reuptake inhibitor (SSRI) antidepressants have achieved high acceptance recently for treatment of depressive disorders, especially for Southeast Asians, because of their lower incidence of side effects and safety in overdosage. About half of our depressed patients are on SSRIs, usually fluoxetine or sertraline. A major disadvantage is that blood levels cannot be measured routinely and, therefore, compliance cannot be monitored. The tricyclics are more sedating and can help with the sleep disorders that accompany depression and PTSD. The majority of patients on SSRIs are on another medicine (usually trazodone) for sleep. The sexual dysfunction side effects of SSRIs are often difficult to discuss with Asians but they are of concern and may prevent a higher acceptance rate. We do not yet have much experience with venlafaxine or bupropion, and the multiple daily dosing results in reduced compliance compared with medicine taken only once a day.

SOCIALIZATION GROUP THERAPY

Asians avoid group therapy because they have little cultural experience with self-disclosure. Although traditional in the United States, those from more reserved cultures find group therapy intimidating, particularly in a setting in which they may be subjected to social criticism, ridicule, or ostracism as sometimes occurs to minority members. Nevertheless, we have found that Asians usually enjoy group therapy that stresses group activities, and it can be very useful. Socialization groups that help Asians learn about cooking and everyday activities in the United States, such as how to shop, rent, obtain insurance, get a driver's license, and so on, have been very beneficial to our patients. Pragmatic and useful, these are also things all patients can relate to. Although oriented to practical activities, they provide group solidarity, reduce loneliness and isolation, and effectively help patients adjust to this country. Most groups have an American and an ethnic professional who work side by side, promoting a bicultural focus. Patients are encouraged to remember and celebrate the culture they came from while accepting and adapting to their new lives in the United States.

Group therapy (Kinzie et al., 1988) successfully supplements the individual's treatment program. Common problems, such as side effects of medicine, continued symptoms, and health maintenance can be addressed in the group setting by skilled professionals. Psychotherapeutic work requires sensitivity and, in our opinion, should not focus too heavily on very difficult, somber material.

We are now also forming socialization groups away from the hospital, run more by American professionals and volunteers, to promote further adjustment to the U.S. lifestyle. This kind of group seems to do better for younger patients, whereas the more traditionally oriented socialization groups prove more helpful for older patients.

Individual psychotherapy with refugees is a complicated phenomenon and requires a great deal of understanding of the patient's culture as well as the therapist's understanding of his or her own culture. An ethnic mental health worker who can bridge the gaps may be needed. Patients need to discuss very personal and private issues, often centered around shameful events that patients have attempted to hide from, or contain within, the family. These events involve spousal abuse, rape, loss of respect by or for children, and the sense of being the subject of community gossip and ridicule. Psychotherapy with a person outside the culture can be very helpful in giving patients a safe place to disclose and work through these difficulties.

The psychiatrist must also recognize the conflict in values that may be inherent in the relationship. American psychiatrists tend to favor autonomy and independence, a relativity in values, and the need to master and control nature. The Asian may hold dear the values of interdependence and traditional family values, the need to have correct social relationships in all situations, and the holistic concept of humans living in harmony with nature (Kinzie, 1985). The psychiatrist must move from the traditional stance of passivity and interact more with the patient and must also consider the patient's values. The patient may not have the ability either to act more independently away from the family or to change a long history of relationships with elders or other people in the hierarchy. Listening attentively and giving patients some options that may be acceptable in their culture can be very useful. Helping patients understand "the American way" may also help defuse some intense value conflicts. Warmth, empathy, and certainly humor greatly decrease the intensity of the sessions and may be valuable in giving a patient great relief from a difficult life.

Ironically, many patients do better in individual treatment without the ethnic counselor present because they may feel that person represents their culture and may, therefore, be more inhibited in thoughts and behavior.

SOME FINAL COMMENTS

Chronic medical problems may develop as the refugee population ages. Diabetes, hypertension, arthritis, and chronic pain syndromes have a medical basis and often need ongoing evaluation. Periodic evaluations of our patients have revealed a number of unsuspected medical illnesses. Providing treatment or referral for these has greatly decreased some patients' symptoms or distress.

Of particular difficulty are conflicts between generations that may increase depression. The older refugee often feels alienated from the native culture, whereas his or her younger children may feel more Americanized and show antipathy toward their culture and background. Family therapy is often very useful, although it is difficult at times to convince the children to participate in treatment. Nevertheless, it should be considered. A home visit by a trained ethnic mental health worker has provided us with important information about our patients as well. An evaluation for potential problems with alcohol, drug abuse, and/or violence whose prevalence in refugee groups is increasing, can be performed during these visits.

In all likelihood, patients will require long-term treatment. Depression in refugees is a chronic process that, despite frequent improvements, often has an exacerbation of symptoms at times of personal or family distress. Constant adjustments to the new life are being made and the vulnerable, depressed person often exhibits symptomatic behavior. The therapist must not become discouraged during these apparent relapses but rather must continue on and provide a steady beacon for the patient during those difficult times.

REFERENCES

Beiser, M. (1988). Influence of time, ethnicity, and attachment on depression in Southeast Asian refugees. *American Journal of Psychiatry, 145,* 46–51.

Brown, G. W., & Harris, T. (1978). *Social origins of depression.* New York: Free Press.

Buchwald, P., Mansen, S., Dingas, E. K., Keane, E., & Kinzie, J. D. (1993). Prevalence of depression among established Vietnamese refugees in United States: Detection in primary case setting. *Journal of General Internal Medicine, 8,* 76–81.

Dohrenwend, B. P., Levav, I., Shraut, P. E., Schwartz, S., Naveh, S., Link, B. G., Shodal, A. E., & Stueve, A. (1992). Socioeconomic status and psychiatric disorders: The causation–selection issue. *Science, 255,* 946–952.

Kinzie, J. D. (1985). Cross-cultural aspects of psychiatric treatment with Indochinese refugees. *American Journal of Social Psychiatry, 1,* 47–53.

Kinzie, J. D., Boehnlein, J. K., Leung, P. K., Moore, L. J., Riley, C., & Smith, D. (1990). The prevalence of posttraumatic stress disorder and its clinical significance among Southeast Asian refugees. *American Journal of Psychiatry, 147,* 7.

Kinzie, J. D., Leung, P., Boehnlein, J. K., & Fleck, J. (1987). Antidepressant blood levels in South Asians. *Journal of Nervous and Mental Disease, 175,* 480–485.

Kinzie, J. D., Leung, P., Bui, A., Ben, R., Keopraseuth, K., Riley, C., Fleck, J., & Ades, M. (1988). Group therapy with Southeast Asian refugees. *Community Mental Health Journal, 24,* 157–166.

Kinzie, J. D., Manson, S. (1983). Five years experience with Indochinese refugee psychiatric patients. *Journal of Operational Psychiatry, 14,* 105–111.

Kroll, J., Linde, P., Habenicht, M., Chan, S., Yang, M., Vang, T., Souvannasoth, L., Nguyen, T., Ly, M., Nguyen, H., & Vang, Y. (1990). Medication compliance, antidepressant blood levels and side effects in Southeast Asian patients. *Journal of Clinical Psychopharmacology, 10,* 279–283.

Lin, K. M., Tazuma, L., & Masuda, M. (1979). Adaptational problems of the Vietnamese refugees: Health and mental health status. *Archives of General Psychiatry, 236,* 955–961.

Masuda, M., Linn, K. M., & Tazuma, L. (1980). Adaptation problems of Vietnamese refugees. II. Life changes and perception of life events. *Archives of General Psychiatry, 37,* 447–450.

Mollica, R. F., Wyshak, G., & Lavelle, J. (1987). The psychosocial impact of war trauma and torture on Southeast Asian refugees. *American Journal of Psychiatry, 144,* 1507–1572.

Moore, L. J., & Boehnlein, J. K. (1991a). Post-traumatic stress disorder, depression and somatic symptoms in U.S. Mien patients. *Journal of Nervous and Mental Disease, 179,* 728–733.

Moore, L. J., & Boehnlein, J. K. (1991b). Treating psychiatric disorders among Mien refugees from Highland Laos. *Social Science and Medicine, 32,* 1029–1036.

Rambaut, R. G. (1985). Mental health and the refugee experience: A comparative study of Southeast Asian refugees. In T. C. Owan (Ed.), *Southeast Asian mental health: Treatment, prevention, service, training, and research.* Rockville, MD: National Institute of Mental Health.

Regier, D. A., Boyd, J. H., Burke, J. D., Jr., Rae, D. S., Myers, J. K., Kramer, M., Robins, L. N., George, L. K., Karno, M., & Locke, B. Z. (1988). One-month prevalence of mental disorders in the United States based on five Epidemiologic Catchment Area sites. *Archives of General Psychiatry, 45*(11), 977–986.

Sue, S., & McKinney, H. (1975). Asian Americans in the community mental health case system. *American Journal of Orthopsychiatry, 45,* 111–118.

17

Assessment and Treatment of Posttraumatic Stress Disorder among Asian Americans

NANG DU
FRANCIS G. LU

Over the past 50 years, Asian peoples have experienced many kinds of traumatic events. These events have ranged from the guerrilla warfare fought for independence against colonialism to World War II when the Japanese Imperial Army invaded Manchuria, Korea, China, and Southeast Asia to the Cold War after 1945 that pitted the Communist against anti-Communist forces. The regional and civil wars in China, Korea, Vietnam, Kampuchea, Laos, and the India subcontinent with their sequelae of atrocity, torture, prison, concentration camps, forced labor, brainwashing, internment, sexual abuse of women, forced migration, and starvation have predisposed survivors to posttraumatic stress disorder (PTSD) and other psychiatric disorders. A great number of these survivors have asked for political asylum in the Western countries, especially in the United States. Even though these survivors have been hypothesized to be at high risk for developing PTSD and other psychiatric disorders, only a few recent studies have investigated this hypothesis.

275

DIAGNOSIS

Psychological consequences of severe traumatic experience have been described since World War I as "combat fatigue" (Southard, 1919), characterized by symptoms of insomnia, startle reaction, overwhelming anxiety, guilt, and depression. American combat veterans of World War II, survivors of concentration camps, and POWs of World War II, the Korean, and Vietnam Wars have also presented with a similar cluster of symptoms (Archibald & Tuddeham, 1965; Eitinger, 1961; Beebe, 1975). According to Horowitz (1986a), intrusive experiences and psychic numbing symptoms are the two major symptoms that lead to the diagnosis of PTSD. PTSD was first officially recognized in the psychiatric nomenclature in the third edition of the *Diagnostic and Statistical Manual of Mental Disorders* (DSM-III; American Psychiatric Association [APA]), 1980). In DSM-IV (APA, 1994), PTSD diagnostic criteria have been more refined; specifically they require the person to be exposed to the event or events that cause threats to physical harm, serious injury, mortal threats, or actual death of self or others with feelings of helplessness, intense fear, or terror. This is followed by at least 1 month's duration of three symptom clusters:

1. *Symptoms of intrusive, persistent reexperiencing of the traumatic event.* In PTSD, a traumatic event is persistently reexperienced by the patient. It intrudes into the patient's thoughts in forms of distressing recollections, daydreams, nightmares, flashbacks, or intense psychological distress at exposure to events symbolizing or resembling an aspect of the traumatic event.

2. *Psychic numbing symptoms.* Psychic numbing or emotional anesthesia is manifested by avoidance behaviors and emotional detachment. The patient would make efforts to avoid thoughts, memories, and activities that remind him of the trauma. He would restrict his affect and interest and gradually become detached and estranged from others (alexithymia).

3. *Hyperarousal symptoms.* Hyperarousal symptoms are evident as hypervigilance, startle response, irritability, outburst of anger, and difficulties of falling or staying sleep.

The disorder is considered acute if the duration of symptoms is less than 3 months. If the duration of symptoms is greater than 3 months, the disorder is considered chronic. When the symptoms emerge within 6 months following the trauma, the prognosis for remission is improved. If 6 months or more have passed between the trauma and the manifestation of the symptoms, the PTSD is characterized as having a delayed onset. The chronic and delayed types are more difficult to treat (Horowitz, 1986a).

When assessing and diagnosing PTSD, it is important to understand that it can coexist with other psychiatric disorders. A high frequency of typically persistent anxiety and affective symptoms has been found in association with PTSD among U.S. veterans of Vietnam, Korea, and World War II (Melliman, Randolph, Mutzer, Flores, & Milanes, 1992). Sierles (1983) found psychiatric disorders including alcoholism, antisocial personality, somatization disorder, endogenous depression, and organic mental syndrome to coexist with PTSD. They recommend that the clinician should screen the PTSD patients for other conditions and treat them when possible. Depressive symptoms and somatic symptoms are prominent among Indochinese patients; in fact, major affective disorder usually coexists with PTSD (Kroll et al., 1989; Mollica, Wyshak, & Lavelle, 1987; Moore & Boehnlein, 1991). Kinzie and Boehnlein (1989) reported seven cases of psychosis among Cambodian PTSD patients. Cambodians with PTSD also had high dissociation scores on the Dissociative Experiences Scale (DES) (Carlson & Rosser-Hogan, 1991).

CULTURALLY COMPETENT CLINICAL ASSESSMENT OF POSTTRAUMATIC STRESS DISORDER

Lee and Lu (1989) outlined four guiding principles when assessing and selecting a treatment approach for PTSD among Asian immigrants and refugees: (1) assessment of traumatic stressors, (2) assessment of the recovery environment, (3) assessment of culturally specific responses to illness, and (4) assessment of PTSD and other symptoms. These evaluation guidelines can be summarized as follows.

Assessment of Traumatic Stressors

Traumatic stressors are assessed by gathering preemigration, emigration, and postemigration histories.

1. Preemigration history reveals stressors and events that may have happened in the patient's homeland. They include the following:

- Local and national catastrophic events.
- External stressful events: life-threatening events, exposure to death and dying situations, torture, destruction of and displacement from home community.
- Personal stressful events: economic loss, medical problems, injury.
- Significant changes in the role of the survivor before, during, and after the traumatic events.

2. Emigration history examines the uprooting process which would include the following:

- The decision to leave: why, when, how, and with whom.
- The escape or emigration experience: degree and type of trauma (e.g., atrocity, rape, hunger, exposure to death).
- The refugee camp experience.
- Separation from and losses of significant others.
- Stress induced by the legal immigration process: uncertainty about sponsorship and the duration of waiting in refugee camps.

3. Postemigration history evaluates stressors during the adjustment process to the new country such as the following:

- Economic stressors: financial responsibility to support the family; pressure or obligation to take care of relatives or send money back home.
- Work stressors: unemployment, underemployment, different work status.
- Acculturation stressors: differences between home culture and the new culture; stress of adaptation to the new culture and often learning a new language.
- Family stressors: change of gender role, family size, family supports, family relationship.

In addition to the assessment of traumatic stressors, it is important to evaluate the impact of the traumatic events on both the patient's individual and family life cycles.

Assessment of the Recovery Environment

Assessment of the recovery environment examines the degree of support the patient can obtain to help him cope with the traumatic stressors listed previously. The assessment would focus on the availability of family support, ethnic community and social supports, and the attitude of the host society and local community.

Assessment of Culturally Specific Responses to Illness

Because of the stigma attached to mental illness, traditionally acculturated Asian patients tend to seek help from a mental health agency only as a last resort. They may present in a state of "crisis" and expect an immediate cure. They may perceive mental illness as a manifestation of either a medical disorder, hereditary weakness, imbalance between *yin* and *yang*, supernatural intervention, or emotional exhaustion caused by external situational factors. The clinician should discuss openly with patients and their family their cultural explanation of the causes of the problems, their past coping strategies, and their expectations of treatment. The coping mechanisms can be functional or dysfunctional. Functional coping could facilitate the patient's adaptation to his or her new environment; for example, belief in fate or karma would help patients endure their misfortune. Belief in the idea that "good fortune follows catastrophic events" would help patients to maintain hope for a better future and to focus on new dreams and new priorities in their new country. Dysfunctional coping would further disable the patient. Asian patients may use somatization, avoidance, and denial to cope with their psychiatric symptoms. These dysfunctional coping strategies prevent patients and their family from seeking appropriate help and support.

Assessment of Posttraumatic Stress Disorder and Other Symptoms

Clinical assessment of PTSD and other psychiatric symptoms would include psychiatric evaluation and medical evaluation.

Psychiatric Evaluation

Asian patients disclose history and symptoms of PTSD only when they trust and feel safe with the therapist. Several authors who work with Asians recommend the use of a bicultural/bilingual clinician or well-trained interpreter who can develop a trusting relationship with the patient and utilize semistructured interview questions to evaluate the patients. The Diagnostic Interview Schedule (DIS) for a DSM-III diagnosis (including PTSD) was used in a pilot study on Vietnamese refugees (Lee & Chan, 1985). Mollica reported on the use of the DIS to evaluate Indochinese patients at the Indochinese Psychiatric Clinic in Boston; the diagnosis of PTSD was 54% among Cambodian psychiatric outpatients, 11% of Vietnamese and 92 % among Hmong patients (Mollica, Wyshak, & Lavelle, 1987). A study of prevalence of PTSD among Southeast Asian refugees at an outpatient psychiatric clinic in Oregon showed that more than 70% of the total patients met criteria for current PTSD: the Mien had the highest rate (93%) and the Vietnamese the lowest (54%) (Kinzie et al., 1990). A very useful, culturally validated scale of depression and anxiety symptoms, the Hopkins Symptom Checklist, was developed by Mollica, Wyshak, Marneffe, Khuon, and Lavelle (1987). The Mollica group also developed the Harvard Trauma Questionnaire, which has been culturally validated as appropriate for the evaluation of Cambodian, Laotian, and Vietnamese PTSD patients (Mollica et al., 1992).

Medical Evaluation

PTSD patients went through physically traumatic experiences including war injury, torture, and starvation. Many of them suffered head trauma and physical injury (Allodi, 1991; Goldfeld, Mollica, Peravento, & Faraone, 1988). The clinician should also be aware of a variety of medical conditions which often occurs in Asian refugees such as tuberculosis reactivity, G6PD deficiency, intestinal parasites, malaria, skin infection, otitis media, thyroid disease, ophthalmologic disorder and hepatitis B (Catazaro & Moser, 1982; Anderson & Moser, 1985; Schwart, Chin, Newman, & Roberts, 1984; Buchward, Lam, & Hooton, 1995). When assessing the patient's somatic complaints, the clinician should be alert to possible medical problems and provide appropriate work-up and treatment rather than simply attributing them to purely psychogenic etiology.

In summary, the assessment and diagnostic approaches to Asian PTSD patients need to be culturally competent. Clinicians should focus on the patient's cultural background and beliefs, traumatic events, process of emigration and adaptation, psychological and medical impacts of trauma, and the common medical problems of immigrants coming from other countries. A complete, thorough assessment would help the clinician to understand the patient's psychodynamics and enable the clinician to select appropriate treatment approaches.

TREATMENT OF POSTTRAUMATIC STRESS DISORDER

The symptoms of PTSD can overlap with symptoms of depression, panic disorder, generalized anxiety disorder, dissociative disorder, and psychosis. The complexity of PTSD requires a thorough biopsychosocial approach to ensure effective treatment outcome.

Biological Approaches

Current biological approaches for treatment of PTSD are based on the clinical studies that indicate that PTSD symptoms are associated with sympathetic nervous system hyperarousal (Brender, 1982; Kosten, Mason, Giller, Ostroff, & Harkness, 1987; Malloy, Fairbank, & Keane, 1983; Perry, Giller, & Southwick, 1987; Krystal et al., 1989), abnormalities of the hypothalamic–pituitary–adrenocortical (HPA) axis (Mason, Giller, Kosten, Ostroff, & Podd, 1986), and endogenous opioid system dysregulation (Kosten & Krystal, 1988; Pitman, van der Kolk, Orr, & Greenberg, 1990). From these clinical studies, a number of biological models are proposed for explanations of PTSD symptoms.

1. *Locus ceruleus hyperactivity model* (Friedman, 1988, 1991; Kolb, 1987; van der Kolk, 1987). The locus ceruleus is a pigmented eminence in the superior angle of the floor of the fourth ventricle. It produces a large amount of norepinephrine in the brain and is responsible for alarm behaviors and emotions of fear and memory. Drugs that stimulate the locus ceruleus, such as yohimbine, would cause PTSD-like symptoms, such as flashback, panic attack, and autonomic arousal. Drugs that downregulate the locus ceruleus, such as tricyclic antidepressants, monoamine oxidase inhibitors (MAOIs), beta-blockers (e.g., propranolol), alpha-2 adrenergics (e.g., clonidine), and possibly serotinergics (e.g., fluoxetine) would improve PTSD symptoms.

2. *HPA axis abnormalities* (Mason et al., 1986; Smith et al., 1989). This hypothesis postulates that a PTSD victim who has been exposed to a prolonged and intense traumatic stimulation would response by producing more corticotropin-releasing hormone (CRH). CRH is an anxiogenic substance as well as a stimulator of ACTH. CRH can also activate the locus ceruleus, which in turn would be responsible for the hyperarousal symptom in PTSD.

3. *Kindling phenomenon model* (Friedman, 1988, 1991; van der Kolk, 1987). The kindling phenomenon is a slow process of changes of the neuroanotomical structures, especially those in the limbic system, following prolonged repeated subthreshold electrical stimuli, which are initially insufficient to produce clear behavioral effects. However, once these structures have been sensitized, further stimulation would lead to grand mal seizure or aberrant behaviors. In the kindling model, the brain of the victim who has been repeatedly exposed to subthreshold traumatic stimulation would ultimately develop its own autonomous excitements and produce symptoms of uncontrollable, repeated flashback or intrusive recollection and aberrant behaviors. Medications, such as carbamazepine, which is effective for reducing the kindling phenomenon, may also helpful in PTSD (Lipper et al., 1986).

4. *Learned helplessness model* (van der Kolk, Greenberg, Boyd, & Krystal, 1985; Krystal et al., 1989). The animal model of learned helplessness to inescapable electrical shock may be applicable to explain PTSD symptoms. This hypothesis postulates that the PTSD victim who is unable to escape from repeated traumatic stimulation would eventually develop nightmares, hyperarousal symptoms, and flashback because the locus ceruleus pathway to the hyppocampus and amygdala has been highly potentiated. This model also suggested that the endogenous opioid system plays an important role in response to traumatic stimuli because the locus ceruleus is inhibited by opioids. This also explains why many PTSD patients have abused opioid drugs to medicate themselves.

Culturally Competent Clinical Applications of Biological Approaches

Based on these biological hypotheses, drugs that reduce the activity of norepinephrine, downregulate the locus ceruleus, or dampen kindling phenomenon may be useful in the treatment of PTSD. Several open clinical trial studies of PTSD treatment with tricyclic antidepressants and MAOIs show reduction in intrusive recollection, nightmares, and hyper-arousal symptoms but little effect on avoidance symptoms (Embry & Callahan, 1988; Friedman, 1991; van der Kolk, 1987). Benzodiazepines, such as alprazolam, have been found to decrease anxiety symptoms only (Braun, Green, Dasberg, & Lerer, 1990). Lithium and carbamazepine are useful in controlling impulsive outbursts, decreasing intrusive symptoms, and improving sleep and mood disturbances (Lipper et al., 1986; Schwartz, 1990; van der Kolk, 1987). Neuroleptics are indicated in paranoid psychotic symptoms, frequent flashback episodes, overwhelming anger, and impulsivity (Friedman, 1988; Schwartz, 1990). Fluoxetine (Prozac) was reported to improve intrusive symptoms, avoidance behaviors, and hyperarousal symptoms (Davidson & Newman, 1991; Nagy, Morgan, Southwick, & Charney, 1993; van der Kolk et al., 1994). However, fluoxetine had minimal effects on improvement of social and occupational functioning (Nagy et al., 1993).

Few studies have been done on medication treatment of Asian PTSD patients. Imipramine and desipramine have been found to decrease depressive symptoms and intrusive symptoms among a group of Cambo-dian PTSD refugees (Kinzie, 1989; Mollica & Lavelle, 1988). Clonidine, an alpha-2 adrenergic agonist, was found to improve depressive symptoms and sleep disturbances and to lessen frequency of nightmares but was ineffective to reduce avoidance behaviors (Kinzie & Leung, 1989).

Most traditionally oriented Asian patients who come to the clinic or hospital will expect to get treatment with medication. However, several cultural issues need to be considered in the pharmacological treatment of Asian patients, especially recent immigrants and those who remain tied to traditional culture.

1. Traditionally oriented Asian patients expect medication to relieve their symptoms in a short period of time. Psychotropic medications would not be considered as "good" medications unless there are immediate therapeutic effects. It is thus important to explain at the beginning of the treatment course that a several-week lag time may be needed for the psychotropics to exert their maximal effects. The patients should also be told which of the targets symptoms can be expected to improve. They will feel more in control when they are able to monitor their symptoms with the psychiatrist. This involvement increases their participation and com-pliance with treatment

2. Traditionally oriented Asian patients believe that Western medicines may be too strong and can cause severe side effects. Several studies have implied that Asians require lower doses of antipsychotics and antidepressants to achieve therapeutic effects (Ananth & Lin, 1982; Bond, 1991; Chien & Katz, 1979; Lin & Finder, 1983). The average textbook dosages can be too much and can cause severe side effects. Suffering from medication side effects has been an important cause of high noncompliance among Asians (Kroll et al., 1990; Kinzie, Leung, Boehnlein, & Fleck, 1987). To avoid unnecessary side effects, the initial dose should be as low as possible with gradual increases to obtain therapeutic effects. To ensure compliance with treatment, the common side effects of the medication should be explained clearly at the patient's level of understanding. Incorporation of cultural beliefs, such as "hot" and "cold" theory, in the explanations would increase the patient's trust and compliance.

3. Traditionally oriented Asian patients think of psychiatric pharmacotherapy as similar to medical pharmacological treatment. They expect the medications to relieve all the symptoms. They will stop the medications when their illness has improved. It is important to explain to the patients the chronic nature of PTSD, which needs long-term treatment and follow-up. The psychiatrist should discuss in an open manner the limitation of current psychopharmacotherapy in PTSD and encourage the patient to participate in other psychosocial treatment modalities which can provide additional symptom improvement.

Psychosocial Approaches

Individual Psychotherapy

The goal of dynamic individual psychotherapy is to help patients integrate traumatic events into their understanding of the meaning of life, self-concept, and world image (Horowitz, 1986a, 1986b; Solomon, Gerrity, & Muff, 1992). However, Western psychodynamic concepts have been found foreign to traditional Asian concepts of medicine (Ciefuego & Monelli, 1983). Western psychology based on Western culture emphasizes individualism, freedom of choice, and mastery of nature. Asian culture emphasizes the values of the extended family group, acceptance of one's own fate due to one's karma, and living in harmony with nature (Kinzie, 1978; Kinzie & Fleck, 1987). Because of the cultural differences, traditional Asian PTSD patients find it difficult to believe that their symptoms would improve by talking out their problems. Confrontation and active exploration of trauma stories in insight-oriented dynamic psychotherapy may increase PTSD symptoms. Moreover, Asian PTSD victims who went through horrible traumatic experiences sometimes of long duration in which they were betrayed, intimidated, and physically and psychologically abused will find it more difficult to entrust their trauma stories to a new and unfamiliar therapist, especially one from another cultural background.

Brief Psychotherapy

Horowitz (1986a, 1986b) outlined a time-limited dynamic psychotherapy in 12 sessions as an early crisis intervention to reduce immediate distress and to prevent delayed and pathological responses. However, most Asian PTSD patients have experienced massive trauma with severe, chronic pathological symptoms without treatment for several years. Kinzie (1989) found that time-limited therapy produced poor results with Cambodian refugees. The brief duration increases the patient's anxiety. The termination after a short period of treatment increases the feelings of being abandoned

Supportive Therapy

Supportive therapy aims to establish a warm, consistent therapeutic relationship without actively exploring the traumatic experiences. This approach has been used effectively at several community mental clinics. Kinzie (1989) suggested a supportive approach combined with medication treatment for Asian PTSD patients which emphasized (1) establishing a long-term trusting therapeutic relationship with the patients, (2) being gentle and patient in handling the patients' trauma stories, and (3) supporting avoidance behaviors that help to suppress intrusive thoughts and to prevent more disruptive symptoms.

Behavior Therapy

Mowrer's two-factor learning theory has been proposed to explain PTSD symptoms. Based on this theory, Keane, Zimmerling, and Cadwell (1985) suggested that a person who has gone through horrible nonhuman life experiences may become conditioned to a variety of neutral stimuli that were presented during the trauma. These neutral stimuli (sound, smell, image, words, thoughts, etc.) became associated with unconditioned stimuli which innately evoke fear and anxiety. Through the process of classical conditioning, higher order of conditioning, and stimulus generalization, these initial neutral stimuli then acquire aversive properties and become capable of producing intense emotional responses when they are encountered later.

Behavior therapy helps PTSD victims reduce their anxiety and fear by repeated or extended exposure to an imaginary or real but harmless feared stimuli. Systematic desensitization and flooding have been used as treatment techniques for PTSD. Keane, Fairbank, Cadwell, and Zimmerling (1989) reported that implosive (flooding) therapy reduced depression, fear, anxiety, and intrusive symptoms of PTSD in 6 months. Cooper and Clum (1989) reported improvement of sleep and "psychotic-like" symptoms 3 months after treatment with the flooding technique. Side effects of the flooding technique have been reported, including exacerbation or recurrence of depression and nightmares and relapse of panic symptoms (Pitman et al., 1991) . In general, behavior therapy is found to be effective for intrusive and anxiety symptoms in PTSD but ineffective for emotional numbing, avoidance, and such other emotional disturbances as anger, shame, and guilt. Literature on behavior therapy for PTSD with Asian patients does not exist.

Cognitive Therapy

Cognitive therapy has been designed to reduce depression, anxiety, and fear by helping PTSD patients develop skills to control or change these emotions. Kilpatrick, Veronen, and Resick (1982) developed a cognitive therapy called stress inoculation training (SIT), which combined techniques of relaxation, breathing control, thought stopping, communication skills, and two most important cognitive techniques: cognitive restructuring (modifying the patient's negative thinking) and stress inoculation (analyzing the patient's stress reactions, developing coping skills, and then rehearsing and testing these skills under similar stressful situations). SIT was found to be effective to reduce anxiety symptoms immediately but was not as effective as flooding after $3\frac{1}{2}$ months (Foa, Rothbaum, Rigg, & Murdock, 1991). There is no literature on cognitive therapy of PTSD with Asian patients.

Group Therapy

Insight-oriented dynamic group psychotherapy has not been successful for Asian PTSD victims because Asians are reluctant to talk about their personal feelings in front of the group. Group "talking" therapy may also remind patients of traumatic "self-criticism and criticism" group meetings, in which they were forced to participate in Communist countries. Kinzie et al. (1988) initiated a socialization group with Southeast Asian refugees which is more activity- than talk-oriented. Such group therapy has helped the patients develop social skills and practical problem-solving skills through traditional, cultural activities. Limited discussion of psychological issues and traumatic experiences occur in the group throughout the activities. At times, the recall of painful experiences can increase PTSD symptoms in the group. Group members are encouraged to give suggestions to suppress these symptoms. Active suppression is considered an effective coping mechanism. More private and painful trauma issues (such as atrocity, rape, and torture) that cannot be expressed in the group are shared with a trusting therapist in individual sessions.

Family Therapy

Several family intervention models are proposed to help the PTSD victim family cope with the crisis situation. Patterson and McCubbin (1983) suggested eight strategies for prevention-oriented intervention that focus on helping the family to be conscious of the crisis, improving the family problem-solving and communication skills, providing psychoeducation for the family on the impact of trauma events, and providing help to the family to connect with social supportive services. Harris (1991) developed a five-step approach intervention: (1) providing an environment where the family can be heard, understood, accepted, and supported; (2) identifying family problem issues and developing family communication and supportive skills; (3) helping family members develop strength to help the victim and themselves; (4) increasing social supports; and (5) increasing family understanding the victim trauma and assisting the family to utilize social resources. These family therapy models emphasize early crisis intervention to provide a safe environment where family members can ventilate their emotions and to develop supports for the patients and families. However, Asian families usually have not been able to take advantage of early intervention for many reasons (e.g., access to appropriate services). Because of the stigma of mental illness, Asian families usually keep PTSD patients at home for a long time before bringing them to get professional help. Several authors (Jung, 1984; Kim, 1985; Lee, 1982) have proposed models of family therapy for Asians. These models emphasize structured sessions that provide psychoeducation, "here and now" problem solving, and social supports for the patients and families members. These approaches are recommended for the Asian family with a PTSD patient (Lee & Lu, 1989).

Culturally Competent Clinical Applications of Psychosocial Approaches

Most of Asian PTSD patients have experienced their PTSD symptoms for several years in their own country and are unlikely to have had much treatment. The repeated, massive, horrible trauma they experienced results in a chronic, malignant disorder similar to a chronic course found in victims of Nazism in World War II (Kinzie, 1989). Psychosocial approaches need to be sensitive to the patient's complex, severe PTSD symptoms and especially to the Asian cultural differences to enhance the effectiveness of treatments.

The Setting. Many Asian patients are new immigrants who are dealing with both the crisis of "loss" after they left their country and the crisis of "load" when they struggle to adapt to the new country. These double crises and the severity of PTSD symptoms require a clinical setting in which the multidisciplinary team can be involved to provide optimal care. Examples of culturally focused clinics for Asians include the Indochinese Refugee Clinic (IRC) in Oregon (Kinzie, Tran, Breckenridge, & Bloom, 1980), Indochinese Psychiatric Clinic (IPC) in Boston (Mollica & Lavelle, 1988), and the New South Wales Service for Treatment and Rehabilitation of Torture and Trauma Survivors (STARTTS) (Reid, Silove, & Tam, 1990). Given the stigma toward mental illness, Asian patients may be referred to mental health clinics from primary care clinics or social services when staff in these agencies pick up on their symptoms. The cooperation between these agencies is very important if they are to provide comprehensive care for the patients.

Culturally Competent Therapy. In general, we recommend a multimodal, supportive, activity-oriented combined individual and group therapy for Asian PTSD patients. The clinical experiences from IRC, IPC, STARTT clinics can be summarized to provide guidelines for therapy:

1. *Initial stage* (building a trusting therapeutic alliance). During the initial stage, the therapy should focus on providing Asian PTSD patients a safe place to interact with the therapist and their peers. To build a trusting therapeutic relationship, the therapist can use traditional cultural activities through which the patients socialize and interact with the therapist and others. During this stage, the therapist should accept and tolerate low levels of expressivity because Asian patients are not comfortable expressing their emotional conflicts in front of the group or strangers. Therapy should focus on "here and now" problem solving and developing communication and social skills. The therapist should take an active role similar to that of a case manager to help the patients stabilize their living situation. Patients appreciate concrete assistance to obtain social welfare supports, appropriate medical referrals, housing, and connection with other agencies. These supportive interventions dramatically relieve the patients from external stress. From the patients' viewpoint, the therapist's assistance symbolizes the fulfillment of their expectations of getting help from the therapist and seeing promises become true. The new experience is in contrast to what they experienced in their traumatic past, when expectations were shattered and promises were betrayed. The therapist is probably one of the few people to provide support to patients who lived in fear for so many years when they were incarcerated, tortured, and humiliated. Trust gradually develops when the patients feel accepted and supported in a safe, therapeutic environment. The first impression during the initial stage is important in terms of facilitating the therapeutic process during later stages.

2. *Therapeutic stage* (unfolding of trauma stories, the centerpiece of therapy (Mollica & Lavelle, 1988). A trusting therapeutic relationship with the therapist and other members in the group will enable patients to open up about their trauma stories. These revelations will slowly unfold out of group activities. Mollica and Lavelle (1988) found that the "trauma story" emerges as a centerpiece of therapy. The emergence of the trauma stories of one or two people will encourage the unfolding of trauma stories from other group members. Members who are feeling vulnerable and cannot tolerate the others' trauma stories are allowed to leave the group. Others may find that their PTSD symptoms resurface when they listen to the trauma stories in the group. Additional individual sessions should be provided to give these patients more support. Behavioral and cognitive techniques can be taught to help the patients control and prevent such PTSD symptoms as intrusive thoughts and anxiety symptoms. These techniques need to be designed sensitively to incorporate the patients' cultures. For example, music is commonly used in Western culture to provide soothing, relaxing feelings. However, music for Asian PTSD patients needs to avoid certain sounds and rhythms that remind them of traumatic experiences. For example, the sound of birds and the accelerating tempo of drums remind them of reeducational camps in the jungle, or the sound of ocean waves reminds boat people of their trauma at sea. Cultural relaxation techniques such as sitting or walking, meditation, praying in church or temple, yoga, or *tai chi* exercises commonly used in Asia are more appropriate for Asian PTSD patients. Psychoeducation during this stage is important to help the patients understand their PTSD symptoms, which have been so bizarre and frightening to them for so many years. The therapist should gently and patiently let patients unfold their trauma stories at their own pace. The patients will choose the appropriate time and setting to bring up their feelings of fear, anger, shame, and humiliation. Appropriate therapeutic interpretation will provide the patients insight into their emotional conflicts and to point out the link connecting the traumatic experiences with their present PTSD symptoms. During the course of therapy, inappropriate countertransparence may occur: (1) the therapist may become fascinated with the different trauma stories and lose track of need for supportive interventions; (2) the therapist may push for more information and aim for catharsis, thus aggravating the patient's PTSD symptoms; (3) the therapist may be overwhelmed by the patient's horrible experiences, thus, leading the therapist to become psychologically numb. Such countertransference feelings and reactions would severely prevent the therapist from getting appropriate information and providing effective treatment. Therapists must be able to recognize their own distress and defense in treatment of PTSD victims.

Family Involvement. Given that the family is considered a basic funda-mental unit of traditional Asian society, family involvement and support are critical in the treatment of Asian PTSD victims. A structured, time-limited, problem-solving, psychoeducational family approach will help the family to understand the patient's symptoms and needs, to facilitate communication in the family, and to provide information of community resources where the family can obtain additional social, economic, and legal assistance.

Community Supports. The loss, suffering, and needs of PTSD victims are great. Social and community supports are necessary to rehabilitate these patients. The Chinese, who have a long immigration history, have created several supportive systems based on the same language dialect (Hakka Association, Jeochiu Association, etc.) or the same surname (Wong Association, Yee Association, etc.). The Vietnamese have organized mutual associations of people who come from the same province and alumni associations. The Vietnamese Veteran Association and recently the Reeducational Detainee Association (Former Political Detainee Associa-tion) have gained tremendous support from the Vietnamese community. The Lao and Cambodians have developed their supportive systems around their Buddhist temples (Canda & Phaobtong, 1992). Religious and traditional ceremonies should be respected and utilized as part of the therapy process to help certain patients go through the grief process, which was suppressed in the past. Participation in cultural activities gives patients a sense of belonging to their own group and helps them regain their social functioning and meaning of life.

CONCLUSION

The assessment and treatment of PTSD have been a challenge for the clinician. Working with Asian PTSD victims has been more difficult and complicated because of the cultural differences and the chronicity and severity of their illness. The current diagnostic formulation of PTSD derives from observation of relative circumscribed traumatic events: combat, disaster, rape. However, evidence exists of a complex form of PTSD in survivors of prolonged, repeated trauma where the victims were in state of captivity, unable to flee and under total control of perpetrators (Herman, 1992). Many Asian PTSD patients have gone through such experiences, including civil wars, prisons, concentration camp detainment, reeducation camp prison, slave labor camp, and captivity by pirates. Their symptoms are more complex, severe, and chronic. Moreover, the symp-tomatology manifested by Asian patients needs to be understood in the context of their culture. Knowledge of therapy for Asian PTSD patients is still very limited. No specific treatment modality alone can provide effective treatment outcome. Medications have been noted to relieve the intrusive recollections (intrusive thoughts and nightmares) and hyper-arousal symptoms (startle reactions, impulsive behaviors, hypervigilant, panic, anxious reactions) but have not been effective in avoidance behaviors or resolving feelings of guilt, shame, anger, and humiliation. However, relief from some of the PTSD symptoms provided by medications enables patients to participate in psychosocial treatment, which helps them to become less withdrawn, less isolative, and more understanding of their emotional experiences. A multimodal, supportive, activity-oriented combined individual and group therapy in a specific Asian-focused clinic setting with a mutidisciplinary team approach and intersocial agency cooperation has been found to improve pychosocial functioning. More study on symptomatology, psychopathology, psychopharmacology, and psychosocial therapy focused specifically on Asian PTSD is needed to provide better understanding on assessment and treatments of this population.

REFERENCES

Allodi, F. A. (1991). Assessment and treatment of torture victims: A critical review. *Journal of Nervous and Mental Disease, 179,* 1-4.

Anderson, J. P., & Moser, R. J. (1985). Parasitic screening and treatment among Indochinese refugees. *Journal of the American Medical Association, 253,* 2229-2235.

American Psychiatric Association. (1980). *Diagnostic and statistical manual of mental disorders* (3rd ed.). Washington, DC: Author.

American Psychiatric Association. (1994). *Diagnostic and statistical manual of mental disorders* (4th ed.). Washington, DC: Author.

Ananth, J., & Lin, K. M. (1982). Physical and ethnic variables in dosage for Asians. *American Journal of Psychiatry, 140,* 490-491.

Archibald, H. C., & Tuddeham, D. R. (1965). Persistent stress reaction after combat: A 20-year follow-up. *Archives of General Psychiatry, 12,* 475-481.

Beebe, G. W. (1975). Follow-up studies of World War II and Korean War prisoners. *American Journal of Epidemiology, 5,* 400-422.

Bond, W. S. (1991). Therapy update: Ethnicity and psychotropic drugs. *Clinical Pharmacology, 10,* 467-470.

Braun, P., Green, D., Dasberg, H., & Lerer, B. (1990). Core symptoms of PTSD unimproved by alprazolam treatment. *Journal of Clinical Psychiatry, 51,* 236-238.

Brender, J. O. (1982). Electrodermal responses in PTSD. *Journal of Nervous and Mental Disease, 170,* 352-361.

Buchward, D., Lam, M., & Hooton, M. (1995). Prevalence of intestinal parasites and association with symptoms in Southeast Asian refugees. *Journal of Clinical Pharmacy and Therapeutics, 20,* 271–275.

Canda, E. R., & Phaobtong, T. (1992). Buddhism as a supportive system for Southeast Asian refugees. *Social Work, 37,* 61–67.

Carlson, E. B., & Rosser-Hogan, R. (1991). Trauma experiences, posttraumatic stress, dissociation, and depression in Cambodian refugees. *American Journal of Psychiatry, 148,* 1548–1551.

Catazaro, A., & Moser, R. J. (1982). Health status of refugees from Vietnam, Laos and Cambodia. *Journal of the American Medical Association, 147,* 1303–1308.

Chien, C., & Katz, M. M. (1979). Transcultural psychopharmacology in depression: East and West. *Psychopharmacology Bulletin, 15,* 24–26.

Ciefuego, A. J., & Monelli, C. (1983). The testimony of political repression as a therapeutic instrument. *American Journal of Orthopsychiatry, 53,* 43–94.

Cooper, N. H., & Clum, G. A. (1989). Imaginal flooding as a supplementary treatment for PTSD in combat veterans: A controlled study. *Behavior Therapy, 20,* 381–391.

Davidson, J., & Newman, B. (1991). Fluoxetine in PTSD. *Journal of Traumatic Stress, 4,* 419–423.

Eitinger, L. (1961). Pathology of the concentration camp syndrome. *Archives of General Psychiatry, 5,* 371–379.

Embry, C. K., & Callahan, M. (1988). Effective pharmacotherapy for PTSD. *VA Practice, 5,* 57–66.

Foa, E. B., Rothbaum, O. B., Rigg, D. S., & Murdock, T. B. (1991). Treatment of PTSD in rape victims: A comparison between cognitive-behavioral procedures and counselling. *Journal of Counseling and Clinical Psychology, 39,* 715–723.

Friedman, M. J. (1988). Toward rational pharmacotherapy for PTSD: An interim report. *American Journal of Psychiatry, 145,* 281–285.

Friedman, M. J. (1991). Biological approaches to the diagnosis and treatment of PTSD. *Journal of Traumatic Stress, 4,* 67–91.

Goldfeld, A. C., Mollica, R. F., Peravento, B. H., & Faraone, S. V. (1988). The physical and psychological sequelae of torture: Symptomatology and diagnosis. *Journal of the American Medical Association, 259,* 2725–2729.

Harris, C. J. (1991). A family crisis intervention model for treatment of PTSD. *Journal of Traumatic Stress, 4,* 195–207.

Herman, J. L. (1992). Complex PTSD: A syndrome in survivals of prolonged and repeated trauma. *Journal of Traumatic Stress, 5,* 377–391.

Horowitz, M. (1986a). *Stress response syndrome* (2nd ed.). Northvale, NJ: Jason Aronson.

Horowitz, M. (1986b). Stress response syndrome: A review of posttraumatic and adjustment disorders. *Hospital and Community Psychiatry, 37,* 241–249.

Jung, M. (1984). Structural family therapy: Its application to Chinese family. *Family Process, 23,* 365–374.

Keane, T. M., Fairbank, J. A., Cadwell, J. M., & Zimmerling, R. (1989). Implosive (flooding) therapy reduces symptoms of PTSD in Vietnam veterans. *Behavior Therapy, 20,* 245–60.

Keane, T. M., Zimmerling, R. T., & Cadwell, J. M. (1985). A behavioral formulation of PTSD in Vietnam veterans. *Behavior Therapy, 8,* 9–12.

Kilpatrick, U. G., Veronen, L. J., & Resick P. A. (1982). Psychological sequelae to rape: Assessment and treatment strategies. In D. M. Dolays & R. L. Meredith (Eds.), *Behavior medicine: Assessment and treatment strategy* (pp. 473–497). New York: Plenum Press.

Kim, S. C. (1985). Family therapy for Asian Americans: A strategic structural framework. *Psychotherapy, 22,* 342–348.

Kinzie, D. J. (1978). Lessons from cross culture psychotherapy. *American Journal of Psychotherapy, 32,* 510–520.

Kinzie, D. J. (1989). Therapeutic approaches to traumatized Cambodian refugees. *Journal of Traumatic Stress, 2,* 75–91.

Kinzie, D. J., & Boehnlein, J. J. (1989). Post-traumatic psychosis among Cambodian refugees. *Journal of Traumatic Stress, 2,* 185–198.

Kinzie, D. J., Boehnlein, J. K., Leung, P. K., Moore, L. J., Riley, C. & Smith, D. (1990). The prevalence of PTSD and its significance among Southeast Asian refugees. *American Journal of Psychiatry, 147,* 913–917.

Kinzie, D. J., & Fleck, J. (1987). Psychotherapy with severely traumatized refugees. *American Journal of Psychotherapy, 41,* 82–94.

Kinzie, D. J., & Leung, P. (1989). Clonidine in Cambodian patients with PTSD. *Journal of Nervous and Mental Disease, 177,* 546–550.

Kinzie, D. J., Leung, P., Boehnlein, J. K., & Fleck, J. (1987). Antidepressant blood level in Southeast Asians. *Journal of Nervous and Mental Disease, 175,* 480–485.

Kinzie, D. J., Leung, P., Bui, A., Ben, R., Keopraseuth, K. O., Riley, C., Fleck, J., & Ades, M. (1988). Group therapy with Southeast Asian refugees. *Community Mental Health Journal, 24,* 157–166.

Kinzie, D. J., Tran, K. A., Breckenridge, A., & Bloom, J. D. (1980). An Indochinese refugee clinic: Culturally accepted treatment approaches. *American Journal of Psychiatry, 137,* 1429–1432.

Kolb, L. C. (1987). A neuropsychological hypothesis explaining PTSD. *American Journal of Psychiatry, 144,* 989–995.

Kosten, T. R., & Krystal, J. H. (1988). Biological mechanism in PTSD: Relevance for substance abuse. In M. Galanter (Ed.), *Recent advances in alcoholism* (Vol. 6, pp. 49–68). New York: Plenum Press.

Kosten, T. R., Mason, J. W., Giller, E. L., Ostroff, R. B., & Harkness, L. (1987). Sustained urination norepinephrine and epinephrine elevation in PTSD. *Psychoneuroendocrinology, 12,* 13–30.

Kroll, J., Habenicht, M., Mackenzie, T., Yang, M., Chan, S., Vang, T., Ly, M., Phommmasouvanh, B., Nguyen, H., Vang, Y., Souvannasoth, L., & Cabugao, R. (1989). Depression and PTSD in Southeast Asian refugees. *American Journal of Psychiatry, 146,* 1592–1597.

Kroll, J., Linde, P., Habenicht, M., Chan, S., Yang, M., Vang, T., Souvannasoth, L., Nguyen, T., Ly, M., Nguyen, H., & Vang, Y. (1990). Medication compliance, antidepressant blood levels and side effects in Southeast Asians: Clinical and cultural implications. *Journal of Nervous and Mental Disease, 175,* 480–485.

Krystal, J., Kosten, T. R., Southwick, S., Mason, J. W., Perry, B. D., & Giller, E. L. (1989). Neurological aspects of PTSD: Review of clinical and preclinical studies. *Behavior Therapy, 20,* 177–98.

Lee, E. (1982). A social system approach to assessment and treatment for the Chinese American family. In M. McGoldrick, J. K. Pearce, & J. Giordano (Eds.), *Ethnicity and family therapy* (pp. 527–551). New York: Guilford Press.

Lee, E., & Chan, F. (1985, August 22). *The use of the Diagnostic Interview Schedule with Vietnamese refugees.* Paper presented at the national convention of the Asian American Psychological Association, Los Angeles.

Lee, E., & Lu, F. (1989). Assessment and treatment of Asian American survivors of mass violence. *Journal of Traumatic Stress, 2,* 93–120.

Lin, K. M., & Finder, B. (1983). Neuroleptic dosage for Asians. *American Journal of Psychiatry, 140,* 490–491.

Lipper, S., Davidson, J. R., Grady, T. A., Edinger, J. D., Hammett, E. B., Mahorney, S. L., & Cavenar, J. O., Jr. (1986). Preliminary study of carbamazepine in PTSD. *Psychosomatics, 27,* 849–854.

Malloy, P. F., Fairbank, J. R., & Keane, T. M. (1983). Validation of multimethod assessments of PTSD in Vietnam veterans. *Journal of Clinical Psychology, 51,* 488–494.

Mason, J. W., Giller, E. L., Kosten, T. R., Ostroff, R. B., & Podd, L. (1986). Urinary free cortisol in PTSD. *Journal of Nervous and Mental Disease, 174,* 145–149.

Melliman, T. A., Randolph, C. A., Mutzer, 0., Flores, L. P., & Milanes, F. J. (1992). Phenomenology and course of psychiatric disorders associated with combat-related post-trauma stress disorder. *American Journal of Psychiatry, 149,* 1568–1574.

Mollica, R. F., Caspi-Yavin, Y., Bollini, P., Truong, T., Tor, S., & Lavelle, J. (1992). Validity of Harvard Trauma questionnaire. *Journal of Nervous and Mental Disease, 180,* 111–116.

Mollica, R. F., & Lavelle, J. (1988). Southeast Asian refugees. In L. Comas-Díaz & E. H. Griffith (Eds.), *Clinical guidelines in cross-cultural mental health* (pp. 262–303). New York: Wiley.

Mollica, R. F., Wyshak, G., & Lavelle, J. (1987). Psychosocial impact of war trauma and torture on Southeast Asian refugees. *American Journal of Psychiatry, 144,* 1567–1572.

Mollica, R. F., Wyshak, G., Marneffe, D., Khuon, F., & Lavelle, J. (1987). Indochinese version of the Hopkins Symptom Checklist-25: A screening instrument for the psychiatric care of refugees. *American Journal of Psychiatry, 144,* 497–500.

Moore, L. J., & Boehnlein, J. K. (1991). Post traumatic stress disorder, depression and somatic symptoms in U.S. Mien patients. *Journal of Nervous and Mental Disease, 179,* 728–733.

Nagy, L. M., Morgan C. A., III, Southwick, S. M., & Charney, D. S. (1993). Open prospective trial of fluoxetine for posttraumatic stress disorder. *Journal of Clinical Psychopharmacology, 13,* 107–113.

Patterson, J. M., & McCubbin, H. I. (1983). Chronic illness: Family stress and coping. In C. R. Figley & H. I. McCubbin (Eds.), *Stress and the family: Vol. II. Coping and catastrophe.* New York Brunner/Mazel.

Perry, D., Giller, E. L., Jr., & Southwick, S. M. (1987). Altered platelet alpha-2 adrenergic binding sites in PTSD. *American Journal of Psychiatry, 144,* 1511–1512.

Pitman, R. K., Altman, B., Greenwald, E., Longpre, R. E., Macklin, M. L., Pinre, R. E., & Steketee, G. S. (1991). Psychiatric complications during flooding therapy for PTSD. *Journal of Clinical Psychiatry, 52,* 17–20.

Pitman, R. K., van der Kolk, B., Orr, S. P., & Greenberg, M. S. (1990). Naloxone-reversible analgesic response to combat-related stimuli in PTSD. *Archives of General Psychiatry, 174,* 145–149.

Reid, J., Silove, D., & Tam, R. (1990). The development of the New South Wales Service for the treatment and rehabilitation of torture and trauma survivors (STARTTS): The first year. *Australian and New Zealand Journal of Psychiatry, 24,* 486–495.

Schwart, I. K., Chin, W., Newman, J., & Roberts, J. (1984). G6PD in Southeast Asian refugees entering the U.S. *Journal of American Tropical Medicine Hygiene, 33,* 182–184.

Schwartz, L. S. (1990). A biopsychosocial treatment approach to PTSD. *Journal of Traumatic Stress, 3,* 221–238.

Sierles, S. F. (1983). Post traumatic stress disorders and concurrrent psychiatric illnesses: A preliminary report. *American Journal of Psychiatry, 140,* 1177–1179.

Smith, M. A., Davidson, J. R., Ritchie, J. C., Kudler, H., Lipper, S., Chappell, P., & Nemeroff, C. B. (1989). Corticotrophin-releasing hormone test in patients with PTSD. *Biological Psychiatry, 26,* 349–355.

Solomon, S., Gerrity, E. T., & Muff, A. M. (1992). Efficacy of treatment for PTSD: An empirical review. *Journal of the American Medical Association, 268,* 633–638.

Southard, E. E. (1919). *Shellshock and other neuropsychiatric problems. Presented in five hundred and eighty-nine cases histories from the war literature 1914–1918.* Boston: W. M. Leonard.

van der Kolk, B. A. (1987). The drug treatment of PTSD. *Journal of Affective Disorders, 13,* 203–213.

van der Kolk, B. A., Dreyfuss, D., Michael, M., Shera, D., Berkowitz, R., Fisler, K., & Saxe, G. (1994). Fluoxetine in post traumatic stress disorder. *Journal of Clinical Psychiatry, 55,* 517–522.

van der Kolk, B. A., Greenberg, M., Boyd, H., & Krystal, J. (1985). Inescapable shock, neurotransmitters and addiction to trauma: Toward a psychobiology of PTSD. *Biological Psychiatry, 20,* 314–325.

18

Substance Abuse Treatment among Asian Americans

DAVIS JA
FRANCIS K. YUEN

Like other minority and dominant-culture groups, Asian Americans are currently besieged by substance abuse, gang violence, and AIDS. Asian ethnic groups, however, typically are not proportionally represented in substance abuse treatment clientele. As demonstrated by the National Drug and Alcoholism Treatment Survey (1989), the percentage of Asians in treatment (0.6%) is unusually low relative to the total Asian population in the United States (2.9%).

Such findings and other reports (Tucker, 1985; Trimble, Padilla, & Bell, 1987) have depicted Asians as not needing substance abuse treatment services as frequently as non-Asians. This notion is reinforced first by the myth of the "model minority" characterization of Asians; second by a lack of data from national surveys (e.g., National Institute on Drug Abuse), which either ignore Asians or subsume these groups under an "other" category; and third by the perception of Asians as a homogeneous cultural group. However, a growing body of literature and information from a number of sources, including treatment providers such as the Asian American Residential Recovery Services (AARRS), have indicated that these assumptions are erroneous and have shown that serious alcohol and drug problems do exist in Asian communities (Ja & Aoki, 1993; Zane & Sasao, 1992).

The notion of Asian Americans as a model minority has been perpetuated by media's portrayal of Asians as being high-achieving and successful immigrants in the United States, both academically and professionally (Ja & Aoki, 1993). Consequently, the dramatization of these successes has contributed to the false belief that Asians do not use alcohol and illicit substances to the same extent as do other ethnic groups. In addition, methodological weaknesses of many study designs involving Asians and the emphasis on biological and genetic factors equally sustain the inaccurate stereotype of Asians as a non-substance-abusing ethnic group (Johnson, Nagoshi, Ahern, Wilson, & Yuen, 1987; Chan, 1986; Suwaki & Ohara, 1985).

The examination of substance abuse within an "Asian American" or "Asian/Pacific Islander" ethnic context is a further aggrandizement of the injustice aimed at these communities. In fact, "Asians" are a heterogeneous group, subsuming at least 32 distinct ethnicities, each with its own languages, culture, traditions, and attitudes toward and patterns of substance use and abuse (Cheung, 1989). It is critically important that substance use and abuse are viewed in accordance with the unique and distinguishing factors of each ethnic group. In fact, studies have shown that the stresses and risk factors associated with immigration—for example, overcrowding, underemployment, separation of families during the immigration process, and intergenerational conflicts—place immigrants/refugees at high risk for substance abuse (Lee, 1990). These factors are evident in the literature showing increased substance abuse rates among Asian populations, particularly immigrants (Wong, 1985).

In an examination of substance abuse treatment issues in Asian populations, critical factors include the (1) linguistic and cultural differences among groups that may inhibit Asians' utilization of traditional treatment modalities, (2) immigrant/refugee status, which places individuals among the highest-risk groups for chemical dependency while interfering with their ability to make use of existing treatment modalities, and (3) cultural factors such as taboo, denial, and "loss of face," which exist among Asian substance abusers, their families, and the greater community. All these factors make it critically important for clinicians to be knowledgeable and sensitive to culturally critical issues to provide treatment services that are both effective and culturally appropriate. Existing treatment approaches, however, often ignore these factors, leaving current treatment modalities inadequate and unavailable for most Asians.

ASIAN POPULATIONS IN TREATMENT

Trimble (1990) reviewed 186 articles published since 1950 on psychoactive drug research on American ethnic minority groups. He concluded that the professional in the field knew little about the patterns and problems of drug use among Asian Americans and Mexican Americans. Even those few who did extrapolate information on specific groups "focus(ed) on prevalence rates and, therefore, shed little light on etiological factors" (p. 152). Among the research on Asian and Pacific Islanders, most has focused on the larger ethnic Asian groups such as Chinese and Japanese Americans. These studies have little ability to generalize their findings to other Asian groups.

Subsequently, there is little research currently available on the drug use patterns or treatment modalities for populations of Asian Americans. What information is available has been summarized previously (Ja & Aoki, 1993; Zane & Sasao, 1992; Sue, 1987; Yu, Liu, Xia, & Zhang, 1985), and much of this information is based on epidemiological research. However, because of the lack of treatment services, little documentation is available on treatment research with Asian populations. Ball and Lau (1966) conducted research on treatment for institutionalized populations, which provided a composite case study description of the Chinese heroin addict. However, this information is obviously inadequate in reflecting the patterns of substance abuse among Asian Americans today. Other, more recent studies (Nemoto, Guydish, Young, & Clark, 1993) provide a brief glimpse of current data regarding Asian populations in treatment. Most other research has used case studies (Westermeyer, 1993) to provide some information on treatment protocols with Asians.

Ball and Lau (1966) examined the admissions records of the U.S. Public Health Service Hospital in Lexington, Kentucky, over a period of 30 years between 1935 and 1964. During this time, they determined that more than 800 male Chinese narcotic addicts were admitted into treatment. After sampling 137 records between 1957 and 1962, they determined that most of the clients were foreign-born and were residents in major metropolitan areas such as New York, Chicago, or other major cities in the United States. All the cases examined were employed at the time of hospitalization, with most involved in laundry work, followed by restaurant work. Their mean age was 53 years, with 31% single, 55% married, and 12% widowed or separated. Almost all the cases (90.5%) were heroin users; the remainder were morphine or opium users. Length of addiction averaged 20 years, with onset of opiate use occurring before the age of 30. Most of the cases were voluntary admissions with financial or health problems or were experiencing difficulties in obtaining opiates.

Nemoto et al. (1993) reviewed the 5-year records of 1,578 Asian Americans admitted to county-funded drug abuse treatment programs in San Francisco between 1986 and 1990. They found that Chinese Americans (n = 499), when compared to Filipino Americans (n = 429), Japanese Americans (n = 213), and other Asian Americans (n = 437), were more likely to take drugs orally, less likely to take drugs by injection, and used sedatives more commonly than other drugs. Chinese Americans were more likely to seek treatment for substance abuse on an outpatient basis (50%) and less likely to enter detoxification programs (36%) than Japanese Americans (53%), Filipino Americans (51%), or other Asian Americans (67%).

A 2-year analysis of 524 of San Francisco's substance abuse-related cases by Darryl Inaba of the Bill Pone Memorial Unit of the Haight Free Clinic indicated that the predominant drug choice of Asian American addicts was cocaine. Breakdown by ethnicity of the Asian Youth Substance Abuse Project in San Francisco showed 49% of the cases to be Chinese, 18% Filipino, 15% other Asians, 13% Japanese, and 5% Pacific Islanders (Office of Substance Abuse Prevention, 1990). A funded outreach program by the Center for Substance Abuse Treatment (COPASA) determined that of 760 Asian drug users who were contacted by staff, most had long histories of drug use (mean = 8 years), and an overwhelming proportion (30%) had used intravenous drugs (heroin, 5%; cocaine, 25%) (Asian American Recovery Services, 1993).

In 1992, I (D. J.) initiated a review of all client and resident charts from the Asian American Residential Recovery Services (AARRS), a long-term 22-bed Asian American residential therapeutic facility located in San Francisco. The AARRS program was established in 1985 and is one of the two residential substance abuse treatment facilities in the United States for Asian Americans. Preliminary data from the AARRS program provide additional information regarding the treatment population of Asian Americans. Of the more than 200 residents treated by the program since its inception, 29.4% were women, and 60.6% of the total 214 residents were Asian.

Of the total AARRS resident population, Chinese represented the highest proportion of Asians with 18.7% (80.5% male, 19.5% female), followed by 12.1% biracial Asians, primarily Asian Africans and Asian whites (57.6% males and 42.3% females). Japanese Americans represented the next largest Asian group at 9.8% (89.9% male, 9.1% female), followed closely by the Filipinos at 9.3% (85% male, 15% female). Southeast Asians represented the smallest group at 3.3% (all males). Including the biracial category, 22% of all Asian residents were female.

Although the majority of the residents were polydrug users, the Asians' primary drug use showed little difference between genders in their drug of choice: cocaine (55% for Asian males, 53% for Asian females), heroin (26% for males, 27% for females), alcohol (6%), and barbiturates (7% for males, 8% for females).

COMMON SUBSTANCE ABUSE TREATMENT APPROACHES

The effectiveness of any treatment modality depends on many variables, including the type of substance abused, the unique characteristics of the clients, and the degree of addiction. Various approaches in the treatment of substance abuse have been developed in the last 30 years. In this section, we briefly review biological treatment, the psychotherapeutic approach, the behavioral approach, group therapy, Twelve-Step programs and therapeutic communities, and employee assistance programs. The Association for Advanced Training in Behavioral Sciences (1989) compiled a comprehensive overview of the various approaches which will serve as the basis for this section.

Many new medications have been developed in the last two decades and used for the biological treatment to assist addicts in facing the challenge of becoming clean and recovering. These medications include disulfiram and methadone, which are used to treat alcoholism and heroin addiction, respectively. When disulfiram (Antabuse) is used with alcohol, it generates aversive symptoms such as nausea and vomiting. These unpleasant consequences along with other treatment approaches are most effective when the alcoholic is at the beginning phase of the treatment or when the sobriety is at risk. However, the risk for relapse is quite high. Methadone (a synthetic narcotic) replaces the craving for heroin and improves clients' overall functioning. However, it also develops clients' dependence on the continuous use of methadone, and its status as a treatment method has been questioned. This medical approach has its proponents but is particularly useful in that it avoids placing the responsibility for abuse on the individual per se.

Psychotherapeutic approaches employ different insight-oriented therapeutic approaches to understand the underlying causes of substance abuse. Substance abase is seen as the symptom of psychological pathology. The success is correlated to whether the clients are verbal, insight oriented, and "psychologically minded." These approaches are usually effective when clients also have other psychiatric disorders.

Behavioral approaches view substance abuse as a learned behavior. Treatment techniques include skills development, training in alternative coping behaviors, environment restructuring, and contingency management. Job training is one example of contingency management. Having stable employment and income is a satisfying reinforcer that will replace substance use and prevent relapse.

Group therapy helps patients gain perspective through contact with other people in the same situation. In discussions led by a trained counselor, patients work on improving their skills in social interaction, communication, and problem solving (Gold, 1991). Group therapy is the most efficient and economical form of treatment. Group pressure and support provide a needed sense of responsibility and belonging for the participants. This approach is particularly useful for clients who have passed the stages of detoxification and do not have formal support systems.

The Twelve-Step program is the core program of Alcoholics Anonymous (AA), which was founded by Bill Wilson and Dr. Bob Smith in 1935. As a self-help group program, the Twelve-Step program has helped millions of people. Predicated on a "moral" model, the program's basic assumptions are that alcoholism is a disease that cannot be cured (Brickman et al., 1982). However, with spiritual guidance and peer support, people can control their alcoholism and achieve total abstinence. Abstinence should be maintained on a day-to-day basis. Although AA and its Twelve-Step program is a successful approach, it also has many critics. Among these criticisms are AA's spirituality orientation, lack of scientific proof of effectiveness, and a high dropout rate. In spite of its critics, the AA model is also used for organizing support and self-help groups for many other types of addictions.

Therapeutic communities provide comprehensive inpatient treatment arrangements for addicts to recover from their substance abuse problems. Although individual, group, and medical therapies are used, the real therapy is the use of the community. Through various therapies, mutual support, and modeling, clients learn to deal with their substance abuse problems and lead a healthy lifestyle.

TREATMENT OF ASIANS FOR SUBSTANCE ABUSE

Traditionally, most Asians view substance abuse as a medical and behavioral problem. It is a situation in which one needs to seek holistic care for both physiological needs and "character rebuilding" or moral education.

A person's substance abuse problems not only indicate an inability to lead a good life but also reflect on the failure of the family to raise a good person for the society. It brings shame and "loss of face" for both the individuals and their families. Shon and Ja (1982) indicate that in the attempt to reduce the potential loss of face, the family may tolerate or deny the existence of the problem, isolate the individual to avoid the issue, or use shame and scolding to try to resolve the issue within the family or community system.

Substance abuse is usually tolerated by family members until it has a severe impact on the proper functioning of the family. Cajoling and nagging are commonly used with the expectation that the individual may "come to his senses." Threats, castigation, and other coercive responses are often used. In some extreme cases, the family may reject or disown the individual. Interventions are usually done within the family and its extended network such as relatives and close family friends. For example, if parents and siblings fail to produce a change in the individual, uncles and other family elders are called on to intervene. Close friends and community elders are involved if interventions from family members are in vain. When all these attempts fail, the family may consider seeking professional help from organizations that are well established and respected by the community.

The fear of social stigmatization keeps many from getting prompt assistance. Often, patients deal with substance abuse problems under the guise of receiving health care from traditional herbal doctors. To bring the substance abuse problem under control and to avoid any disgrace, the family and the individual may seek confidential medical treatment from herbalists and acupuncturists.

CLINICAL AND THERAPEUTIC CULTURAL FACTORS

Immigrant Asians often face the conflicts between the native world values of familism, hierarchical relationships, and social conformity and American values of individualism, egalitarianism, and independence. They face these issues in the various interactions with mainstream society—school, work, and peer networks—but also at home. The cultural dissonance that immigrant youth experience is compounded by the intergenerational conflicts present in their families.

Consequences of these cultural conflicts may include low self-esteem, depression, fearfulness, anxiety, and anger. Unfortunately, some of these younger immigrant Asians lack the cognitive and social skills to resolve these conflicts. Other sources of stress are related to linguistic isolation and lack of familiarity and access to systemic resources.

In times of crisis in the old world, the family, community, and social structure are usually able to alleviate conflicts. However, in the new environment in which immigrant youth find themselves, not only are the old-world structures unavailable, but they are not appropriate. One of the results of immigration is the breakdown and reconstruction of the family structure. Often, the extended family is left behind or dispersed. Support from the extended family is no longer available, and the common hierarchical family structure that presupposes traditional values in problem solving does not adequately address the demands of an unfamiliar and imposing culture. In addition, many parents are underemployed and must take on two or three jobs to support their families.

The stress immigrant Asians feel and the breakdown of the family and community support system often leave them vulnerable to such social risk factors as delinquent behavior, truancy, dropping out of school, gang activity, unemployment, and drug use. These risk factors and the difficulties of emotional stress and family distress, along with the loss of many traditional protective factors, drive many of these youth and adults to use and abuse drugs.

Asians who came as immigrants and refugees face the problems described previously, but American-born Asians, despite being acculturated, also face cultural identity crises. Unlike their first-generation counterparts, they struggle with their place in a society in which they are seen as "foreign." In part because American-born Asians are more acculturated, they are more aware of and therefore more susceptible to institutional racism. Because of the newness of immigrants, and particularly refugee youth, to this country, they are less aware of these subtler forms of discrimination.

Immigrant and refugee Asians may rely on traditional values to perceive the world and manage personal crises, but this is not an option for American-born Asians. This is partly because of the collective assimilation of many third- and fourth-generation Asian Americans, resulting in a loss of Asian traditions values. This existential dilemma is especially acute for American-born Asian youth who face the dual pressures to excel academically as "Asian" students and to be socially accepted by their mainstream peers.

There are differences in the perception of substance abuse treatment services between Asian Americans. For example, American-born Asians or those who have been in the United States for a substantial period of time are more receptive to the traditional substance abuse treatment processes such as the disease concept, therapeutic community, and psychotherapy. Foreign-born Asians who have recently arrived in this country prefer the traditional approaches from their native countries to the Western approach. However, because these native approaches are often not available in the United States, many recent immigrants are left without any services. Further discussions in this chapter focus on issues that apply primarily to these recent arrivals.

A good understanding of these new immigrants and refugees' native culture, migration experience, and experience in the United States is necessary for the establishment of a productive and trusting working relationship. There are marked differences among American-born Asians, immigrants who came to the United States under mostly favorable conditions, and refugees who settled in the United States.

Many new Asian immigrants and refugees arrived in this country under severe hardship, fleeing poverty and political persecution, often risking their lives and their families. "Making it" in this newly adopted country is a second chance for many adults and the beginning of hope for a better future for their children. Barriers to success, however, exist in many forms. Lack of employment and economic opportunities, insufficient English-language and American cultural skills, uncertainty of immigration status, and the loss of family and other formal support networks are some of the factors that, according to many Asian service providers, contribute to many problems—including substance abuse—among Asians.

"Recent Asian immigrants [who] experience stress in adjusting to a new culture may turn alcohol and other drugs. . . . [These] problems may be greater than what is reported in survey" (Office of Substance Abuse

Prevention, 1990). In California, special programs were developed to address the increase of substance use among Asian refugees. "The fact that many of these new residents are refugees makes their problems of assimilation unique and even more poignant than those faced by immigrants in general. Because of these stresses, alcohol and drug abuse is increasing in this population" (Senate Bill No. 2392, 1992). Yee and Nguyen (1987) asserted that the increase of drug and alcohol abuse among Asian refugees and immigrants is a symptom of psychological distress that "creates enormous health risks for a population already at greater risk than the general American population."

Several culturally appropriate substance abuse treatment programs have been developed in several cities that have high concentrations of Asian refugees and immigrants. Among them are the Asian American Drug Abuse Program in Los Angeles, the Bill Pone Center and Asian Americans Recovery Services in San Francisco, Asian Americans for Community Involvement in San Jose, Southcove Community Health Center in Boston, and the Asian Counseling and Referral Services in Seattle.

A culturally competent substance abuse treatment service for Asian Americans should consider the following factors: (1) accessibility, availability, and acculturation; (2) one-stop service center that serves as a less stigmatized point of entry; (3) the family as well as the individual as the units of intervention; (4) extensive one-on-one contacts in client's environment to allow the building of a productive working relationship; and (5) culturally appropriate assessment and treatment procedures.

Accessibility refers to both geographical and cultural relevance as well as difficulties in service delivery. Ideally, the service delivery location is within reach of the target population. Transportation is a common barrier that keeps new refugees and immigrants from getting services. Furthermore, whether clients can culturally and linguistically gain access to or communicate with the service provider often determines their desire to use the service. Bicultural and bilingual workers who are respected by their ethnic community are vital to bridge this gap. Availability refers to the existence, recruitment, and retention of service, clients, and qualified service providers. It is a factor that is closely related to accessibility. Acculturation refers to the quality and extent of exposure to the dominant American culture and the degree of social functioning in the dominant culture. Differential assessments of clients' extent of acculturation help plan the most appropriate treatment plan for the client.

RECRUITMENT AND ASSESSMENT IN TREATMENT

Because Asians view substance abuse as a medical problem and turn to herbal or family doctors for help, it is best to recruit these clients through health care services. In fact, many Asian substance abusers have difficulty accepting the fact that they may be substance abusers. Often, unless legal or criminal pressures from criminal justice systems exist, they resist treatment unless they have "bottomed out" or exhausted all resources for their addictive behaviors, including family and friends. Subsequently, any recruitment process is much more effective if the treatment service is linked to a general health care and human service facility. This link allows treatment to be perceived as a continuation of the health and human services. Furthermore, if the facility provides education, general health care and screening, and other human service activities for the community, it will be even more effective in serving as a less stigmatized point of entry that can effectively identify and refer potential clients.

Many Asian clients use complaints of physical discomfort to express problems that they are unable to identify or are too embarrassed to report. Counselors should be sensitive to this type of cultural expression of symptomatology and provide services that not only reduce the symptom but also lead clients to explore the underlying problems.

As discussed earlier, it is not until internal resources have been exhausted that Asians seek outside help. At that point, the outside help is usually highly recommended by friends or relatives. Once a professional working relationship is established, these service providers are considered experts and are well respected. Consequently, clients usually expect expert direct advice or guides. Counselors should be sensitive to these expectations and guide the clients to define their problems and needs without becoming paternalistic.

Individual interviews and family conferences are usually useful in gathering necessary information and soliciting support for the treatment process. During the interviewing process, particularly for immigrants, a key factor is to assume the professional stature of a helping professional. For example, because many Asians will respond to an authority figure, along with the belief in a medical model, the service provider with a fairly direct approach may have a better opportunity to establish some trust and to guide the client through questions regarding drug history.

Because of the shame and guilt often associated with substance abuse, it is also important to identify with the client culturally. For example, an informal exchange of familial or cultural history allows the client to build a bridge to the provider and begin sharing information otherwise difficult to obtain. However, it may prove more difficult to elicit information from clients under legal obligation for treatment because the possibility of resentment and anger exists. In these cases, at times, clients may have high levels of denial. Among American-born Asians, empathic and shared histories often facilitate the assessment process. Interpretation of the denial and confrontation of their denial with certain clients may in fact produce more honest responses.

As part of the assessment process, a critical activity is the comprehensive assessment of the relationship between family members and the clients. The degree of "healthy" and "unhealthy" codependency, different culturally specific communication approaches, and parental or spousal conflicts are often important issues among seriously addicted substance abusers. In addition, for the clients themselves, a physical or sexual abuse history as well as a history of generational substance abuse are crucial factors to explore. At AARRS, more than 40% of the clients have had some experience with prior physical or sexual abuse. Finally, vocational and educational histories are important because many Asians perceive their self-worth through their earning ability.

TREATMENT

When designing service programs for recent Asian immigrants and refugees, providers should take into consideration the Asian view that all aspects of life are interconnected. An individual's substance abuse problem is not an isolated individual problem. Intervention should include the client's family and immediate support network. It should also consider the economic, social, and other well-being factors of the client.

Asian substance abuse clients see drug and alcohol use as both a behavioral and a medical problem. Many believe that the effective way to treat substance abuse is to teach abusers a healthy lifestyle, find them good employment, restore their place in the family and the community, and provide activities that encourage them to live a "proper" life.

Practicing *tai-chi* (an ancient Chinese martial art), having a proper and an "ecologically well-balanced" diet, and using herbal medicine and acupuncture are some of the common approaches for promoting healthy physical condition and lifestyle. Vocational and other job skills training are not only critical for future employment but also prepare clients to develop self-confidence and provide the means by which they can regain their acceptance in the community. Meanwhile, working with the community to prepare for the return of the substance abuse clients is equally important for the service provider to pursue.

AARS is a multiservice human service agency in San Francisco. Through its many years of outstanding services with the Asian American communities, it has enjoyed a good reputation and is well respected by the target communities. In AARS's substance abuse treatment program, volunteering in community works and service projects is part of the treatment process. The clients' participation in service projects positively reinforces both the clients and the communities. Service projects keep clients in contact with their community in a positive way and assist them in regaining "face" and rebuilding their own place in the community. They are identified as "good people" who help out community projects instead of "bums" who adversely affect or destroy the community.

As for the treatment process itself, it should include an extensive one-on-one contact in the client's environment. This allows the building of trust and the motivation to continue participation in the treatment program. Treatment programs for Asian Americans should therefore incorporate a blend of individual, group, and family interventions. Many Asian service providers (Tung, 1985) also suggest that successful services to Asian Americans should be tangible, goal oriented, time limited, directive, and—most important—culturally appropriate.

The high dropout rate and underutilization of mental health and substance abuse treatment programs among Asian Americans are well documented (Mokuau, 1991). The stereotypes that Asian Americans are a "model minority," are successful and enterprising, have few problems, and have strong family support have led to the neglect of their service needs. The nonassertiveness of some Asian clients, however, may be misread as a lack of commitment to the treatment process, and consequently service is terminated. Although it is important to be sensitive to the cultural characteristics of different Asian American groups, it is even more important to recognize the uniqueness of each ethnic group and individual and that differential assessment of each person is necessary.

The Twelve-Step program is an effective and successful program that has saved the lives of millions of people. However, the application of the Twelve-Step program among Asian clients may require further adaptation. Most Asian clients do not have difficulty with the spiritual foundation of the Twelve-Step program, but many have problems accepting the public self-disclosing helplessness approach. Substance abuse continues to be seen as a social taboo among Asians that should be handled privately and confidentially.

Total abstinence from alcohol and absolute freedom from relapse for Asian clients after the treatment process are culturally difficult. Controlled drinking is quite prevalent and is culturally acceptable. It may be a more realistic goal to ask alcoholic clients to prepare themselves for the relapse: "If I slip, it is a relapse, and it is okay." They should try again, and it is their responsibility to control their drinking habits, not someone else's.

CONCLUSION AND RECOMMENDATIONS

Human service providers need to first understand the substance abuse issues from the Asian clients' and their community's perspectives. How one views or defines the problem directly affects how one conceives alternatives and solutions.

Particularly in working with new immigrant and refugee communities, because of the small size and closeness of these communities, individual and community lives are interwoven. Consequently, any interventions for an individual will more likely be effective if these interventions have the "buy-in" or sanction from the community.

Individuals who have different degrees of acculturation will differ in the extent of their receptiveness to various treatment modalities. Human services providers should be cognizant to these differences, assess each client individually within his or her social and cultural context, and apply the most effective intervention strategies. Human services providers should also be self-conscious about their own culture and belief system. A helping relationship in a multicultural context, as Gross (1995) described, is a "learning as they go along" process and the client and the service provider only "have each other's perceptions and resources to work with and nothing more" (p. 212).

Among the Asian communities, work is considered more than gainful employment. It is also perceived as a reflection of one's morality and ability to lead a productive and purposeful life. Vocational training, employment assistance, and community volunteering along with substance abuse treatment provide an avenue for reentry and acceptance for clients and their communities.

Finally, human services professionals should learn how to be effective in finding funding and other resources to support such culturally specific services. They should be effective as culturally competent service providers, advocates, program planners, and evaluators.

REFERENCES

Asian American Recovery Services. (1993). *Competence through transitions biannual report* (H86-SPO4968). Washington, DC: U.S. Department of Health and Human Services, Center for Substance Abuse Prevention.

Association for Advanced Training in Behavioral Sciences. (1989). Substance abuse. In *Preparation for the social work examination* (Vol. 2). Santa Monica, CA: Author.

Ball, J. C., & Lau, M. P. (1966). The Chinese narcotic addict in the United States. *Social Forces, 45*(1), 68–72.

Brickman, P., Rabinowitz, V., Karuza, J., Coates, D., Cohn, W., & Kidder, L. (1982). Models of helping and coping. *American Psychologist, 37,* 368–384.

Chan, A. (1986). Racial differences in alcohol sensitivity. *Alcohol and Alcoholism, 21,* 93–104.

Cheung, Y. (1989). Making sense of ethnicity and drug use: A review and suggestions for future research. *Social Pharmacology, 3*(1/2), 55–68.

Gold, M. (1991). *The good news about drugs and alcohol: Curing, treating and preventing substance abuse in the new age of biopsychiatry.* New York: Villard Books.

Gross, E. R. (1995). Deconstructing politically correct literature: The American Indian case. *Social Work, 40*(2), 206–213.

Ja, D., & Aoki, B. (1993). Substance abuse treatment: Culture and barriers in the Asian American Community. *Journal of Psychoactive Drugs, 25*(1), 61–71.

Johnson, R. C., Nagoshi, C. T., Ahern, F. M., Wilson, J. R., & Yuen, S. H. L. (1987). Cultural factors as explanations for ethnic group differences in alcohol use in Hawaii. *Journal of Psychoactive Drugs, 22,* 45–52.

Mokuau, N. (Ed.). (1991). *Handbook of social sciences for Asian Pacific Islanders.* New York: Greenwood Press.

Nemoto, T., Guydish, J., Young, M., & Clark, W. (1993). Drug use behavior among Asian Americans in San Francisco. In L. Harris (Ed.), *NIDA Research Monograph* (Series 132, p. 290). Washington, DC: National Institute on Drug Abuse, U.S. Department of Health and Human Services.

Office of Substance Abuse Prevention. (1990). *Prevention resource guide: Asian and Pacific Islander Americans.* Washington, DC: U.S. Department of Health and Human Services.

Shon, S. P., & Ja, D. Y. (1982). Asian families. In M. McGoldrick, J. K. Pearce, & J. Giordano (Eds.), *Ethnicity and family therapy.* New York: Guilford Press.

Sue, D. (1987). Use and abuse of alcohol by Asian Americans. *Journal of Psychoactive Drugs, 19*(1), 57–66.

Suwaki, H., & Ohara, H. (1985). Alcohol-induced facial flushing and drinking behavior in Japanese men. *Journal of Studies of Alcohol, 46,* 196–198.

Trimble, J. (1990) Ethnic specification, validation prospects, and the future of drug use research. *International Journal of the Addictions, 25*(2A), 149–170.

Trimble, J. E., Padilla, A. M., & Bell, C. S. (1987). *Drug abuse among ethnic minorities* (DHHS Publication No. ADM 87-1474). Washington, DC: National Institute on Drug Abuse.

Tucker, M. B. (1985). U.S. ethnic minorities and drug use: An assessment of the science and practices. *International Journal of the Addictions, 20,* 1021–1047.

Tung, T. M. (1985). Psychiatric care for Southeast Asians: How different is different? In C. T. Owan (Ed.), *Southeast Asian mental health: Treatment, prevention services, training, and research.* Washington, DC: U.S. Department of Health and Human Services.

Westermeyer, J. (1993). Substance abuse disorders among young minority refugees: Common themes in a clinical sample. In *Drug abuse among minority youth: Methodological issues and recent research advances* (NIH Publication No. 93-3479, pp. 308–320). Washington, DC: U.S. Department of Health and Human Services.

Wong, H. Z. (1985). *Substance use and Chinese American youths: Preliminary findings on an interview survey of 123 youths and implications for services and programs.* San Francisco: Youth Environment Services.

Yee, B., & Nguyen, T. (1987). Correlates of drug use and abuse among Indochinese refugees: Mental health implications. *Journal of Psychoactive Drugs, 19*(1), 77–81.

Yu, E. S. H., Liu, W. T., Xia, Z., & Zhang, M. (1985). Alcohol use, abuse and alcoholism among Chinese Americans: A review of the epidemiologic data. In *Alcohol use among U.S. ethnic minorities* (NIAAA Research Monograph 18, pp. 329–342; DHHS Publication No. ADM 89-1435). Washington, DC: U.S. Department of Health and Human Services.

Zane, N., & Sasao, T. (1992). Research on drug abuse among Asian Pacific Americans. *Drugs and Society, 6*(3–4), 181–209.

19

Anxiety Disorders of Chinese Patients

HUNG-TAT LO
GODWIN LAU

This chapter on the anxiety disorders and their management is primarily based on our experience with the Chinese population in Toronto. In Toronto, the Chinese constitute one of the larger and more visible minority groups, composed of recent immigrants from all over the world, although the majority are from Hong Kong. Because of the universal access to the health care system in Canada, as well as the availability of Chinese-speaking professionals, we have been able to see many patients suffering from anxiety disorders. However, our observations should also be useful to readers interested in other Asian Pacific populations.

The fourth edition of the *Diagnostic and Statistical Manual of Mental Disorders* (DSM-IV; American Psychiatric Association, 1994) lists the following conditions under anxiety disorders: panic disorders with or without agoraphobia, agoraphobia without history of panic disorder, specific phobia, obsessive–compulsive disorder, posttraumatic stress disorder, acute stress disorder, generalized anxiety disorder, substance-induced anxiety disorder, and anxiety disorder due to a general medical condition.

Our comments generally refer to the group as a whole. We highlight certain specific conditions when necessary.

EPIDEMIOLOGY

There are no epidemiological data on the Asian population in North America. Thus, we have looked at two studies done in Hong Kong and Taiwan, respectively, for comparison with the epidemiological study in the United States (see Table 19.1). The difference is slight, with the Chinese figures somewhat lower than the American data except for the high figure for generalized anxiety disorder in Hong Kong. Kuo's (1984) study on depression revealed significant level of symptomatology among the Chinese in the United States. Our impression in Toronto also shows that the level of anxiety disorders among the Chinese is as high as the mainstream population. Future epidemiological study in North America should yield interesting data in this area.

TABLE 19.1. Comparative Epidemiological Data on Anxiety Disorders

	ECA (United States)[a]	Hong Kong[b]	Taipei[c]
Generalized anxiety disorder	2%–5% (both sexes)	7.7% ± 0.55% (males) 11.11% ± 0.99% (females)	2.39% (males) 5.4% (females)
Panic disorder	1.4%–1.5% (both sexes) 0.6%–1.2% (males) 1.6%–2.1% (females)	0.2% ± 0.08% (males) 0.34% ± 0.1% (females)	0.12% (males) 0.28% (females)
Simple phobias	3.8%–14.5% (males) 8.5%–25.9% (females)	0.96% ± 0.2% (males) 3.16% ± 0.51% (females)	2.2% (males) 5.0% (females)
Agoraphobia	1.5%–5.2% (males) 5.3%–12.5% (females)	0.61% ± 0.17% (males) 0.84% ± 0.26% (females)	0.77% (males) 1.46% (females)
Social phobia	0.9%–1.7% (males) 1.5%–2.6% (females)	N/A	0.24% (males) 0.95% (females)
Obsessive–complusive disorder	1.9%–3.0% (both sexes) 1.1%–2.6% (males) 2.6%–3.3% (females)	0.87% ± 0.16% (males) 1.22% ± 0.18% (females)	0.81% (males) 1.07% (females)
Posttraumatic stress disorder	1%	0.57% ± 0.15% (males) 0.66% ± 0.13% (females)	N/A

[a]Robins, Helzer, and Weissman (1984).
[b]Chen, Wong, and Lee (1993).
[c]Hwu, Yeh, and Chang (1989).

SPECIAL DIAGNOSTIC AND ASSESSMENT ISSUES

The anxiety disorders are a heterogeneous group with anxiety as a predominant symptom. However, anxiety as a symptom is also found in many other disorders, including neurasthenia, somatoform disorder, and depression. The overlap is unavoidable in our current diagnostic system.

Among the Asians, language and cultural barriers can lead Western-trained professionals to misdiagnosis or underdiagnosis. In contrast to psychotic disorders, anxiety disorders are more influenced by sociocultural factors in terms of how the disorders are diagnosed and treated (Good & Kleinman, 1985). It is thus more variable in different cultures, and a cross-cultural perspective is even more important. The case of social phobia is a good example (Tseng, 1992). It is more prevalent in the Asians, particularly Japanese, but has often been misdiagnosed as paranoid psychosis, personality disorders, and other disorders leading to mismanagement (see case example).

Another difficulty has to do with the lack of appropriate psychometric instruments in assessing the appropriate symptoms. Although certain instruments such as the Symptom Checklist (SCL-90-R) and General Health Questionnaires (GHQ) have been translated into different languages, the overall validity of the instruments applied in various ethnic groups has yet to be documented. Furthermore, Asian Americans comprise a very diverse population covering different ethnic groups with many generational, educational and cultural differences among themselves. Therefore, it is hard to generate any uniform diagnostic criteria across this population.

The common tendency to somatize their emotional difficulties may present diagnostic problems. The differential diagnosis between anxiety disorders and various physical diagnoses is important, as shown in the case of panic disorders. Some might be related to such conditions as mitral valve prolapse, but many such disorders are psychogenic and elaborate investigations can add to the anxiety of such patients.

The coexistence of anxiety and depression is a common phenomenon, and it is not uncommon for patients to present anxiety symptoms or somatic complaints instead of depressive symptoms. This is particularly so with the Chinese, who may have a lower awareness, and perhaps even a more limited vocabulary, to express such symptoms.

Anxiety can also present in the form of family conflicts, work problems, and other behavioral manifestations. It is important, then, for social services workers to be able to identify such conditions and refer for the appropriate treatment.

Asian Americans also tend to seek simultaneous treatment from Western and traditional practitioners. They may not reveal such practices to the physician, but the physician should be aware because medications prescribed by the different practitioners may have negative interactions. Moreover, some herbal tonics prescribed for the presumed weakened patients might lead to excessive sympathetic activities such as palpitations. Both patients and clinicians might misinterpret these activities as symptoms of anxiety.

Finally, a phenomenon in the immigrant population occurs in their adjustment to new culture, weather, and language. Some new immigrants tend to stay home and refuse to venture out, leading to a situation not unlike agoraphobia.

SYMPTOMS, PROBLEMS, AND THEIR CAUSES, AS PERCEIVED BY FAMILY

A traditional view of the anxiety disorder attributes the problem to a combination of depletion of body functions because of constitutional deficiencies, unhealthy lifestyle, and personality traits triggered by stress or physical illness. Specifically, weak nerves are seen as a constitutional deficiency, just as weak lungs make the person more prone to cough and to other respiratory problems. Smoking, drinking, gambling, sexual indulgence, and masturbation have all been thought to be behaviors indicative of a negative lifestyle. These behaviors are seen to lead to an upset of the internal equilibrium. Anxiety symptoms are manifestations of this imbalance. As far as personality dispositions are concerned, high anxiety traits and high dependency on parents are all thought to be related to anxiety symptoms. A cultural view of the significance of stress is also well developed. Stress may arise in the context of emotional trauma and social network disruption such as immigration, but also after such physical trauma as high fever or head injuries.

Furthermore, students who have been under both family and school pressures are also prone to experience nervousness. Asian American students in the United States have demonstrated on surveys that they tend to display more neurotic/anxiety traits (Sue & Kirk, 1973).

Nevertheless, anxiety problems are not always viewed as medical/psychological problems per se, and the causal factors are often attributed to environmental stresses as opposed to the intrapsychic conflicts suggested in the Western literature and theories.

HELP-SEEKING BEHAVIOR AND INDIGENOUS TREATMENT

The help-seeking pattern of the Chinese has been described in other populations, for example, the mentally ill in Vancouver (Lin, Tardiff, Donitz, & Goresky, 1978) and the college students in Hong Kong (Cheung,

1989). None so far has focused on the so-called minor psychiatric disorders, including anxiety disorders. However, we believe that the help-seeking behavior of this group of patients is similarly influenced by the explanatory models of their "illness," and the services available to them.

Because somatic symptoms are so common in anxiety disorders, medical practitioners are often the first to be consulted when self-management has not worked. Self-management may be in the form of dietary changes or supplements, including herbs. Other techniques may include some lifestyle changes, especially the avoidance of stress. However, because Canada has free medical service, patients use medical practitioners quite readily. Many are also referred to psychiatrists, unless they are concerned about stigma. But when the condition does not respond quickly to treatment, and particularly after the condition has become chronic, many Chinese do not hesitate to consult traditional practitioners, some of whom even advertise to specialize in treating different anxiety symptoms (neurasthenia, impotence, etc.). Treatment offered by these practitioners may include herbal prescriptions, acupuncture, and massage. Other indigenous methods include *tai chi*, *qi-gong*, and other exercise types of treatment. Some patients may even consult *feng-shui* masters (who are skilled in geomancy and offer various advice from the rearrangement of furniture to the alteration of one's schedule) or other fortune-telling types of practitioners. In Canada, Chinese patients also consult chiropractors and other Western practitioners (reflexologists, etc.). Chinese patients are quite pragmatic and often follow various methods of treatment at the same time. Doctor shopping is not uncommon. At times, patients get confused because of the many different explanatory models proffered by so many different practitioners. It is thus wise for mental health professionals to explore their treatment history while assuring the patient that they are open to different schools of thoughts.

The Christian churches are very active in the Chinese immigrant population (as well as the Korean population), and they are also a common source of assistance to people with emotional problems.

TREATMENT EXPECTATIONS

The mental health professions are still shrouded in some mystique, and those who venture to consult these professionals have uncertain expectations but often come because they have not been helped by the other practitioners. Still, some of them expect nothing less than immediate cure. Physicians and therapists are usually seen as authority figures and are respected for their education and social status. This respect could enhance a rapid positive transference, which could be therapeutic or harmful depending on how it is managed in therapy.

The expectation also varies with the patient's understanding of his or her condition. Thus, the negotiation of explanatory model (Katon & Kleinman, 1981) is an essential first step in treatment. Often we would modify the folk model in a way that would naturally lead to our treatment plan. When the model is accepted by the patient, the rationale of the treatment and its expected result follow. This extra effort goes a long way in ensuring compliance and subsequent improvement.

EFFECTIVE TREATMENT STRATEGIES

In the first session with Chinese patients with anxiety disorder, it is important to clarify their own explanatory models, past treatment, and current expectation. Some immediate relief is often expected, and if they are not satisfied, they drop out readily (Lo, 1992). A psychoeducational approach consisting of the explanation of the pathophysiology of anxiety, especially in panic disorders, is necessary because of the general low level of mental health knowledge and the presence of various folk beliefs. It is also effective because of the readiness of the Chinese to adopt a learning mode. They can be helped to see their condition with less shame and more hope.

As we look at the psychodynamics of such patients, insecurity is the predominant theme. In the background, certain cultural factors are often present (Lo, 1992). The patient may have had a strict upbringing, at times with a lot of physical discipline; or the patient may have suffered parental neglect because of a large number of children or overworked, unavailable parents. At the other extreme, overprotection can also lead to a child's being unprepared for the stress of daily life. High expectations to achieve, especially in study, were alluded to earlier. Other factors include the emphasis on social approval and suppression of negative affects and morbid thoughts, particularly in relation to one's elders. The hectic and competitive lifestyle in such places as Hong Kong also contributes in some cases.

Insecurity is also a common theme in the adjustment of new immigrants. The availability of adequate support in the community becomes an important preventive factor as well as a valuable treatment resource. Helping patients to gain access to and use such resources is often a necessary part of the treatment, though not all therapists feel comfortable in doing so.

The work environment may be one source of insecurity. The work ethic of the Chinese make work environment an important part of their lives. Yet, as newcomers, baffled by the subtle cross-cultural differences in work habits, many Chinese feel unsure of themselves and may even feel discriminated against. Racism does exist but often gets exaggerated in the context of high anxiety. We have found that emotional support and assertiveness training are both necessary to help the Chinese to unlearn the submissiveness they have acquired in their own culture. They need to understand this learning as part of the acculturation process. The acculturation framework put forward by Ramirez (1991) and his theory of cognitive and cultural flex are relevant here. Ramirez describes the varying ability of people to operate in a bicultural situation and sees the goal of therapy as the enhancement of the cognitive and cultural flex in the particular patient. Often, the framing of the patient's problem in the light of acculturation stress also frees the patient from the guilt and shame associated with his or her emotional problem and places his or her problem in a more normative context.

Another source of insecurity arises from tension in the family unit, which is the most significant social unit in the Chinese culture. If at all possible, it is helpful to involve family members in the treatment. If they are not helping the process, they would be hindering it. Most Chinese patients agree to such involvement, and the issue of confidentiality is more often a reflection of the uneasiness of the therapist to be involved with the whole family system. In such work, the subsystem intervention described by Lee (1982) has been found to be useful. She suggested separate interventions with different subsystems of the family (e.g., parents alone), keeping in mind the hierarchy and taboo involved in the family dynamics. At times, we have also successfully employed role-play and psychodrama techniques to help the patients come to terms with absent family members.

Relating to the therapist can also be a source of insecurity because the therapist represents an authority figure. Some may have been traumatized by such a relationship in the past, and management of the transference can be an important part of the therapy. However, it may be difficult for patients to express their feelings, and they may somatize or act out. Observation and interpretation of the nonverbal communication are other avenues the therapist may employ.

Cognitive-behavioral treatment has been used effectively for anxiety disorders among the Chinese. The cognitive aspect is in keeping with the rational approach preferred by the Chinese culture, but a certain experiential component is still desirable though harder to attain with certain Chinese who are very unaware of their feelings.

The issue of somatization may seem to preclude the use of psychotherapy. We believe this is more a problem for therapists because of their ethnocentric training rather than a deficiency on the part of the patient (Kirmayer, 1987). The therapist needs to acknowledge the distress of the patient even though it is couched in somatic idioms. If patients feel understood and accepted, they will be more open to further intervention. If an alliance is established, the exploration of the psychosocial context of the patient's life will readily provide the therapist with further psychody-namic understanding. Such can then be presented to patients in an explanatory model they can understand. This process may require patient negotiation, which can only proceed with trust and respect.

Group therapy is another effective treatment modality. The dynamics of the group has several benefits to the Chinese patient. First, it reduces the shame and isolation felt by most patients. They are often more ready to divulge their feelings after they start to trust the group. Second, Chinese are accustomed to the group situation because of their upbring-ing and their outside situation, even though the nonjudgmental and supportive nature of the group will be very different from their other group experiences. Third, for immigrants, who are often very isolated, the group can be a very significant second family where a corrective emotional experience can occur.

Relaxation training is another valuable modality of treatment, but it needs to be customized for the individual patient. Some may never have experienced relaxation consciously in their lifetime. Their lifestyle and their previous environment may have precluded them from such experi-ence. They may have thought of it as mere idleness. On the other hand, indigenous relaxation methods also exist, as in meditation, *tai chi* and *qi-gong*, but the latter method, which has certain features likened to hypnosis, can at times lead to further aggravation of the condition. In fact, psychogenic psychotic states have been seen in China as a result of such exercise (H. C. Lo, personal communication, 1990).

Finally, sharing the same cultural background does not necessarily ensure a perfect match (Lin, 1983). At times, sharing a cultural back-ground can even be a handicap because of concern about lack of confidentiality, social sanction, and "conspiracy" to avoid certain shared cultural taboos. The insight of a therapist from a different culture can be very therapeutic if it is explored in a trusting atmosphere (Cheng & Lo, 1991; Tyler, Sussewell, & Williams, 1985).

MEDICATION ISSUES

The pharmacokinetics of various psychotropic medications particularly the antipsychotics, but also the antidepressants, have been found to vary with different ethnoracial populations. Generally, a lower dosage range is used in the Asian populations. There are fewer studies with ben-zodiazepine and other anxiolytics, and the findings are inconclusive. Clinically, there does not seem to be any major difference. However, the difficulty in the use of such agents is the marked ambivalence about them. Patients, reinforced by the popular media, and their relatives often see the use of such agents as a sign of weakness and likened it to "opium" for addiction potential or damage to the body systems. The guilt and shame patients may have about their emotional problems are thus aggravated further by similar feelings about their treatment. This is particularly so for the anxiety patients who already have conflicts about dependency.

When anxiety is mixed with depressive symptoms, an antidepressant is indicated and often relieves the anxiety symptoms as well as the depression. However, the use of antidepressants has been difficult for the Chinese patients because of their proneness to side effects. Those that make them feel dizziness or other discomfort in the head are especially unwelcome. They may also discontinue or reduce the dose without telling the physician, leading to a poor treatment outcome. Fortunately, the new wave of antidepressants, such as the selective serotonin reuptake inhibitors (SSRIs) and the reversible inhibitors of monoamine oxidase (RIMAs), have a much lower incidence of such side effects and have been found to be much better tolerated by the Chinese patients.

CASE EXAMPLE

May is a 30-year-old Chinese female from Hong Kong who chose to further her education in a university in Newfoundland, where there are few other Chinese. She had already worked for 10 years as a teacher in Hong Kong but finally accumulated enough savings to support herself to go through this university education, which she had always wanted for herself.

While in school, she was bothered by the other Chinese male students looking at her and talking to her during class, she being the only Chinese girl there. Then, she developed a fear that she was blushing, thus indicating that she was interested in the boys. This feeling gradually generalized to all men she encountered, and she felt she could not go out of the house. She also became fixated with rings on any man's fingers. She found that she had to stare at them, and later she would look for such rings even when she did not see them.

May was diagnosed as suffering from a paranoid psychosis and treated with Haldol. The stiffness and other side effects rendered her even more "psychotic," and she was in a poor state when she came out to Toronto to stay with her sister.

Upon assessment, she was rediagnosed as suffering from social phobia and taken off all her medications. We also discovered that she never had any heterosexual relationship. She liked a boy in high school but never managed to tell him. Later, while teaching, she became the center of attention of the principal, a married man. She enjoyed the attention but was rebuked by her colleagues for being so "shameless." The attention of the boys in her class aroused a lot of unresolved feelings around this area. The fixation on the ring also sprang from the fact that some of the boys had rings, signifying that they were already in a relationship.

The formulation of a social phobia was presented to May as a reaction to the tremendous pressure she experienced in the university where she studied very hard, partly because of her limited English and partly because of the isolation she imposed on herself. At the same time, we solicited her collaboration in working on her symptoms, thus putting her in active control over her treatment.

We employed behavioral techniques of exposure and desensitization with success, making use of May's motivation and habit of hard work. She had to look at a ring for some 2 hours to achieve the desensitization. The treatment was also supported by her father, who flew from Hong Kong to visit with her. We explored May's ambivalence about her own sexuality in a gentle manner. She was encouraged to socialize more while in Toronto, and she enjoyed it.

By the third session, most of May's symptoms were gone, and she was ready to return to St. John to study, but she was advised to conduct her life in a different manner and instructed as to how she could deal with any symptom that might recur.

CONCLUSION

As more Chinese and other Asians settle in North America, they will also make increasing demands on the mental health system. Conditions as prevalent as anxiety disorders will need to be treated more effectively. This chapter reflects some of our clinical experience in this area, and we hope it will encourage more research and study which are needed to address this emerging need.

REFERENCES

American Psychiatric Association. (1994). *Diagnostic and statistical manual of mental disorders* (4th ed.). Washington, DC: Author.

Chen, C. N., Wong, J., & Lee, N. (1993). The Shatin Community Mental Health Survey in Hong Kong: II. Major findings. *Archives of General Psychiatry, 50,* 125–133.

Cheng, L., & Lo, H. T. (1991). On the advantages of cross-culture psychotherapy: The minority therapist/mainstream patient dyad. *Psychiatry, 54,* 386–396.

Cheung, F. M. (1989). The indigenization of neurasthenia in Hong Kong. *Culture, Medicine and Psychiatry, 13,* 227–241.

Good, B. J., & Kleinman, A. M. (1985). Culture and anxiety: Cross-cultural evidence for the patterning of anxiety disorders. In J. Maser (Ed.), *Anxiety and the anxiety disorders*. Hillsdale, NJ: Erlbaum.

Hwu, H. G., Yeh, E. K., & Chang, L. Y. (1989). Prevalence of psychiatric disorders in Taiwan defined by the Chinese Diagnostic Interview Schedule. *Acta Psychiatrica Scandinavica, 79,* 136–147.

Katon, W., & Kleinman, A. (1981). Doctor–patient negotiation and other social science strategies in primary care. In L. Eisenberg & A. Kleinman (Eds.), *The relevance of social science for medicine*. Hingham, MA: Reidel.

Kirmayer, L. (1987). Languages of suffering and healing: Alexithymia as a social and cultural process. *Transcultural Psychiatric Research Review, 24,* 119–136.

Kuo, W. H. (1984). Prevalence of depression among Asian Americans. *Journal of Nervous and Mental Disease, 172*(8), 449–487.

Lee, E. (1982). System approach to assessment and treatment for Chinese American families. In M. McGoldrick, J. K. Pearce, & J. Giordano (Eds.), *Ethnicity and family therapy*. New York: Guilford Press.

Lin, E. H. (1983). Intraethnic characteristics and the patient–physician interaction: "Cultural blind spot syndrome." *Journal of Family Practice, 16*(1), 91–98.

Lin, T. Y., Tardiff, K., Donetz, G., & Goresky, W. (1978). Ethnicity and patterns of help-seeking. *Culture, Medicine and Psychiatry, 2,* 3–13.

Lo, H. T. (1992). *Psychotherapy for Chinese Canadians*. Paper presented at Psychotherapy for Chinese, Hong Kong.

Ramirez III, M. (1991). *Psychotherapy and counselling with minorities*. Pergamon Press.

Robins, L. N., Helzer, J. E., & Weissman, M. M. (1984). Lifetime prevalence of specific psychiatric disorders in three sites. *Archives of General Psychiatry, 41,* 949–958.

Shear, M. K. (1993). A psychodynamic model of panic disorder. *American Journal of Psychiatry, 150,* 859–866.

Sue, D. W., & Kirk, B. A. (1973). Differential characteristics of Japanese and Chinese American college students. *Journal of Counselling Psychiatry, 20,* 142–148.

Tseng, W. S. (1992). Diagnostic patterns of social phobia—comparison in Tokyo and Hawaii. *Journal of Nervous and Mental Disease, 180,* 380–385.

Tyler, F. B., Sussewell, D. R., & Williams, J. (1985, Summer). Ethnic validity in psychotherapy. *Psychotherapy, 22*(Suppl.), 311–320.

Part IV

Treatment Modalities in Working with Asian Americans

20

Psychoanalytic Psychotherapy with Chinese Americans

NADINE M. TANG

The applicability of psychoanalytic psychotherapy to members of non-White cultures has been a matter of some dispute for some time (e.g., Sue & Zane, 1987; Hsu & Tseng, 1972). The argument has ranged from the notion that psychoanalytic therapy is about intrapsychic processes and relationships and thus no modification of technique is necessary to the complete dismissal of psychoanalytic theory for other than middle-class European Jews. My own view is that psychoanalysis has much to offer and provides a framework for both theory and technique in working with Chinese Americans. Because there are specific differences between Chinese culture and values and those of European Americans, a better understanding of the interplay between Chinese culture and specific intrapsychic phenomena in Chinese Americans may be helpful in informing clinical work. To provide a context for the clinical setting, I first examine the guiding philosophies of Chinese culture that define the values and aspirations Chinese have for themselves and their children and how these describe the ideal man. This philosophy influences childrearing practices, and there are psychological consequences of such beliefs and practices. (These issues are discussed in greater detail in Tang, 1992.) I examine Chinese attitudes toward male versus female children and how such attitudes can lead to different paths of identification in the broader American culture. Finally, I apply these observations to changes one might make in clinical practice with Chinese Americans. Though this discussion is confined to Chinese, it has some relevance to those who are from other Confucian-influenced cultures (i.e., Japanese, Korean, and Vietnamese).

CHINESE PHILOSOPHICAL INFLUENCES

The most important philosophical influence in China was that of Confucius. His was a set of ideas that valued harmony in relationships above all else. Confucius believed that harmony is maintained by observing clear lines of authority, respecting the status of others, and subordinating oneself to the needs of the family. There is no such thing as an equal relationship. He discouraged the expression of feelings because it only applies to an individual and is an infringement on the harmony of others. Besides, not to be in control of one's own feelings is thought to promote poor judgment. To maintain familial and social harmony, Confucius discouraged assertiveness. Rather, it is considered a mark of maturity to be able to agree publicly with something with which one privately disagrees. Confucius also stressed education as a means of character development. Scholars and teachers maintained the highest social status in China.

Taoism's contributions included the basic law that "when a thing reaches one extreme, it reverts from it" (Chinese saying). This fundamental law is evident in the apparent modesty with which Chinese greet their accomplishments or those of their families and their subdued expressions of feelings over joyful events. To be joyful or boastful is to encourage a reversal of fortune. A further tenet is that the true understanding of the Tao or the Way would make feelings unnecessary. Thus, both Confucianism and Taoism discourage the expressions of emotions.

Buddhism is the third major influence on the Chinese and was most likely introduced to China in the latter half of the first century A.D. Indian Buddhism interpreted with Taoism became the synthesis that was known as the "Ch'an" sect, or Zen in Japan. There is no requirement for belief in any one individual god, and many Chinese simply incorporate all three philosophies in their lives. The Taoist influence supported the notion of nonaction, and if one is truly enlightened, one loses the cravings and possessiveness that lead to the baseness of feelings. Buddhism's contribution was also in the area of the compassion for all beings, and social conscience. It provided a framework for the idea of divine retribution, which was seen to apply on a family basis and worked through a chain of lives.

In summary, what do these philosophies tell us about the ideal man in Chinese culture? Clearly, a major value is in the ability to keep one's feelings to oneself. Taoism discourages the pride that comes with one's achievements or those of one's family, for this would invite failure. Self-restraint in all things is highly encouraged. In a society that values age and men, it is assumed that the patriarch knows what is best. True maturity is shown by fulfilling one's duties to one's family, including putting the family's needs before one's own. A case in point is that of a 30-year-old Chinese man whose father died. As the only son, he was expected to provide a home for his mother. Though the situation was very trying, it did not occur to him to have her live elsewhere. All individuals, by their very existence, are in a contractual relationship. Roles are clearly defined so that parents in fulfilling their duty have the right to expect that their children will fulfill theirs by being respectful and obedient. This holds true in a broader sense so that employers expect loyalty from workers, teachers from students, and so on.

CHILDREARING PRACTICES

Children are greatly indulged for the first 4 to 6 years of life, usually longer for boys. Parents express this indulgence by meeting every physical need the child may have, often including having the child sleep with them. Children are encouraged to be dependent in areas such as feeding themselves and physical exploration. What is forbidden, however, is physical aggression. In one study comparing Chinese American and European Americans mothers, 74% of the Chinese mothers made no demands for aggression even in appropriate situations. This was compared with a majority of American mothers who expected aggression and who said they would punish children who ran home for help (Sollenberger, 1968). Chinese mothers rely more on the values of sharing, noncompetitiveness, and setting good examples for younger siblings. Wolf (1978) observed, in a village setting in Taiwan, that the older son was expected to cater to every demand of the younger son in childhood. This expectation is then reversed when the older son becomes the head of the household. Thus, a traditionally raised child was taught to be a dependent and passive person. These are qualities that are often viewed as somewhat feminine in European American culture

As the Chinese philosophies discourage the expression of feelings, children are expected to fit into their places within the family and little interest is shown in how a child might feel. The words used to describe feelings are all somatically related. To have feelings is to have an imbalance in some part of the body, so that depression is "pressure on the heart," psychosexual difficulty is "weak kidney," and rage is "fire in the liver" (Cheung, 1985). The absence of curiosity about children's feelings is poignantly demonstrated in the novel *China Boy* (Lee, 1991). The main character, Kai, loses his mother to cancer when he is 6 years old. When his mother falls ill, she denies anything is wrong, and her hospital stay is portrayed as a visit to friends. When death is near, Kai is sent to live with another family for a month. Because of his age, both the adults and his older sisters refuse to tell him of his mother's death to protect him. When he returns home, Kai's questions about his mother's whereabouts remain unanswered so that he wonders whether he has done something wrong. Not only are his feelings and questions ignored, but they are also forbidden to be expressed. Later, when his uncle sees Kai and learns obliquely that all is not well between Kai and his new stepmother—in fact, she is terribly abusive to him—his uncle's response is, "This is a very wonderful opportunity for you. Having a new mother is like facing a very stern examination. An examination of the mind and spirit, your *chi,* your essence" (Lee, 1991, p. 234). In other words, the ability to withstand bad situations is what builds character. Besides, it is clear that rebellion is absolutely forbidden for "the authority of the parent cannot be disturbed" (p. 236).

When feelings are not expressed, and are indeed viewed as a sign of weakness and poor judgment, how is it that love is expressed? It is my impression that love is conveyed in physical ways, not by affection but by catering to the child's physical needs. This is especially clear in areas of food and in gifts. Again, Lee (1991) notes of his mother that "she carefully extracted and then placed the valued fish's cheek on my plate. I smiled, for this meant that she loved me" (p. 41). I think Chinese families work hard to be able to provide a tremendous amount for their children, buying them things and supporting them as much as possible. I have been struck by the difference in attitudes between European Americans and Chinese when it comes to providing for their offspring. A European American father I observed was proud of his son's ability to pay for his own skateboard. When I described this to a Chinese friend, she was appalled that such should be expected. Chinese families more clearly bind their children to them in this "giving," for it leads all the more to the sense that one cannot make it without one's family. It can also contribute to feelings of guilt if one is disobedient. To disobey and to do what one wants is often labeled selfish. The opposite is encouraged in an American family and children are rewarded for being self-reliant. However, the compliance and obedience so characteristic of well-raised Chinese children are often derided in U.S. classrooms, where such obedient children are labeled "brown nosers" and "teacher's pets."

This ability to bind children to the family is accomplished in other ways as well. Toddlers who try to feed themselves are discouraged from doing so, and spoon feeding can continue until the child is 3 or 4. It is in the area of physical exploration that the admonishment to stay close and safe is particularly noteworthy. Whereas a European American parent might encourage daring attempts at climbing a jungle gym, a Chinese parent I watched remained glued to a toddler who was trying to balance on a plank, her hands barely an inch away from the child. She kept saying, "You're going to fall," and made noises designed to startle the child, causing him in fact to lose his balance. It is not surprising that in a study done by Kagan, Kearsley, and Zelazo (1978) at Harvard, Chinese mothers described their children as staying close to their mothers and being afraid of the dark. Caucasian mothers chose talkativeness, laughing, and activity to characterize their children. It is part of the Confucian belief that to hurt oneself is unfilial because "the body with its hair and skin is received from parents; do not cause it harm" (*Hsiao Ching,* 1908, p. 16).

Although children are physically indulged, a great deal is also expected from them, especially after the age of 5 or 6. Children are taught to address their elders correctly and to be respectful, neat, and clean. Discipline takes the form of scolding, spanking, or shaming. Threats to abandon the child are used effectively. The focus is to teach the child impulse control and proper behavior toward others. There is little interest in the child's expression of opinions, creativity, or independence. Indeed, in a study of San Francisco Chinese (Lum, 1979), respondents expressed a clear belief that mental illness was a result of character weakness, a lack of will power, and dwelling on morbid thoughts. Chinese parents want a child who will "become a strong healthy adult who is obedient, respectful, and capable of supporting them in their old age" (Wolf, 1978, p. 224). Parents show little affection to children, for to let children know that you love them is was to risk losing control of them.

Finally, praise is used in a particularly striking manner in the Chinese mode of childrearing. A number of Asian American patients report feeling belittled not only by the lack of recognition for their accomplishments but also by the amount of praise heaped on other people's children. The combination left them with the feeling that nothing they ever did was good enough, and, more important, it contributed to their feeling that *they* were not good enough. This stands in sharp contrast to my observations of Western childrearing practices, in which a child's self-esteem is a matter of concern and is enhanced by the use of praise. Those of you familiar with *Mister Rogers' Neighborhood* will recognize the degree to which Mr. Rogers tries to make children feel special.

Praise is limited not only when it is within the family, but also when it comes from people outside the family. One 19-year-old Chinese American woman complained that when others told her father that she was pretty, he would respond, "No, no, she is not pretty. But your daughter is really beautiful." She wondered plaintively why he could not have just said thank you for once. A moving example of the reluctance to acknowledge and praise positive attributes within the family is provided by

Kingston (1976) in *The Woman Warrior,* in which as an adolescent, she flares up in anger at her mother, saying:

> "And it doesn't matter if a person is ugly; she can still do schoolwork."
>
> "I didn't say you were ugly."
>
> "You say that all the time."
>
> "That's what we're supposed to say. That's what Chinese say. We like to say the opposite." (p. 203)

CONFLICTS FOR CHINESE IN AMERICA

To understand the potential problems that arise for many Chinese Americans, it is helpful to examine the world views that Chinese and Americans espouse. Balint (1955) provides a useful model for understanding the differences. He argues that there are two defensive responses to the trauma of the recognition that one is separate. One is to view the world as essentially a safe place with some areas of danger that one can overcome by relying on one's own resources. I believe this describes a more typically American world view. The other is to see the world as a dangerous place in which one's safety lies in clinging to objects. The Chinese view is that the world is basically a dangerous place, but islands of safety are to be had within one's family and community. The Chinese show a tremendous reluctance to venture abroad, and it is discouraged in the saying, "At home you will find things go smoothly for a thousand days, but once you go out you will quickly come across difficulties" (Yee, 1940/1953, p. 187). The traditional Chinese family has been described as providing a "relatively warm atmosphere in which the individual found not merely economic security but also the satisfaction of most of his social needs. Beyond this warm atmosphere lay what the traditional individual considered the cold and harsh world wherein his treatment and fate became unpredictable " (Yang, 1959/1972, p. 11).

The American view is that the world is mostly a friendly place dotted with some dangerous and unpredictable people. To survive in this world, one must rely on one's own resources and is encouraged to stand alone. As far back as the 1830s, de Tocqueville noted that "the citizen of the United States is taught from infancy to rely upon his own exertions in order to resist the evils and the difficulties of life" (1835/1945, pp. 198–199). The famous lines from Thoreau express this admirably when he wrote, "If a man does not keep pace with his companions, perhaps it is because he hears a different drummer. Let him step to the music which he hears, however measured or far away" (p. 374). A properly raised Chinese child would consider such behavior outrageous and dangerous.

I do not think it is an accident that one of the ways Chinese parents attempt to control their children is by using threats to disown or abandon them. Such threats are most effective if one sees one's safety as residing entirely within the family. Unfortunately, this view can lead to a dependence on the family, which is often misinterpreted as timidity and fear of dealing with the world.

One of the conflicts posed for Chinese children growing up in the United States is the assumption that the family and not the individual is the basic unit of society. The actions of children reflect not just on themselves but also on their entire family, past, present, and future. Under such circumstances, one does not take risks lightly. Also, privacy is for the family, not the individual. This contrast is clearly demonstrated in the way that traditional Chinese homes differ from those in the United States. The Chinese home is usually hidden from public view behind a high wall. Once inside, however, there are no doors to close. The American home is full of windows to the outside world yet with internal doors that often lock. As Hsu (1981) so aptly put it, "since the remotest of times, the Chinese have said that their individual successes derived from the shadow of their ancestors and that their individual successes, in turn, shone upon their ancestors" (p. 249). This view of individuals as being unimportant is in direct contrast to what American culture holds most dear.

These differences in world view, in childrearing practices, and in what are considered valuable personality traits can lead to conflicts for Chinese in the United States. These conflicts, by their very nature, have a different impact on men and women. Broadly speaking, I believe that Chinese world view, values, and childrearing practices tend to lead to the formation of what most Americans view as feminine characteristics.

One factor that needs to be mentioned is the generally smaller physical stature of Asian men in general. This disadvantage is clearly addressed in *China Boy,* when Lee (1991) describes himself as "blessed with a body that made Tinker Bell look ruthless" (p. 4). Thus, he is a target for bullies and finds himself constantly being beaten up. His uncle admonishes him to "use reason" (p. 299) and to eschew fighting and become a scholar instead. When this physical disadvantage is coupled with the prohibition against aggression, many Chinese boys appear to Westerners to be "wimps." The value of self-restraint so prized by Confucian societies is not appreciated here or in the workplace, where tremendous value is placed on being able to speak one's mind and put forth one's ideas clearly and aggressively.

In an individualistic society like the United States, the child is encouraged to express his feelings, thoughts, and ideas. A child who is creative is praised. This stands in marked contrast to the traditional Chinese education in which the child's ideas are of little interest. Rather, it is the child's task to learn what others have to teach him, often in rote form. Chinese children are taught not to be assertive in putting forth their own ideas but to be quiet and respectful. Those who were reared simply to perform their tasks and not put themselves forward are at a distinct disadvantage here.

Communication is an important area that sets apart more tradition-ally raised Chinese. Children are schooled from early on to be aware of their place in any given hierarchy. In general, they are to defer to those who are older and in authority. Questioning orders, putting one's own notions forward, or challenging someone else are all forbidden. The primary concern is to maintain harmonious relationships, and this is more important than any business that may get transacted. It is only on a foundation of a trusting relationship that any business can be done at all. There are several ways in which the wish to promote a good relationship with someone is communicated in the Chinese culture. It is important to assume a "one down" position so as not to appear too stuck up and to enhance the status of the other party, often by soliciting their opinions. In a society that values free and open expression, this style of communi-cating can be misconstrued as a sign of insecurity, unimaginativeness, or simply dull-mindedness. If there are any disagreements, they can only be raised indirectly and respectfully. It is perfectly appropriate to resort to compromise and evasion to avoid any conflict. For example, one young woman dealt with her parent's objections to a man she liked by increasing her acts of filial piety rather than arguing for her cause. She attended most diligently to their every need until they were forced to give up their objections because she had proven herself to be such a good daughter.

Although these various styles of communication show an admirable use of self-restraint and modest bearing, they can be and often are interpreted as signs of weakness. In fact, Tannen (1990), a psycholinguist, makes it clear that the concern for preserving relations and the means we use in conversation to do so are the way that women most often communicate. Girls are more apt to try to compromise or evade an issue when there is a dispute. Boys are more likely to carry on a direct conflict. In her own experience, she found that men were more likely to want to challenge an expert, viewing this as a way of promoting constructive interchanges. Women, on the other hand, were much more supportive in their questions and did not come across in an adversarial manner. Indirect communications are often experienced as covert, somewhat sneaky, and as evidence of powerlessness. Yet there are many cultures in the world that value indirectness. Only in modern Western societies is so much value placed on being direct.

As in many Asian cultures, girls in this society are admonished to "stay in the background; never brag; always do your best" (Tannen, 1990, p. 223). Thus, it is a decided disadvantage, at least in U.S. culture, to communicate in a way that would be approved of in a traditional

Confucian family, because this is viewed as feminine in Western society and therefore weaker. It is not the way to enhance and display one's leadership and authority, which are also linked to more masculine ways of conversing in the United States, by being direct, confrontational, and challenging.

It is clear from the descriptions of the Chinese world view that individuals are expected and encouraged to stay close to and even live with their family for as long as possible. This expectation often includes the period after college and before marriage except for the case of oldest sons, who are expected to care for their aging parents and to provide a home for them in their old age. A number of Asian students have confided that the only way they received permission to live away from home while going to college was to plead that the proximity of a dorm room to the library would help them do better academically. Once they graduated, however, they were expected to return home to live. In a country that values independence from one's family and the ability to make it on one's own, this apparent closeness to and dependence on the family make maturity and competence somewhat suspect.

Related to this is the loyalty that many Chinese have to their families. This includes an injunction against criticizing one's parents and elders in general. Conversely, American children are expected to be creative and independent thinkers, even if this means being critical of their parents. For the more traditionally raised Chinese, in matters of conscience, it is vital to consider the impact of one's actions on one's family in deciding what is right and wrong. In an effort to be loyal, it is imperative that children not confront their parents and superiors. Even if the parents do or say something with which the child disagrees, out of a sense of respect the child agrees. There is no expectation in Chinese culture for consistency between actions and inner convictions. Although this might be viewed as hypocritical in the United States, it is considered a mature response among the Chinese. In the *Analects* (1938), Confucius makes it clear that one's first loyalty is always to one's family. Indeed, he chastises a son who turns his father in to the authorities for stealing a sheep. Such a conscience can be criticized for being weak in a country that values rigid standards of right and wrong.

CHINESE MEN AND CHINESE WOMEN

The impact of being Asian in America is different for males and females. Let us first examine the disparate roles and expectations for each in traditional Chinese families.

Women in Chinese culture are less than highly valued. As Confucius wrote back in 500 B.C., "Women and people of low birth are very hard to deal with. If you are friendly with them, they get out of hand, and if you keep your distance, they resent it" (Book XVII, 25). Historically, the lot of women was always one of subservience. Wolf (1985) discusses "the Three Obediences by which women were to be governed: as an unmarried girl a woman must obey her father and her brothers; as a married woman she must obey her husband; and as a widow she must obey her adult sons" (p. 2). With conditions of poverty and starvation not uncommon in much of China, girls were often unwanted additions. In the words of one old lady who explained why she had gotten rid of her daughters, "Why should I want so many daughters? It is useless to raise your own daughters. I'd just have to give them away when they were grown, so when someone asked for them as infants I gave them away. Think of all the rice I saved" (Wolf, 1968, p. 40). The degree to which women were denigrated is most clearly demonstrated by the practice of foot binding, which remained in fashion for 1,000 years. With such attitudes toward women, it is no surprise that many Chinese women would have preferred to have been born male. I believe that such attitudes contribute to feelings of unworthiness and low self-esteem. Women are expected to be quiet and obedient and concerned with doing things for other people. In a strictly hierarchical society such as China, women were clearly at the bottom of the heap. They were viewed as being outside the family almost from birth, and their separation from the family was always expected. Girls became the family of their husbands. This attitude is clearly described in *A Daughter of Han* (Pruitt, 1945): Mrs. Lao explains that when a son is born, the afterbirth is buried in the house to symbolize the expectation that he will remain home. When a girl is born, the afterbirth is buried outdoors.

Lee (1991) provides an example of how sons are valued over daughters. Kai's mother reacts hysterically when he eats a peanut, terrified that he will choke himself. His sister wonders why it is all right for her to eat peanuts and not for her brother.

I believe these attitudes are changing, for there is a great deal expected from girls as well in providing for their families. However, historical and cultural attitudes persist to varying degrees and contribute to the Chinese girl's sense of relative unimportance, poor self-confidence, and confusion as to how to be. A patient described her own experience in which she was supposed to do well in school but was discouraged from being smart at home, especially compared to her older brother. For many years, she sat through meetings and conferences, painfully convinced that anything she might have to contribute was either obvious or stupid. When invited to speak to groups, her automatic, reflexive response was to defer such an honor to a male colleague I have since learned that many Chinese women report similar feelings.

To do well in U.S. society requires the traditionally raised Chinese to make a transition to becoming more forthright and outspoken. However, such a transition is not without its costs. The feeling of being somehow inferior is hard to overcome. To do so means risking the loss of one's family and the approval one has learned to value and depend on. In a sense, Chinese patients report feeling that they are losing their identities as Chinese, and that this would be an irreparable loss. Some Chinese women worry that no Chinese man could possibly by attracted to them because they are too outspoken. They are afraid that by becoming more confident, they no longer fit into the Chinese community in which they were raised. At the same time, many believe that being female in such a community is not such a great deal, and that they would feel better if they were able to become more integrated into the dominant culture. But they are also unclear as to the degree to which they would be accepted by the larger society. A young Chinese woman recalled a close white male friend of hers casually saying that he could never imagine dating someone who was not white.

In rebelling against the accepted female role, a number of Chinese women experience a new sense of themselves as unique, something that they see as being very important in U.S. culture. Because these women have less to lose than a favorite son, it makes it easier to rebel. Chinese women have learned roles that are less discordant with the demands of U.S. society and have an easier time fitting in.

In a traditional Confucian family, being a boy was hard to beat. A boy is treated as someone of value, or as Lee (1991) is told by his uncle, "You are the only living son in your father's line. This is very special, very grand!" (p. 4). It is only with the birth of a son that the family's, and therefore one's own, continuity was assured. Of tremendous concern traditionally was the state of being after death. Without sons, one's plight after death was hopeless. There would be no one to tend to an individual's grave or to acknowledge the individual's existence, and this would result in a loss of continuity of being. A man without sons was pitiful indeed.

But what of the expectations of the sons? Together with the fact that they are highly valued, Chinese sons, especially the oldest son, are burdened with the future of the family's fortunes. Whereas daughters may disgrace the family, sons can destroy it. They are expected to take care of their parents in their old age. How their characters develop, what they choose for careers, whom they marry, and how and where they decide to live are all open to family intervention and instruction.

The denigration of women and the idealization of boys result in a rather interesting relationship between Chinese mothers and their sons. A woman comes to her husband's home as a stranger and "has no status in that family until she bears a son, but even then the comfort of her declining years is not assured unless she can bind that son to her with the ties of gratitude and affection" (Wolf, 1968, p. 127). This is not difficult to do, particularly given the father's prescribed role in childrearing, so aptly described by Lord (1990): "The good father was aloof, strict and authoritarian. To befriend a son was to be a bad father, neglecting one's duties. Conversely, to thrash a son, to order him about, to command his awe, to decide what was good for him were the acceptable forms of paternal caring" (p. 94). A son is also expected to demonstrate his love and respect by being able to "sense" his parent's needs without their having to state them. An illustration of this is the third of the *24 Examples of Filial Piety* (*Hsiao Ching,* 1908) in which a son who is away from home is able to "feel" his mother's distress across the distance and hurries home to assist her. Such dynamics can lead to somewhat different solutions to the Oedipal conflict, as described by Tang and Smith (1996).

Thus, a male in Chinese culture commanded a special place within the family and was cherished and spoiled. The price is the tremendous sense of responsibility to and for the family, the requirement that the boy be completely obedient and remain close and loyal to the family. A female was a second-class citizen, at times unwanted, expected to be obedient to any males in the family and yet not really belonging to the family at all. A male had little choice about his life because the father dictated the son's choices for the benefit of the entire family. I think this partially accounts for the pressure many students feel to major only in potentially lucrative fields. The male risks losing a great deal if he chooses not to comply with what the family is deemed to need. The demands may be great but so are the rewards.

Paradoxically, Chinese females have less to lose in being disobedient. Although a great deal is expected of the female, the entire well-being of the family does not hinge on her actions. In a sense, she is freer to pursue her own goals. Being viewed as separate from the family from birth allows a smoother and less frightening separation from the family nest. In a country like the United States, more appreciation is accorded a woman's achievements, and many women learn that they have something of value to offer when they begin school. Suddenly, they are in an environment that openly praises them for good work. The very traits that make Chinese men feminine are exalted and idealized in Chinese women, who are often viewed as the epitome of femininity. Ironically, the experience of being viewed as separate from the family from the beginning results in greater independence for Chinese women. In my view, Chinese men have a more difficult and conflictual experience trying to reconcile their cultural values with those of America. Chinese women may be stereotyped and seen as submissive, but they have different conflicts to overcome in living in the United States.

In short, Chinese men in the United States often come from families that treated and view them as special, but they are not admired in the larger society. Chinese women, on the other hand, can feel unappreciated and unwanted within their families yet find their sense of self-worth outside the family setting.

PSYCHODYNAMIC IMPLICATIONS

As a result of the degree to which Chinese families bind their children to them and impart the view that the world is a dangerous place and their safety lies within the family, it is not surprising that the encouragement toward independence is largely absent. In a culture that values dependence on and responsibility to one's family, the push toward separation and individuation is likely to be actively discouraged. Especially during the rapprochement phase (Mahler, Pine, & Bergman, 1975), in which the mother must encourage the child to move away, a Chinese mother is more likely to keep the child close to her and to discourage the child's attempts to explore. It is easy to see how the need to prevent active toddlers from physically hurting themselves necessitates a watchful eye and maintenance of closeness on the mother's part. It is within the bounds of being a good Chinese mother that she prevents any injuries and safeguards the physical well-being of the child. Given such a prescription, there is a longer separation and individuation process, and the form it takes may be less in terms of a physical distancing than in the relative emotional distance that is maintained. Because feelings are neither shared nor elicited, children have a sense of separateness in their own thoughts and feelings.

There is also a difference in the way a Chinese person might experience a sense of self because there are essentially two sets of private selves as it were: the individual self and the family self. The family self is often the more compelling and can override what an individual might want. This is illustrated in many cases by college students who feel bound to major in family-prescribed lucrative fields of study even if the subject matter is of no interest to them. The good of the family must come first. Although there is a relative lack of sin and guilt in Chinese culture, not living up to the family's needs can unleash a great deal of guilt.

In a society that values relationships above all else, it is not surprising that shame plays a more important role in shaping a child than guilt. Shame implies the failure of the ego to live up to an ego ideal and can result in the loss of self-esteem and depression. This definition contrasts with guilt, which is a transgression of the ego that conflicts with the superego (Piers & Singer, 1953). Moreover, the anxiety related to guilt is castration, whereas with shame, it is the threat of abandonment.

Because individual feelings are considered unimportant but close attention is paid to physical needs, it is not surprising that Kleinman (1986), in his work in mental health clinics in China, found large numbers of patients who had been diagnosed with neurasthenia were actually suffering from dysphoric symptoms. Many often presented with somatic complaints. It is in this way that depressive feelings can be expressed, and, indeed, those patients were often given reduced workloads and were treated better by their spouses or parents when they were perceived to be physically ill. It is not unusual in the clinical setting to have Chinese patients give accounts of their physical symptoms as a way of describing their distress. In a world view that makes no distinction between the mind and the body, it is the body that carries the "illness" in a socially acceptable way and without the shame that goes along with mental weakness.

Given the prohibition against anger, the discouragement of the expression of affects in general, and the expectation for individuals to be dutiful and respectful to their parents no matter how mean or cruel the parents are, reaction formation is an important defense. This defense is often manifested in an oscillation between a ready compliance to authority and murderous, antiauthoritarian rampages such as occurred during the Cultural Revolution from 1966 to 1976.

CLINICAL IMPLICATIONS

It is my contention that Chinese Americans can benefit from psychoanalytic psychotherapy, just as many others in the population can. There is much to be gained from examining and understanding how childhood experiences, history, and cultural heritage contribute to an individual's personality formation. I do not agree with those who have suggested a more problem-solving approach with Chinese American patients (Hsu & Tseng, 1972). At times, some argue that those who are more recent immigrants and therefore more traditional can benefit only from a more focused therapy that relies on giving a "gift" to enhance the relationship (Sue & Zane, 1987). In thinking about my own clinical experience, I was struck by how capable some new immigrants are of plunging into the work of analysis, freely discussing parental influences and childhood events. These patients include one woman from the People's Republic of China and another from Malaysia. Conversely, I have also seen second- and third-generation Chinese Americans who were far more resistant to the idea of an examination of their families and were ashamed of seeking help. I had hoped to present a case that would provide a clear example of some of the issues I have already raised, but every case proved far more complex, refusing to fit neatly into any category or to be perfect for the application of any particular technique.

However, certain issues need to be approached carefully and with an eye toward understanding some of the psychological issues already discussed. For example, it is crucial to recognize the roles of shame and reaction formation in the therapy. The danger of interpreting shame is to exacerbate an already unbearable feeling by calling attention to it. This contrasts with the interpretation of guilt, which the patient usually experiences as relieving. It is important, therefore, for the therapist to distinguish carefully between these two affects in any given clinical situation.

The very act of seeking out a psychotherapist carries a tremendous burden of shame. It is viewed as being disloyal to one's family, because it involves the disclosure of the "family self" as well as the individual self to a stranger's scrutiny. Moreover, it is an implicit statement that the family is not enough so that the individual then risks the dangerous world of nonfamily objects. As Lum (1979) discovered in his research, talking about "morbid thoughts" was believed to contribute to mental illness. Given this, it is not surprising that a certain amount of testing of the therapist is to be expected. In the transference, a Chinese American patient is likely to see the therapist as someone who is potentially intrusive, a person with authority who is therefore powerful and dangerous. It is not unusual for such a patient to seek advice and to work hard at pleasing the "authority" and to agree with whatever the therapist says. I have had consultations with Chinese American patients which I thought went extremely well, only to find that they were not interested in returning. My impression is that any dissatisfaction or disagreement is not expressed, mostly as a matter of preserving face for both the patient and myself.

Consequently, it is important to maintain a fairly neutral stance and not to exhibit too much curiosity about the patient or his or her family. Therapists need to present themselves as someone who is authoritative, warm, and supportive. Given how important the issue of shame is for most Chinese American patients, they are likely to be highly sensitive to criticism and the therapist must be careful not to make comments that can be construed as disapproving or judgmental.

Those of us who were trained in the United States cannot help but pick up some of the values of this culture. Dependence is seen as practically sinful in U.S. culture, and this attitude accounts for the relatively poor treatment accorded those in the society who are most helpless (i.e., children, the elderly, and the chronically ill). This attitude stands in sharp contrast to a Confucian-based culture in which the dependence of the child is encouraged, and in which the care of the elderly is assumed as part of one's responsibility. It is not surprising that a young Chinese man's failure to leave home is often seen as a sign of pathology in this culture. However, it is important to keep the context of such behavior in mind, because it should be clear that a great deal of the oldest son's self-esteem lies in the proper fulfillment of his duties, which include living with his parents and seeing to their needs. Though such demands may be placed on a younger son and the daughters, there is less pressure on them to comply. In my experience, patients who are female or are a younger son often make greater strides toward more independence from family.

The choice of a therapist can sometimes indicate the direction in which a Chinese patient may wish to go. Most of the literature on cross-cultural therapy has been written with the assumption of a Chinese patient and a Caucasian therapist dyad. However, because of the growing number of Asian mental health professionals, we are also learning what it means for an Asian patient to choose an Asian therapist. When such is the case, the patient initially explains that a fellow Chinese or Asian will understand better just what his or her family and family expectations were like. I wonder whether there is also an implicit belief that such values will also be respected by the therapist and less open to challenge, so that the patient is able to preserve his or her role in the family. When a Chinese patient selects a Caucasian therapist, he or she may wish for greater autonomy and permission to become more independent. Such a choice may also represent the wish to confide in someone "outside," which may be experienced as less disloyal than seeing someone within the community. Possibly, it may reflect a Chinese American who is much more assimilated in U.S. culture. Regardless of the racial mix, I have been struck by the importance of forming a connection so that there is a sense of relatedness, even if only in a superficial fashion. Many Chinese invite the therapist to become part of the family. As a Chinese therapist, I am often asked about my region of origin in China or what dialect I speak. Though this may seem to be a personal question, and inappropriate to answer, it is my belief that such questions are an attempt by patients to place me relative to themselves and to find some common ground from which to work. If such questions persist, however, I understand them to be an attempt to show interest in me, an attempt by patients to put themselves in a one-down position and not to presume on my time. This is not to say that a certain amount of resistance is not also extant, but given the importance accorded to relationships, such groundwork is essential.

As discussed in the philosophy section of this chapter, it is clear that Chinese Americans are not encouraged to verbalize or even to experience feelings. This holds true for introspection as well. It is therefore confusing to Chinese patients when they are asked how they felt about a particular event. Rather than viewing the lack of responsiveness to such a query as resistance, it is important to consider whether patients are able to recall feelings when they have had little or no experience in doing so. If the therapist is going to inquire about affects, it is less threatening to do so in fairly general and benign ways, especially when referring to anger or aggressive impulses that were prohibited in childhood.

CASE EXAMPLE

A case vignette illustrates the points discussed earlier. The case is one I supervised in which the therapist was a Caucasian intern at a low-fee clinic. Mr. W was a 38-year-old Chinese American male, the older of two sons, who worked full time in a white-collar job while living with his parents.

His mother was a chronic schizophrenic who was maintained on psychotropic medication and had her own room. The father was suffering from a degenerative disease that made him increasingly dependent on this son. The younger son had recently moved out into an apartment of his own, leaving Mr. W solely responsible for his parent's care. His daily schedule involved waking up early to make breakfast for himself and his parents, commuting to work and back, then doing the grocery shopping, cooking and cleaning, and getting to bed late at night, only to start all over again. He sought treatment on the advice of his physician because he was complaining of exhaustion.

When he was seen in an initial consultation, Mr. W seemed devoid of affect, and his therapist described his communicative style as robotic, with no inflections in his voice. As Mr. W described his routine, the therapist asked him how he felt about the degree of responsibility he carried for the family. He seemed puzzled by the question and did not respond other than to continue an account of his day. At this point I suggested to the intern that she should not expect him to come up with feelings but instead should concentrate on forming some connection with him. An opportunity presented itself when Mr. W was chronicling the demands his father made that he drive some distance to buy a special kind of mushroom for a particular dish. Mr. W went on to describe his way of preparing beef and mushrooms. I encouraged the intern to inquire more about the recipe and to try to talk to the patient in terms to which he could relate. In a culture that values relationships, communications are considered important, not for the information that is imparted but for what it indicates about how one person feels about the other. For this reason, there is also likely to be a fair amount of indirect communication from which we learn to infer where one the other stands. The inquiry about food proved to be a good beginning because Mr. W became quite engaged in the description and was gradually able to build his relationship with the therapist. At least in the first year, they did not discuss feelings in direct terms, but Mr. W increasingly expressed his frustration with his home situation.

At one point during the first year of treatment, Mr. W began to present material that indicated the development of a sexualized transference. Though it was clear to the intern that such feelings were surfacing, we agreed that it would be wiser not to confront these transference themes to avoid placing Mr. W in an embarrassing and potentially shameful situation. To have done so might have disrupted the treatment and made it too painful for Mr. W to return.

During this year, Mr. W was offered a job opportunity that involved a move across the country. Though it was clear this would be a move he might want, Mr. W could not make it at the cost of abandoning his parents. He chose to stay but gradually sought domestic help to relieve himself of some of the burden. He was also committed to continuing in therapy beyond the 2 years allotted and was able to make good use of therapy to help in dealing with the conflicting demands on his life.

This case example illustrates some of the ways in which some modification in thinking and working may be useful in a therapeutic relationship with a Chinese American man. The importance of establishing a relationship is paramount and may require the therapist to explore what appear to be superficial subjects. However, patients may interpret the interest in such matters as an expression of curiosity about and goodwill toward them. An insistence on revealing feelings would have proved frustrating to both patient and therapist and would have left the patient with the feeling that he had failed to conform. It is also crucial to view this man's "dependence" through a different lens. In the Chinese culture, he was doing what mature and worthy individuals do—that is, carrying out his duty to his parents. Though to many this would appear to be unhealthy, it is also what defines a worthy Chinese individual.

The therapist's neutrality about the choices in Mr. W's life allowed Mr. W a safe place in which to express his conflicts, even if in an oblique way. An issue that raised shameful feelings for him was wisely sidestepped, and because it was so indirectly raised, both therapist and patient could save face and not risk embarrassment or humiliation. Mr. W was able to make use of the relationship with his therapist to express whatever frustrations he was feeling at home, and over time he was less "exhausted" and depressed. The use of the therapy as a repository for his more negative feelings about his parents contributed to his ability to fulfill the demands of his role as the eldest son and therefore to maintain his self-esteem as a filial son. To some degree doing so upheld his charge of loyalty to the family and was in keeping with his "family self." That this was most likely a reaction formation against the anger he may have felt at the excessive demands placed on him was not interpreted in this phase of the therapy because Mr. W might well have experienced it as an assault on his self-esteem.

SUMMARY

In this chapter, I tried to demonstrate the importance of psychoanalytic understanding of the consequences of Chinese childrearing practices in work with Chinese Americans. The values of dependence and responsibility to family and the discouragement of individual expressions of affect lead to a different version of the separation individuation process and to different views of the self. These views have certain implications for transference issues in both same-race and mixed-race therapeutic dyads and require some modifications in technique.

REFERENCES

Analects of Confucius. (1938). (A. Waley, Trans.). New York: Vintage.

Balint, M. (1955). Friendly expanses—horrid empty spaces. *International Journal of Psycho-Analysis, 36,* 225–241.

Cheung, F. M. (1985). An overview of psychopathology in Hong Kong with special references to somatic presentation. In W.-S. Tseng & D. Wu (Eds.), *Chinese culture and mental health* (pp. 287–304). New York: Academic Press.

de Tocqueville, A. (1945). *Democracy in America* (Vol. 1). New York: Vintage. (Original work published 1835)

Hsiao Ching. (1908). (I. Chen, Trans.). London: John Murray.

Hsu, F. (1967). *Under the ancestors' shadow.* Stanford, CA: Stanford University Press. (Original work published 1948)

Hsu, F. (1981). *Americans and Chinese* (3rd ed.). Honolulu: University of Hawaii Press.

Hsu, J., & Tseng, W.-S. (1972). Intercultural psychotherapy. *Archives of General Psychiatry, 27,* 700–705.

Kagan, J., Kearsley, R., & Zelazo, P. (1978). *Infancy.* Cambridge, MA: Harvard University Press.

Kingston, M. H. (1976). *The woman warrior.* New York: Knopf.

Kleinman, M. H. (1986). *Social origins of distress and disease.* New Haven, CT: Yale University Press.

Lee, G. (1991). *China boy.* New York: Dutton.

Lord, B. B. (1990). *Legacies.* New York: Knopf.

Lum, R. (1979). *Impact of mental illness in Chinese families.* Unpublished doctoral dissertation.

Mahler, M. S., Pine, F., & Bergman, A. (1975). *The psychological birth of the human infant.* New York: Basic Books.

Piers, G., & Singer, M. (1953). *Shame and guilt.* Springfield, IL: Charles C Thomas.

Pruitt, I. (1945). *A daughter of Han.* Stanford, CA: Stanford University Press, 1967.

Sollenberger, R. (1968). Chinese-American child-rearing practices and juvenile delinquency. *Journal of Social Psychology, 74,* 13–23.

Sue, S., & Zane, N. (1987). The role of culture and cultural techniques in psychotherapy. *American Psychologist, 42,* 37–45.

Tang, N. (1992). Some psychoanalytic implications of Chinese philosophy and child-rearing practices. *Psychoanalytic Study of the Child, 47,* 371–389.

Tang, N., & Smith, B. (1996). The eternal triangle across cultures: Oedipus, Hsueh and Ganesa. *Psychoanalytic Study of the Child, 51,* 562–579.

Tannen, D. (1990). *You just don't understand.* New York: Ballantine Books.

Thoreau, H. D. (1983). *Walden.* New York: Penguin. (Original work published 1854)

Wolf, M. (1968). *The house of Lim.* New York: Appleton-Century-Crofts.

Wolf, M. (1978). Child training and the Chinese family. In A. Wolf (Ed.), *Studies in Chinese society* (pp. 221–246). Stanford, CA: Stanford University Press.

Wolf, M. (1985). *Revolution postponed.* Stanford, CA: Stanford University Press.

Yang, C. K. (1959). *Chinese Communist society: The family and the village.* Cambridge, MA: MIT Press. (Original work published 1959)

Yee, C. (1953). *A Chinese childhood.* London: Methuen. (Original work published 1940)

21

Neuropsychological Assessment of Monolingual Chinese-Speaking Patients

SHIAO-LING JUDY HSIEH

This chapter provides a brief introduction to contemporary neuropsychological assessment. The chapter reviews when and why to make referrals for neuropsychological evaluation and what to expect in terms of findings. In addition, the chapter explores common clinical issues of particular concern regarding neuropsychological assessment for adult monolingual Chinese-speaking patients. This chapter is not intended to review all aspects in neuropsychology relevant to the monolingual Chinese-speaking population but, rather, to provide an overview and introductory discussion of neuropsychology to clinicians interested in working with this specific population.

A GENERAL INTRODUCTION TO NEUROPSYCHOLOGICAL ASSESSMENT

Clinical neuropsychology examines the relationship between brain and human behavior in both cognitive and emotional domains. By observing and examining particular behaviors, the neuropsychologist is able to understand and make inferences regarding specific brain functions and dysfunctions and to identify behavioral strengths and weaknesses. Neuro-psychologists then can make informed recommendations about the need for follow-up or rehabilitative services.

Clinicians can conduct neuropsychological examinations for a variety of purposes: (1) to provide a differential diagnosis between organic (brain-related) and functional (emotional) influences on psychological functioning, (2) to assess cognitive strengths and limitations and to establish a baseline of neuropsychological functioning for later compari-son and follow-up evaluation, (3) to provide constructive recommenda-tions for case management that are specifically designed to accommodate patients' limitations, teach new coping skills, establish appropriate expec-tations, and make pertinent referrals for therapy and rehabilitation; and (4) to provide consultations in forensic work on issues related to compe-tence to stand trial, mental state at the time of offense, personal injury, worker's compensation, and so on.

People of all ages can benefit from a neuropsychological examination. Common problems that warrant neuropsychological assessment include traumatic events such as head injury, Cerebral Vascular Accident, brain tumor, and a variety of chronic medical conditions such as vascular disease, metabolic disorder, AIDS, and alcoholism. In addition, a neuro-psychological assessment can aid in rendering complex differential diag-noses such as depression versus dementia.

A typical neuropsychological assessment evaluates cognitive functions in a wide range of areas: intellectual ability; language and communication skills; motor performance; sensory function, including auditory, visual, and tactile sensation; visual, spatial, perceptual, and constructional abili-ties; attention, concentration, and memory; and higher conceptual and executive functions, such as capacities for maintaining and shifting sets, practical judgment, abstraction, self-monitoring, problem solving, and planning.

A complete battery of neuropsychological tests usually examines cognitive as well as emotional functioning and carefully evaluates the relationships between them. In addition to assessing the many cognitive abilities listed previously, a complete battery also addresses personality functions.

To understand human behavior, the neuropsychologist collects data through clinical interviews with the patient and family, review of medical records, medical staff and clinician consults, and administration of neuropsychological tests. A clinical interview with patients and family members usually covers family history, educational and occupational background, medical history, history of head injury, current list of medi-cations, and past and current substance use.

The extent of a neuropsychological examination depends on a num-ber of issues, including referral questions, the patient's level of deficits and limitations, language capacity, age, education, level of premorbid functioning, and cultural background. Assessment can be brief. For example, when impairment is readily obvious but the level and extent of dysfunction need further delineation, assessment may take the form of a simple screening test. Assessment can also be elaborate and detailed, as might be necessary when the presenting problem involves more subtle impairments.

Neuropsychological tests for monolingual Chinese-speaking patients are limited in terms of the number of appropriate tests and in norms derived specifically for this population. In addition, careful efforts must be directed toward selecting a testing battery that is relevant to the patient's own life experiences and repertoires. Tests appropriate for a 70-year-old retired Chinese cook who spent the last 20 years living in Chinatown would be quite different from those for a recent Chinese immigrant who, prior to a head injury, had been attending a local college.

However, even when testing items are carefully chosen, they may still be irrelevant. For example, I tested a head-injured Chinese male who recently immigrated to the United States from Vietnam. When I showed him an American-made comb; he was unable either to identify it or to describe its function. His wife, present during testing, later told me that she was not surprised when her husband did not recognize the comb: he had never seen one in Vietnam, and his head injury occurred prior to immigrating.

The following is a list of neuropsychological tests that I selectively use when evaluating monolingual Chinese-speaking patients. Lezak (1995) provides a detailed description of these tests:

1. Neurobehavioral Cognitive Status Examination (NCSE)
2. Mini-Mental Status Examination (Chinese version)
3. Wechsler Adult Intelligence Scale—Revised in China (WAIS-RC)
4. Test of Nonverbal Intellligence (TONI-2) (Brown, Sherbenou, & Johnsen, 1990)
5. Test of Variables of Attention (TOVA) (Leark, Dupuy, Greenberg, Kindschi, & Corman, 1996)
6. Wechsler Memory Scale—Revised (WMS-R), selected subtests
7. Fuld Object-Memory Evaluation (FOME)
8. Rey–Osterrieth Complex Figure Test
9. Animal Naming Test, Fruit, Vegetable and Food Naming Tests
10. Peabody Picture Vocabulary Test—Third Edition (PPVT-III)
11. Raven's Colored Progressive Matrices and Raven's Standard Progressive Matrices
12. Reitan–Kløve Sensory-Perception Examination
13. Finger Tapping Test
14. Grooved Pegboard Test

15. Hand Dynamometer Test
16. Tactual Performance Test (TPT)
17. Draw a Clock Test
18. Bender–Gestalt Visual–Motor Scale (copy phase)
19. Hoope Visual Organization Test (VOT)
20. Trail-Making Test, Parts A and/or B
21. Color Trail Test, Parts I and II
22. Symbol Digit Modalities Test (SDMT)
23. Seashore Rhythm Test
24. Wisconsin Card Sorting Test (WCST)
25. Category Test

CASE EXAMPLES

The following cases demonstrate several possible issues addressed in a neuropsychological assessment.

Case Example 1

Mr. X is a 74-year-old monolingual Chinese-speaking man who is right-handed, married, and a retired restaurant owner. Mr. X was referred by his internist for evaluation of cognitive and emotional functions and for treatment recommendations. His medical history included hypertension, gastric and duodenal peptic ulcer disease, possible past mild cerebral vascular accident with right-side weakness, hyperlipidemia, and hyper-cholesterolemia. The patient presented to his internist with chronic symptoms of vertigo, disequilibrium, recurrent headache, poor appetite, rapid weight loss, insomnia, and depressed mood. His current medical work-up included an echocardiogram, Holter examination, computerized transaxial tomography (CT scan), electrocardiogram, carotid ultrasound, tests on thyroid function and peripheral vestibular system, and an extensive clinical neurological examination. Findings on all these investigations were essentially negative. Current psychosocial stressors included Mr. X's wife's placement in a convalescent hospital 6 months earlier, following the most recent in a series of cerebral vascular accidents over the past 2 years.

Neuropsychological testing revealed average performance in a variety of domains: passive attention, Chinese-language function (auditory comprehension, repetition, naming, verbal fluency, and spontaneous speech), motoric function, arithmetic ability (addition, subtraction, multiplication, and division), and short- and long-term auditory memory. The patient demonstrated no problems in storage, encoding, or retrieval of memory.

On the other hand, testing data indicated impaired performance in sustained concentration and mild cognitive impairments in visual/spatial/constructional functions. More notable problems were evident in reasoning/frontal/executive functioning (i.e., abstraction, similarity, and set shifting). The overall pattern of this patient's neuropsychological evaluation was consistent with a severe affective problem and the presence of some less severe organic features.

Mr. X was referred to individual psychotherapy for reactive depression in the wake of his wife's cerebrovascular accidents and nursing home placement. Given Mr. X's concrete performance on neuropsychological tests, the evaluater suggested that therapy focus on direct, problem-solving strategies, psychoeducation, relaxation techniques, and cognitive reframing and that a more insight-oriented focus be avoided. The patient was further referred to a senior center for social activities, to a dietician for consultation on proper diet, and to a psychiatrist for antidepressant medication evaluation.

By the patient's report, after 3 months in psychotherapy, his depression lifted and many somatic symptoms, including insomnia, weight loss, dizziness, and headaches, were gone.

This case demonstrates how neuropsychological evaluation can assist in differential diagnosis, particularly in the absence of other positive medical findings, and how it can aid in selecting appropriate therapeutic interventions geared directly toward the patient's cognitive strengths and weaknesses.

Case Example 2

Mrs. Z is a 69-year-old widowed, right-handed, monolingual Chinese-speaking female, referred for a neuropsychological evaluation to obtain suggestions for treatment intervention. Mrs. Z exhibited behavioral and affective problems, such as screaming and crying, in the convalescent home where she resides. Mrs. Z, an immigrant to the United States 14 years earlier, had no formal education and had worked as a restaurant dishwasher for more than 10 years. Her medical records indicated a history of hypertension, renal osteodystrophy, and a recent cerebral vascular accident, which resulted in with dysarthria and right hemiplegia.

On clinical observation, Mrs. Z exhibited affective instability, loud crying spells, recurrent outbursts of rage, and paranoid ideation. For example, she insisted that a staff member at the nursing home had pinched her and caused bruising on her leg. She frequently expressed the belief that she was being mistreated and responded with uninhibited loud crying spells and verbal assaults on her imagined enemies. In addition to a language barrier, which placed her in an even more unfortunate situation, Mrs. Z had difficulty with articulation (dysarthria) as a result of a recent cerebrovascular accident. This problem further handicapped her ability to communicate with the nursing staff, causing additional frustrations for both patient and staff. The patient became extremely agitated when her needs were not met. To communicate her needs, Mrs. Z either yelled for help or made incessant demands. These behaviors caused significant discomfort for other residents in the nursing home, who resented her disruptions.

The results of the neuropsychological evaluation revealed significant overall deterioration and mild to severe diffuse impairment in a variety of cognitive functions Mrs. Z's deficits were in the areas of language functions (auditory comprehension, repetition, word fluency, and word finding), arithmetic functioning, reasoning/frontal/executive functioning (abstraction, similarity, self-monitoring, set shifting, and practical judgment), and concentration and memory (both short- and long-term memory and problems in storage, encoding, and retrieval). As such, the neuropsychologist saw the problems resulting from Mrs. Z's generally deteriorated cognitive functioning as being further exacerbated by her severe impairments in concentration and comprehension. Given her illiteracy and limited job history, the neuropsychologist estimated that Mrs. Z's premorbid intellectual functioning was also limited to the low-average and borderline range. The results of the neuropsychological evaluation suggested the presence of moderately impaired multi-infarct dementia with organic personality features.

Based on the neuropsychological findings and the identification of Mrs. Z's cognitive strengths and weaknesses, intervention for Mrs. Z could then proceed. The neuropsychologist consulted with the nursing home staff and Mrs. Z's family on effective communication and management techniques (i.e., keeping phrases and sentences brief and distracting the patient with different tasks when she exhibited disruptive behavior). It was suggested that a Chinese calendar be placed on the wall of Mrs. Z's nursing home room in order to promote her orientation to time. A recommendation was further made to obtain a psychiatric consult for medication evaluation, to address her paranoid ideation. Mrs. Z was also referred to a bilingual speech therapist for help in designing a "picture board" to improve her communication, which was hindered both by the language barrier and because of her cognitive impairments.

COMMON CLINICAL ISSUES ENCOUNTERED WHILE WORKING WITH MONOLINGUAL CHINESE-SPEAKING PATIENTS

Establishing Rapport and Soliciting Cooperation

When making a referral for neuropsychological assessment, comprehensible explanations must be given to the patient and family. Rationales need to be simple and direct. I usually tell the patient and the family that I will be assessing brain functions nonintrusively to identify their strengths and

weaknesses and to make recommendations for improvements. Neuropsychological testing can be frightening to some Chinese patients who have
never encountered a psychologist. Just as many Chinese patients have
particular fears and misconceptions about seeking psychotherapy, some
are resistant to neuropsychological assessment as well. An anxious Chinese patient may respond to such a referral with, "My brain is fine. I have
no problems." In this case, I explain to the patient that everyone has
strengths and weaknesses. Weaknesses can be improved on by using
strengths to help out. I emphasize that I am here to work with the patient
to reach this goal together. Importantly, I avoid using the term "testing,"
as in Chinese language, it represents a pass/fail concept that can be quite
threatening to many Chinese patients. Instead, I find that using the term
"examination" is more acceptable, as in Chinese, it is perceived as
investigation and inquiry, similar to a "medical and physical examination."

Further, "craziness" and "brain-related problems" tend to be interpreted synonymously in Chinese language. As such, monolingual Chinese-
speaking patients may be fearful and resistant about being assessed. I have
had patients angrily tell me that they are not "crazy." In these situations,
patients need reassurance that brain dysfunctions are often caused by
medical conditions and do not imply mental illness.

In working with Chinese patients, it is particularly important to show
a genuine interest, respect, and patience, especially with the elderly.
Chinese culture emphasizes respect for the elderly and for their wisdom,
authority, and contributions, particularly within the family system. Illness,
accidents, or debilitation do not change an individual's cultural beliefs
and values. A gentle greeting, some verbal compliment, and nonverbal
welcome gestures can promote rapport, enhance feelings of acceptance,
empower ego strengths, and maximize motivation during the testing
process.

I often begin clinical interviewing with a somatic inquiry. Usually
patients are more than willing to describe bodily symptoms, such as headaches, dizziness, or insomnia. After establishing a therapeutic rapport with
patients in this less threatening way, it is then easier to begin to address
emotional and affective experiences. In my experience, relative to the
English-speaking population, drug and alcohol problems are rather uncommon among monolingual Chinese-speaking patients. However, to be thorough, I routinely take a drug and alcohol history with all testing patients.
To prevent possible protest, I emphasize that all questions are part of a
"standard" interview and ask each question in a matter-of-fact manner.

Administering the Test

When working with monolingual Chinese-speaking patients, flexibility
and adaptability in test administration are particularly important. For

example, frequent breaks during testing for elderly patients are impera-tive to avoid fatigue. Anxious patients can benefit from deep breathing and relaxation techniques when their anxiety threatens to interfere with their performance. Generally, certain tests should not be interrupted before being completed, but exceptions may need to be made. For example, one of my patients complained about a headache during testing. He took some medicine, napped for 20 minutes, and resumed testing after he woke up. Similarly, in the middle of a Rorschach administration, another patient became extremely anxious and needed to take a walk, resuming the test a half hour later, after calming down. As Lezak (1995) suggests, a flexible approach is needed to "tailor the examination to the patient's needs, abilities and limitations" (p. 98) and to promote the patient's best welfare.

Involving the Family

Most of the time, family members are asked to wait outside the testing room during testing. Occasionally, however, I let a parent or relative sit in the testing room, particularly when working with child and elderly patients. As a rule, I ask for permission from the patient in advance. If the patient expresses hesitation, I do not allow a family member to sit in. When family members are to be included, I prepare them before the testing not to interfere. I selectively allow a family member to be present during testing administration for two reasons. First, because Chinese parents are usually very involved in many aspects of their youngsters' lives, younger children may feel more comfortable with them present. Second, the presence of a significant family member (e.g., a spouse or, in the case of the elderly, an adult child) sometimes facilitates fuller participation from the patient.

Using an Interpreter

Many major medical facilities do not provide neuropsychological exami-nations to monolingual Chinese-speaking patients unless a bilingual neuropsychologist is available. Other facilities, lacking access to bilingual neuropsychologists, rely on interpreters, who primarily assist in screening tasks and generally do not administer in-depth batteries.

Use of an interpreter depends on the individual's cultural sensitivity, familiarity with testing procedures, educational background, training, and experiences. Cultural sensitivity of the interpreter is even more important at times than language fluency. The ability to recognize certain subtle behaviors relevant to a specific Chinese ethnic group and not to misinter-pret culturally acceptable behavior is a critical challenge that both the interpreter and psychologist must face. For example, monolingual Chi-

nese-speaking patients may not express their opinion. This behavior can
easily be interpreted by an inexperienced interpreter or psychologist as
representing impairment in comprehension. I have had Chinese patients
tell me that they did not understand an examiner's verbal directions but
pretended to understand so as not to lose face or to embarrass the other
person. Language assessment, even for fluent Chinese speakers, can be
difficult. It is unlikely that an interpreter is trained or skilled enough to
identify specific language problems or diagnostic signs such as persevera-
tions, common in frontal lobe dysfunctions. In addition, interpreters may
be overenthusiastic, adding their own verbatim instructions or elaborating
on the patient's verbal responses, and thus may invalidate test scores. For
example, it is easy for an interpreter to provide more explanation than
necessary on testing items (e.g., those on the PPVT-III) and thus produce
skewed responses on the test. Finally, information obtained by observing
the qualitative aspects of a patient's testing behavior, an important part
of the neuropsychologist's testing repertoire, would be limited at best with
the use of an interpreter.

Modifying the Tests

The scarcity of culture-relevant and norm group-referenced tests is an
ongoing problem in neuropsychological testing with Chinese-speaking
patients. Even when Chinese patients speak English fluently, they may be
at a distinct disadvantage with certain tests, such as the Comprehension
or Information Subtests on the WAIS-R, which are quite culture-bound.
A specific example of cultural test bias was noted in a recent study of
bilingual and monolingual Chinese American children (Hsieh & Tori,
1993). An item in the Riddles subtest of the Kaufman Assessment Battery
for Children (K-ABC) asks, "What is made from beans, is brewed, and is
often drunk by grownups at breakfast?" In responding, a number of
bilingual children gave the culturally relevant answer, "soybean milk,"
rather than the technically correct response, "coffee."

Strictly speaking, there is no such thing as a culture-free test.
Modification of American-normed tests may be necessary when working
with monolingual Chinese-speaking patients. Choice of testing materials
and techniques for administration must take the patient's cultural context into consideration. For example, an item on the NCSE requires a
patient to explain how a rose and a tulip are similar. Because tulips are
not popular flowers in China, this item may not be clear to some
Chinese patients. In this case, "lily" may replace "tulip." An additional
item assessing a patient's response to an emergency situation asks,
"What would you do if you came home and found that a broken pipe
was flooding the kitchen?" This item may not make sense to a Chinese
patient residing in a small, cluttered Chinatown rooming house with

only the barest kitchen facilities. An alternative to modifying the testing items described earlier would include either or both of the following: developing new tests which are culturally relevant to this specific population or empirically deriving new norms for currently used tests which are specific to Chinese-speaking patients.

Hsieh, Zhang, and Riley (1996) have been working toward this goal by developing new norms on some of the neuropsychological tests. Following their initial collection of Chinese norms, Hsieh and colleagues collected data on a group of attentionally related tasks, including the Color Trails Test; Trail-Making Test, Part A; SDMT; and Digit Span Subtest of the WAIS-RC. Importantly, they extended the age range of subjects, and were able to stratify Chinese norms by age, sex, and educational level. Also in progress is a normative study for neuropsychological performance in children. In collaboration with Manuel Sedo, data are also being collected for the Five Digit Test. This test in an analog of the Stroop procedure, modified in a manner that allows administration to non-English-speaking populations.

Providing Feedback

Providing feedback from a neuropsychological assessment to the patient and family can be challenging. The amount of information the clinician should give depends on the patient's level of education and need. Most people do not like to hear about their own deficits; as such, a patient's strengths should always be addressed, regardless of his or her level of impairment. A review of strengths might include such things as the patient's compliance during testing, residual ability to write his or her own name, ability to take a bus on familiar routes, or good family support. I employ a "sandwich" approach, which begins with an introduction emphasizing the patient's strengths. Then I address limitations and provide recommendations to accommodate these limitations. I close the feedback session with a recap of strengths. My goal is to provide the patient and family with hope and to offer specific guidelines which the family and the patient can pursue together.

Frequently, at the conclusion of a neuropsychological evaluation, the clinician makes treatment or referral recommendations: to a day treatment center for social skills retraining; to a physician for medical consultation; to an individual, group, or family therapist; or to a rehabilitation facility for cognitive rehabilitation, behavioral management, and/or speech therapy. Clinicians need to anticipate resistance to these suggestions on the part of the patient or family. For example, the son of a testing patient responded to recommendations in the following way: "My father has always been like this. There is nothing wrong with him. I don't believe that what you suggest would help him." It is critical that resistance to recommendations be addressed and explored. In the previous case, the son revealed that he believed that he had been abused by his father during childhood. In addition, the patient's son felt he was being discriminated against by mainstream U.S. culture. As a psychologist trained in the United States, I was a target for his projected anger. Despite my ability to speak Chinese, he believed that I was incapable of understanding his pain. Only after the clinician addresses resistance can constructive therapeutic goals be agreed on and followed.

CONCLUSION

Neuropsychology has been recognized as a clinical subspecialty in the field of clinical psychology. Proficiency requires years of training, ongoing consultation, and continuing education to keep abreast of new developments. Neuropsychological skills include the ability to identify cognitive impairments quantitatively and qualitatively, to recognize obvious as well as subtle deficits, and to make appropriate recommendations specifically tailored to patients' needs and available resources.

In summary, when working with monolingual Chinese-speaking patients who reside in the United States, it is important to engage these patients' full cooperation, to solicit family members' participation, to monitor the testing process carefully (particularly when an interpreter is being used), to select relevant testing materials, to make appropriate modifications in test administration, to maintain a flexible approach in the testing room, and to provide feedback effectively. In addition, clinicians must be culturally aware and sensitive, taking into account a given patient's cultural context.

Although there is an urgent need for culturally relevant and empirically normed tests, specifically designed for monolingual Chinese-speaking patients, it will take a long time to accomplish this goal. In the meantime, it is necessary to address the current level of need for neuropsychological assessment within this population. I hope that suggestions made in this chapter will be helpful to clinicians seeking to address this goal.

REFERENCES

Brown, L., Sherbenou, R. J., & Johnsen, S. K. (1990). *Test of Nonverbal Intelligence* (2nd ed.). Austin, TX: PRO-ED.

Hsieh, S. J., Zhang, Y. C., & Riley, N. (1996). *Normative performance in the People's Republic of China: Preliminary data for five tests.* Poster presentation at the 16th annual conference of the National Academy of Neuropsychology, New Orleans.

Hsieh, S. L. J., & Tori, C. D. (1993). Neuropsychological and cognitive effects of Chinese language instruction. *Perceptual and Motor Skills, 77,* 1071–1081.

Leark, R. A., Dupuy, T. R., Greenberg, L. M., Kindschi, C., & Corman, C. L. (1996). *Test of Variables of Attention.* Los Alamitos, CA: Universal Attention Disorders.

Lezak, M. D. (1995). *Neuropsychological assessment* (3rd ed.). New York: Oxford University Press.

22

The Dynamics of Cultural and Power Relations in Group Therapy

PHILIP TSUI

There are two significant impediments to conducting effective psychotherapy with culturally different clients. One is the failure on the part of the therapist to recognize cultural differences and apply therapeutically appropriate interventions. The other, which is more insidious and detrimental to the therapeutic process, is the tendency for therapists (and other clients in the case of group work) to project their subconscious cultural stereotypes onto clients. Such projections, coupled with clients' reactions to them, set up a vicious cycle of confusion, frustrations, and unspoken resentment between therapists and clients, inevitably undermining any chance of therapeutic rapport and success in treatment. Nowhere is this kind of vicious cycle more evident and its effect more pernicious than in group psychotherapy. This chapter outlines how such an antitherapeutic process can take place; using Asian clients as a case in point. It also discusses how therapists can avoid, or break, such vicious cycles.

CULTURAL DIFFERENCES AND POWER RELATIONS

In my experience running both homogeneous Asian groups and mixed groups with a majority of Caucasians and a small Asian minority, Asian clients in the homogeneous groups report having benefited from the group therapy as much as Caucasians in mixed groups. These homogeneous Asian groups include American- and foreign-born Chinese, Filipinos, and Vietnamese with various levels of acculturation to U.S. society. Asian clients in the mixed groups reported less benefit from the group process in comparison to Asians in homogeneous groups and to their fellow Caucasian group members. The Asian clients in the mixed group are the only ones who seem to vigorously question the value of their involvement in groups.

One of the major differences between the two types of groups is that in the homogeneous Asian groups, the therapist has to provide a bit more direction and structuring of the group process in the early phase of the therapy experience. This difference can be accounted for by the fact that although the group process is not at all alien to many Asian cultures, as evidenced by the existence and the vibrancy of village councils, mutual aid societies, and Asian cultural enclaves in almost every metropolitan area in this country, these groups often operate under the acknowledged leadership and direction of authority figures selected on the basis of expertise, seniority, position, or status. Many Asian clients find alien the ambiguity in "Western" therapy groups when there is an authority figure (the therapist) and yet the group is run in a quasi-democratic manner with the therapist implicitly in charge but rarely explicitly acknowledging himself or herself as being in charge. Once the homogeneous Asian groups receive the clear message that the therapist is in charge, and are given some guidelines regarding the purpose and the ground rules of the group, the group members seem to carry on quite well. One of the explicit ground rules is that the therapist is the boundary keeper and moderator, as well as a participant observer.

The ambiguity surrounding who is in charge in Caucasian-dominated groups is often the source of discomfort and anxiety for Asian members who are less acculturated to U.S. society. Because many Asians have already experienced the imbalance of power, wealth, and status vis-à-vis Caucasians in the larger society, the therapy group as a microcosm of U.S. society further accentuates, if not amplifies, such an imbalance (Tsui & Schultz, 1988). The lack of clear definition of authority in the group, in fact, causes Asian clients to worry about who will guard the interpersonal boundaries between them and the more powerful group members, who will protect their rights as a member of a small minority, and who will mediate the interactions between them and the more powerful others.

THE ISSUE OF SAFETY IN GROUPS

Compounding this problem is the reality that many of the Asian clients lived under the rule of Communism, where groups were used as instruments of social control, and where the group leader was often a Communist Party official and an informant was planted in every social or work group in every factory, village, or neighborhood association. Group criticism was often dreaded because it could lead to deprivation of social status, loss of job, public humiliation, exile, imprisonment, or physical harm. Given the lack of role clarity, the reflective style of many psychodynamically oriented therapists may appear duplicitous to Asian clients. The therapist, on the other hand, can easily regard the lack of participation and the constricted affect of these clients as expression of "resistance," a defensive maneuver which the therapist needs to confront and interpret (Flapan & Fenchel, 1987). Clients experience such confrontations and inappropriate interpretations, no matter how cautious, as forms of intrusion and persecution. Such a pernicious dynamic understandably might prevent many Asian clients from participating fully and comfortably in either homogeneous Asian groups or mixed racial groups. Adding this dynamic to the issue of power imbalance in mixed racial groups, as mentioned earlier, would make Asian clients doubly guarded and withdrawn in such groups.

The social withdrawal and guardedness of Asian clients often trigger cultural stereotypes in the minds of some therapists and other group members that Asians are intrinsically quiet, inscrutable, and clannish. After a few attempts by the therapist to engage Asian members with marginal success, the nonresponsiveness or silence of the Asian members may become a source of frustration and even annoyance for the rest of the group. Without much feedback as to how the Asian clients are feeling about and experiencing the group process, the therapist and other clients can easily feel that they must walk on egg shells and watch their words, and that the Asian clients are passing silent judgment on their every utterance.

This kind of situation is difficult to tolerate over a long period. The therapist may become anxious and decide to redouble his or her efforts to engage the Asian clients. Some clients may verbalize their resentment of the Asian clients as being noncontributing to the group process. Some group members may even project anger, hostility, and frustrations, sometimes more related to their own previous failure in relating to others than to the silence of the Asian clients, by accusing the Asians of being silently judgmental. The assertiveness of the therapist in engaging the Asian clients in this context ends up setting the stage for these clients to be derogated and scapegoated. Sensing the onslaught of attacks, some Asian clients may become more withdrawn, feeling that their earlier concern about group persecution based on their experience living under Communism has indeed been validated. Fearing that outright verbal defense on their part might lead to their annihilation by the group, they might respond to the others' comments tangentially or obliquely. The Asian clients might also divert the conversation to a safer, often intellectual subject, or they might even engage in superficial self-disclosures just to keep the others at arm's length.

Some self-acknowledged "culturally sensitive" group members often play peacemaker at this point, rescuing the group by bringing up cultural concerns and engaging both Asian and non-Asian clients in intellectual discussions on issues such as global cultural understanding, findings of anthropological studies, and history of intergroup relations in the United States. Well-intentioned therapists, eager to demonstrate their cultural competence, might express pervasive concern and hovering curiosity about the Asian clients' cultural backgrounds. Such excessive and ambivalent cultural curiosity, as Gorkin (1987) pointed out, is actually a significant countertransference problem on the part of the therapists. Nevertheless, in the end, peace and order in the group are restored. Group members and therapists alike may even congratulate themselves for making progress in mutual understanding when, in reality, no productive therapeutic work has been accomplished.

ANTITHERAPEUTIC IMPLICATIONS OF LINGUISTIC MISUNDERSTANDINGS

A significant problem in both individual and group therapy when the therapist does not speak the native language of the Asian clients is misunderstanding. Many Asian clients for whom English is their second language do not think in English; they often formulate their thoughts in their native tongue, and then translate them into English before expressing them. Many Asian languages are a lot more metaphorical in nature than the English language, with the expression of thoughts embedded in metaphors, idioms, proverbs, and imageries. The more educated the Asian clients in their native language, the more frequently they adopt such metaphorical modes of expression. Without an understanding of the historical, cultural, and linguistic contexts of such expressions, the therapist and other group members may find them "awfully concrete," "odd," "crazy" or "off the wall." Somewhat stunned and confused by such "unusual" or "weird" utterances, non-Asian members of the therapy group may choose to avoid and ignore such comments and move on as if nothing has been said.

One common response of both group members and therapists to interpret the Asian client's statements based on their own cultural experience. Thus, I have seen the therapist and a few of the more "psychologically sophisticated" clients in a group interpret a female Chinese client's comment about having "heart pain" after the departure of both of her sons to college as a form of somatization, which then require them to assist this client to come up with some insight on the subconscious cause of such disorder. Others hurried to speak for the client and discussed among themselves as to what the client could have meant. With "heart" in Chinese being conceived metaphorically as the seat of all emotions, all the client was saying was that she was experiencing emotional distress as a result of the loss of and separation from her sons. However, the responses of the group and the therapist left the client feeling unheard, confused, and attacked. I should point out that the phenomenon of non-Asian clients coming to the rescue of "fragile," "meek" Asian females by speaking for them and by impatiently interpreting what they could have said occurs frequently in the group process.

PITFALLS OF CULTURAL SIMILARITY

The cultural similarity of Asian therapists to their clients creates different set of issues in the treatment process. The Asian therapist may evoke the memory of persecution in groups while the Asian clients were living under Communism more so than a Caucasian therapist would. Also, the Asian therapist is more easily tempted to use his or her own cultural and acculturation experience in North America as the cultural norm, the yardstick in evaluating the validity of the client's experience without careful understanding of the client's feeling within the proper group and relational contexts. This form of projection on the part of the therapist is often more difficult to identify and to recognize and may be perceived, at best, as benign authoritarianism—more of what the client experienced in his or her home country.

To understand the dynamic of the interaction of the Asian therapist–Asian client pair, an analysis of the "minority identity development model," as summarized by Sue (1981), in the context of group therapy would be helpful in elucidating the complexity of the issue. I believe that this model is applicable to both Asian immigrants and Asian Americans.

In the "conformity" stage of the client's struggle to form a new self-identity vis-à-vis the majority culture the client tends to have a strong preference for the majority culture and to use Caucasian Americans as a reference group. Clients identify the majority culture as good because it holds the promise of a better life and liberation from the victim position they often experience. These clients may act out their cultural ambivalence in groups by siding with Caucasian clients excessively, denigrating what other Asian clients have to say, and often competing with the Asian group therapist to demonstrate to themselves that they are more acculturated in the majority culture than the therapist is. The therapist's interpretation of such behavior in groups only encourages more defensiveness on the part of these clients. The therapist should patiently allow the group process to evolve without engaging these clients in unnecessary arguments. The building up of resentment by other Asian clients who are on the receiving end of these projections and the confusion on the part of the Caucasian clients regarding these clients' overidentification with them will eventually provide opportunities for discussion on these issues, allowing the possibility for these clients to own up to their projections and gain some insight into their own struggle to forge a new identity within the dominant culture.

Sue (1981) calls the next stages "dissonance" and "resistance and immersion." Clients at these stages often question the value of the majority culture, possess some insights regarding the seamy side of the racial and cultural stratification in U.S. society, and have renewed motivation to get in touch with their cultural roots. Such clients can conceivably become quite withdrawn and often maintain a quiet, cynical attitude toward the Asian therapist as a representative of the oppressive majority culture, a "sellout" to the white establishment. They may also become zealous in imposing what they understand as valuable in the "Asian cultures" on what other Asian clients have to say, while ignoring the real content of what the other clients are expressing. Direct confrontation or interpretation of their behavior by the Asian therapist would only further polarize the group in a nonproductive and divisive manner. The Asian therapist needs to role model for the whole group his or her respect for all cultural backgrounds and maintain focus on the "here and now" issues (Yalom, 1985), staying with the current feelings evoked by the interpersonal dynamic of the group rather than being drawn into political polemics with these clients. By assisting other Asian clients and non-Asian clients to safely express their sentiments pertaining to these clients and by acting nondefensively, the Asian therapist can help them come to terms with the agony related to their cultural confusion and uncertainty about their self-identity.

At the third and fourth stages of the minority identity development model (the "introspective" and "synergetic, articulation, and awareness" stages), these clients, having examined carefully over time—through intellectual understanding and life experience—the merits and problems of their cultural heritage, as well as that of the majority culture, have come to terms with the cultural conflict within themselves. They have achieved a certain degree of cultural integration in their world views and personality structures. The pitfall for an Asian therapist and this type of Asian client is the tendency for them to overidentify with each other. The Asian therapist may succumb to the temptation of allowing these clients to assume the role of "co-therapist" vis-à-vis the other Asian clients, thus avoiding and neglecting the personal issues that these clients might have brought with them into the group. The sense of "we-ness" between the therapist and these clients can easily generate feelings of envy, jealousy, competition, and rivalry within the group. To avoid these problems, the Asian therapist needs to consciously maintain an appropriate boundary with this type of client without severing the empathetic bond between therapist and client. Yet, steadfastly, the therapist should focus these clients' attention on their own interpersonal issues and the content of the feelings afloat in the group context.

INTERGROUP COMPARISON

Three possible group contexts exist for group therapy with Asian clients. The first is groups with Asian clients in the minority and non-Asian clients (primarily Caucasians) in the majority. The second is homogeneous Asian groups, and the third is homogeneous Asian groups of one particular ethnic background (e.g., all Chinese or all Cambodian). Both the homogeneous Asian groups and the homogeneous Asian ethnic groups present with specific benefits and pitfalls.

As mentioned earlier, the mixed Asian/non-Asian groups often create role confusion and the associated anxiety for the Asian clients. Homogeneous Asian groups have the tendency to replicate the more clearly defined role differentiation of status, class, and gender in the members' cultures of origin. Although such replication offers clients a certain degree of comfort with the familiar, it often impedes in-depth discussion of clients' sentiments because many clients feel that it is "inappropriate" for them to act outside their role expectations. An open discussion of such "inappropriate" feelings might well be most important because one of the central issues of treatment is how such Asian clients can define themselves as part of the larger society and at the same time retain a certain degree of cultural identity and a consolidated sense of self. In this context, Asian clients could easily bring up and analyze the significant issue of redefinition of being Asian, being American, and being themselves with their own sense of who they are and their own "personal" set of problems, issues, and identity. It is beneficial for Asian clients to discuss such issues of cultural and personal identity in group where there is automatic and implicit understanding and shared concern. However, how are group members expected to discuss their resentment of being repressed by the authoritarian nature of the informal power structure of the Vietnamese community and their dependency on the same power structure for support and guidance in negotiating with the mysterious white society with all its unwritten cultural and bureacratic rules when their former commanding general in the South Vietnamese army is a member of the group? How is a Japanese woman going to express her anger toward her husband and his family for keeping mistresses and neglecting family support when she knows that many of the Asian men in the same group have similar attitudes as her husband and their cultures of origin often tolerate or grant implicit support to such attitudes? It is extremely difficult to feel safe, not to mention trusting, under this set of circumstances. What is it like to be a Korean woman who was forced into the role of "comfort lady" by the Japanese army during World War II with Japanese men of her same age range sitting in the group?

This issue of confidentiality and boundaries is even more acute in groups in which all members have the same ethnic background. Many Caucasian group members can return to their own respective walks of life and, consequently, disappear into anonymity, but a Cambodian group member will have to face the same Cambodian group members on almost a daily basis given the small size of the community and his or her ongoing reliance on this community for support and nurturance. How is a former Vietnamese civilian going to deal with a group member who is a former South Vietnamese official without experiencing retraumatization when her central issue was her brutalization and torture by former government officials who suspected she was a Vietcong spy?

Group therapists must have a heightened sensitivity to such issues. Working through these issues in the group process is precisely the reason for the existence of such groups, because it will enable group members of similar or identical cultural backgrounds to genuinely support each other and to confront, reconcile, and overcome many of the issues they face in their own interpersonal relationships and in their relationships with others in U.S. society.

However, creating such homogeneous groups in itself is a difficult task. It is often necessary to start the group with a concrete focus, assisting group members to work on an issue of common concern (e.g., the citizenship application process). Only when group members experience each other in an instrumental role as helpful persons and as people rather than actors in certain roles can the therapy group have a chance of becoming more process-oriented. I recommend such a beginning because jumping into a discussion of personal issues and past traumas right away can either turn the group into a seminar on some universal theme (e.g., injustice in the world) or turn it into a terribly uncomfortable situation to which group members will not return for further treatment.

It is also important for the group therapist to assume a more "authoritarian" role in dictating the rule of confidentiality and enforcing the boundaries of the group. Once the group is formed, it is important to avoid the admission of new members until an extended period of time has elapsed. A specified open-enrollment period in the future can be determined ahead of time and communicated to the group members so that they have an idea of how much time they will have to work with each other until their newly developed "envelop of safety" is broached. Although there is no practical way to prevent what is discussed in the group from becoming "gossip" in the various Asian communities, the group therapist needs to bring up this issue of breach of confidentiality whenever it is brought to his or her attention. Bringing up a specific breach of confidentiality in the group does not mean confronting specific group members in public. Outright shaming of a group member for his or her "misdeed" is clinically counterproductive and destructive to the group norm of safety and trust. Discussing the violation of confidence as a group norm with reference to certain incidents provides the appropriate and necessary group sanction and generates the kind of support the "victim" of such violation feels is due him or her and restores to some degree his or her faith in the group process. Some therapists might object to such an approach, fearing that it will reenact the more rigid role definitions in many Asian cultures and, consequently, impede free-flowing conversations of emotional content. I have found that such a move has a paradoxical effect on the group process. When the group therapist in a homogeneous group exerts such a sense of control, it actually frees the group members from the need to stick to the security of their own perceived cultural roles.

SOME GUIDELINES FOR GROUP THERAPISTS

It is quite clear that cultural similarity does not exempt a therapist from an in-depth understanding of the evolution of the development of cultural identity and from safeguarding against the significant issues of countertransference resulting from cultural affinity. It is important in working with Asian clients in groups to focus on the idea that the group is a laboratory for social learning, because this idea is quite consistent with many Asian cultural values that view group experiences as an educational process. At the same time, the therapist must acknowledge on an ongoing basis these clients' concern for personal safety and act assertively to protect these clients from the aggressive acting-out behaviors of their fellow group members, be they Asian or non-Asian. Allowing the reenactment of the horrible experience of "group criticism" some of these clients have experienced under Communist or other authoritarian regimes would be very detrimental to the group process and would inappropriately retraumatize these clients. It is also quite clear that, especially in racially and culturally mixed groups, truly culturally sensitive therapists must become assertive enough to prevent themselves and group members from speaking for the Asian clients, from projecting their personal issues and cultural biases on to the Asian clients as the result of the group's and the therapist's anxiety generated by the cultural differences. Cultural sensitivity does not include treating Asian clients as if they are fragile by nature and need to be treated with excessive caution. Unnecessary avoidance or protection of a client commonly arises from the therapist's own sense of vulnerability or the activation of his or her stereotype of Asians being helpless, fragile, and inarticulate. The therapist's impatience, excessive confrontation, and overinterpretation of the Asian client's behaviors might be the projection of the therapist's own sense of frustration, helplessness, loss of control, and fear of the exposure of his or her own cultural ignorance. Such behaviors on the part of the therapist end up encouraging other group members to ignore or to devalue the Asian members.

The group therapist needs to understand that any racial and culturally mixed group, especially one with Caucasians in the majority, is a microcosm of the larger society, with its unequal distribution of power among different racial and cultural groups. Allowing group norms to evolve while remaining passive amounts to permitting the development of a group process characterized by dominance of the majority—with neither the majority nor the minorities making any therapeutic gains.

In this chapter, Asian clients are used as a case in point to illustrate how cultural differences and the power dynamics of intergroup relations in U.S. society can be played out in the group process, in the absence of the active intervention of the group therapist.

Whether the therapist is working with a homogeneous Asian group or a mixed racially and cultural group, it is important to set ground rules at the onset that clearly define the therapist's benevolent authoritative role. It is necessary to provide active intervention to prevent or to understand the projection of cultural stereotypes and personal issues activated by such stereotypes. Asian therapists need to guard vigilantly their own cultural projections on to or overidentification with their Asian clients. These are the essential tasks of a therapist in working with Asian or other minority clients in the group context.

REFERENCES

Flapan, D., & Fenchel, G. H. (1987). *The developing ego and the emergence of self in group therapy.* New York: Jason Aronson.

Gorkin, M. (1987). *The uses of countertransference.* New York: Jason Aronson.

Sue, D. W. (1981). *Counseling the culturally different.* New York: Wiley.

Tsui, P., & Schultz, G. (1988, January). Ethnic factor in the group process: Cultural dynamics in multi-ethnic therapy groups. *American Journal of Orthopsychiatry, 58,* 136–137.

Yalom, I. (1985). *The theory and practice of group psychotherapy* (3rd ed.). New York: Basic Books.

23

Psychological Testing of Monolingual Asian American Clients

JENNIE YEE

This chapter examines the testing issues presented by adult monolingual Asians who are immigrants and living in the United States. The specific subgroups of Asians I discuss are the Chinese, Vietnamese, Cambodian, and other Southeast Asians. I do not discuss children and adolescents. Critical issues, theories, and suggestions expressed in this chapter are primarily based on my 14 years of experience with psychological testing of monolingual Asians. Because I have tested large numbers of Chinese, more of the discussion covers this group. This chapter examines some of the assessment research pertaining to this group and explores problems in the process. Testing procedure and evaluation rely on a broad and culturally unique approach, encompassing the preparation process, development of rapport, selection of tests, and their application and interpretation. The emphasis during testing is on how to analyze subtle complex confounding variables. Specifically, this chapter reviews such factors as the clinic and testing culture, motivation, test content validity, and styles of learning.

Cross-cultural variation in psychological assessment of intelligence, psychopathology, and personality has been researched and reported for many minority groups, especially Hispanic/Mexican Americans and African Americans. However, the meaning behind the differences is not as clear. Less research has been conducted with Asians and Asian Americans, especially monolingual Asians. Because of the swelling numbers of the Asian/Pacific Islander population since 1980, it is now compelling for psychologists to engage in this type of research and testing. Historically, whites have been ranked as worthy versus not especially in white versus black research (e.g., Noh, Avison, & Kaspar, 1992; Frydman & Lynn, 1989). Other races also are judged by the standards of the majority society and are not given the benefit of being measured against their own reference groups. For instance, Western cultures stress intellectual achievement and problem solving over social/interpersonal skills (Sattler, 1974). Jones and Thorne (1987) point out how minorities have been considered psychologically deficient in intellectual performance, personality, and social functioning. Perez-Arce (1992), as well as other psychologists, has raised the question of whether the constructs used in tests are equivalent and fair. For example, schizophrenia and depression are considered universal psychiatric disorders and diagnostic categories; how these symptoms manifest may vary across cultures. Because Asians are a very heterogeneous group, they present universal disorders in different frequencies and patterns. An example of how Asian groups tend to describe depression in their own lexicon highlights this problem. What Western culture describes as "sad or feeling down" may be expressed as "problems with sleeping, eating, feeling tired, numb, irritable, low in spirit and having headaches or stomachaches" for Asians. These symptoms are primarily somatic and clinicians have complained about being stymied in diagnosing the client as depressed, psychosomatic, or physically ill. Brandt and Boucher (1986) call these clusters "depression-type words." Thus, norms need to be developed for different cultural groups as a function of the validity and reliability of a test. It is also imperative that clinicians not misdiagnose or ignore specific meaningful clusters of symptoms.

CONSTRAINTS OF TESTING

It is an enormous task to assess monolingual adults because of the constraining and moderating variables of language, age, education, socio-economic status, immigration stress, and amount of exposure to a new cultural and educational environment. Asian community mental health centers serve populations in the lower economic stratums who endure multiple environmental/adaptational problems of poverty, unemployment, and language limitations. Adult and elderly immigrants have diverse language and cultural backgrounds. Educational achievement may range from zero to college level, clustering more on the low end. Often, their previous work may have been restricted to more basic and practical skills, such as farming, fishing, and other nonintellectual professions. With little education or opportunity to learn, their ability to initiate and complete the test protocol would be remarkable because lower education produces lower performances on these tests. Many protocols are partial, adjusted for the particular client with educational, language, and visuomotor limitations. In the setting where I work, multiple Asian groups immigrate from all over the world and speak diverse languages. Measuring the language and verbal functions of monolingual Asians can be particularly frustrating and challenging because literacy differs from urban to rural regions, with illiteracy more prominent in the former (Lezak, 1976; Sattler, 1974). Also, specific speech problems are hard to discern when the dialect can be one of hundreds. Without linguistic facility, immigrants cannot adequately obtain everything they need for basic survival in the new country. Thus, large numbers of refugees and immigrants are unable to gain access to employment and fall prey to severe depression, posttraumatic disorders, and other psychiatric disorders.

PROBLEMS WITH TRANSLATED TESTS

Few bilingual Asian American psychologists who conduct psychological testing are available to the low-income immigrant population. Even when a bilingual psychologist can conduct the assessment, he or she may not be reading literate in, for example, Chinese, or may speak a dialect such as Mandarin or Shanghainese, not common in the low-socioeconomic-status community. Translated tests that are applicable for general intelligence and for emotional functioning need to be standardized and normed with monolingual and bilingual Asians. Translated versions of standard tests are scarce and limited. Following are some of the traditional adult tests that have been translated into Chinese:

>   Wechsler Adult Intelligence Scale (WAIS). There is a mainland Chinese version (Wechsler, 1955) and a Cantonese translation (Chan et al., 1977, 1979), WAIS-RC, revised for China (Gong, 1982).

>   Minnesota Multiphasic Personality Inventory (MMPI). There is a Chinese revision developed for China by the National MMPI Coordinating Group (1982) and tested in Hong Kong and China.

>   Beck Depression Inventory (BDI). This test has been translated into multiple languages by the Psychological Corporation.

>   Rorschach and Thematic Apperception Test (TAT). A Chinese translation has been reported by Abel and Hsu (1949) and a Japanese translation has been reported by De Vos (1955). These tests can easily be translated into other languages.

Rotter's Incomplete Sentences (Rotter & Rafferty, 1950). This test can be translated into Asian languages.

Wide Range Achievement Test (WRAT). The arithmetic section can be used for Asian cultures that have learned the Western numerical system.

Other tests such as the Bender–Gestalt Visual–Motor Test (Bender, 1938), the Benton Visual–Motor Retention Test (BVRT; Benton, 1963), and Raven's Standard Progressive Matrices (SPM; Raven, 1938) test have been easily translated because less verbal or written instruction was required.

Many of these tests have been revised, but the original tests are used because translated versions exist.

USE OF TRANSLATORS

When using translators, the clinician should consider several factors: The translator, who is usually the client's therapist or another clinician, is rarely a psychologist. Often, the translator is the only person available who can speak the specific dialect required. An inexperienced person who lacks familiarity with test materials, procedures, and style of test prompting may contaminate the examinee's responses and test results. The translator should be well-trained prior to testing and should be made aware of the constraints of the structured test format and instructed not to aid the examinee with verbal cues or gestures on specific tasks. I usually ask translators to write down verbatim what the client is reporting and when possible I do the same. Then I match what I have written with their version. The translator and the psychologist/tester can both report nonverbal reactions and verbal side remarks.

Translators help in the process of obtaining test results that offer at least some indication of the patient's problems rather than none. Multiple dialects complicate the process of obtaining an appropriate translator. Again, the clinician must weigh the pros and cons according to how important and necessary the psychological assessment will be for treatment decisions and/or to help the client qualify for appropriate resources (social security disability insurance, medical treatment, occupational rehabilitation, neuropsychological testing, etc.).

CULTURAL DIFFERENCES AND BIASES IN TESTING

A therapist's biases and cultural world view can contribute to how he or she rates a client in diagnosis and severity of disturbance. A study

comparing white and Chinese American therapists' empathy and perceptions of normality found differences between these two groups and how
they rated the same clients. More White therapists rated Chinese American subjects higher on a Depression/Inhibition cluster and lower on a
Social Poise/Interpersonal Capacity cluster in comparison to white subjects (Li-Repac, 1980). The same dynamics can occur in the testing
process.

Biases in tests occur when expectations of similarities across culture
operate under false assumptions. Diverse Asian groups from all parts of
the world transport to the United States their own beliefs, rituals, and
practices, which are often considered primitive and odd by some Americans. For example, many Asian subgroups practice what is called "coin-
ing," *cao gio* or *gat sah,* a specific healing technique where you rub the
skin energetically with a coin or spoon. Adults and children have been
mistakenly identified as physically abused because of the red marks on
their body caused by this treatment. Misinterpretations can lead to
dramatic and unwarranted results. Other beliefs include folk healing with
use of herbal medicines and acupuncture and religious or philosophical
beliefs in ancestor-worship, reincarnation, ghosts, and possession involving ablution rituals.

However, the culture of psychological testing is experienced as
atypical and very novel by many Asians. Factors such as interactional
behavior (with examiner), appearance, and sense of time can be very
different and unique. There is such a phrase known as "Chinese time,"
whereby the client arrives at the clinic 1 hour late. The phrase is typically
made in jest but nevertheless captures the concept that punctuality and
speed are not considered important for Asians under certain circumstances, so timed and speeded tests often cause anxiety and at times
paralysis. Many Chinese clients have told me that they find the Americans'
"rush-rush" lifestyle puzzling. Urbanized Asians may fare better with
cognitive tasks than their rural cohorts because of their opportunity to
obtain education and to become more familiar with structured intellectual
tasks. This experience does not hold true with projective personality tests,
which are discussed later.

As a result of long-term oppressive political experiences in their
countries of origin, Southeast Asian refugees and other immigrants may
have developed a natural suspicion toward authorities who work for the
government agencies. Thus, their test-taking attitude may appear more
skewed and pathological, especially with projective tests. By the same
token, Western society assumes that writing and drawing are similar
natural skills for all cultures, but in reality the bases are structurally and
stylistically different. In place of the alphabet system, Chinese and many
other Asians practice a symbolic character system in which 3,000 characters must be visually memorized to have a working vocabulary. The writing

layout starts spatially from the right to the left side of the page. In addition, many words have multiple tones, each with a different meaning. What they are asked to write or draw (e.g., geometric shapes) may not be within their realm of knowledge. The Hmong, who are a subgroup of the Laotian and are from a mountain region, have a specific visual experience and perspective that does not include familiarity with pens and paper for writing and drawing, so that when they are tested they may not perform well. Skills such as these may not be sufficiently learned or practiced and can produce a test profile with a lot of scatter subject to misinterpretations (Sattler, 1974). Also, Western society often stresses intellectual tasks over manual skills; thus, rural subcultures suffer on cognitively oriented tests.

With projective tests, reluctance, resistance, anger, or verbal constriction may surface because a testing or learning context does not usually stress creativity and imagination. In China, control over emotions and compliance to the norm are dictated. If an individual is too deviant or spontaneous, he or she is thought to be losing equilibrium within society. When personal or family issues are raised, again reluctance and feelings of shame or suspicion may be aroused because these concerns are considered very private, not to be expressed in public.

RESEARCH ON PSYCHOLOGICAL TESTS WITH ASIANS

A review of the literature for the past 15 to 20 years found few studies on tests used with monolingual Asians. Some of this research and the premise for using conventional tests are discussed. Many psychologists have debated the value of measuring intellectual capabilities for the purpose of defining overall competence (McClelland, 1973; Goleman, 1981; Yee, 1983). They feel that intelligence tests were unfair to minorities and that "competencies" would be better in predicting occupational placement and job performance. Others argue against that premise. Disputes around how to estimate intelligence range from looking at the combination of genetics and environment (Eysenck, 1991; Scarr & Weinberg, 1978) to emphasizing its malleability to environmental factors, such as the quality of education and the home situation (Angoff, 1988; Eysenck, 1991; Gould, 1981; Tuddenham, 1948. Gould (1981) debunks the idea that intelligence can be ranked as a single entity. His argument is that research can be subjective and based on the majority social, cultural, economic, and political context. He continues to remind us that Binet stressed using tests as a way of defining the areas of learning difficulty and of offering supplemental help. What can we deduce from these theories? Certainly that intelligence tests are still being used and many times misused. Often teachers and testers may have a "self-fulfilling prophecy" attitude which prejudges a student/client and, therefore, provides lower-quality instruction or limited or skewed interpretations. Jones and Zoppel (1979, cited in Jones & Thorne, 1987) feel that "standard assessment instruments are more valid for minorities who [have] achieved middle-class status than for the working-class or poor" (p. 490). Thus, diagnosticians and researchers need to use universal and standardized criteria effectively by considering the appropriate moderating variables for proper comparative cross-cultural studies (Mann et al., 1991).

Creating specific tests for specific races and cultures can be daunting. Jones and Thorne (1987) suggest that the "construction of new norms for conventional measures or the development of new, culture-specific instruments" (p. 488) must be critically examined in conjunction with using the personal and narrative accounts of subjects. Current test materials have been modified to adjust to the cultural texture and climate of Asians. Many modified and newly constructed tests for Chinese and Southeast Asians have found that certain somatic and physiological symptom clusters represent the universal construct of depression and for a specific constellation, posttraumatic stress disorder (Dao, 1991; Kinzie, Frederickson, Ben, Fleck, & Karls (1980); Kinzie, Manson, Vinh, et al., 1982; Kinzie, Manson, Ades, & Do, 1982; Lin, Masuda, & Tazuma, 1982; Mollica et al., 1986; Chan, 1991). When using standardized and modified tests, caution and care in the interpretation and recommendations are emphasized. Some nonverbal tests have been used for bilinguals and monolinguals (e.g., the Leiter International Performance scale). However, many psychologists feel these tests are still bound to culture and not really culture-fair. Sattler (1974) thinks they measure the middle-class cognitive style of logical and analytical reasoning rather than relational thinking. Problem solving and perception of achievement may also be different in lower-socioeconomic-status groups.

CONVENTIONAL COGNITIVE ABILITY AND PERSONALITY TESTS

The methodological and conceptual reasoning behind intellectual and personality research with Asians has been sharply criticized (Kokka et al., 1975). Can the results convey the "nature of the Asian American sense"? asked Sue and Morishima (1982). A few studies of Asian subjects are discussed here.

Intelligence Tests

A recent cross-cultural study in China used the WAIS-RC developed by Gong (1982) to compare sex differences and intersubtest scatter of Chinese with standard American samples. When the Chinese scatter range was compared to the American, Ryan, Dai, and Paolo (1992) found similar patterns. However, an inverse relationship between years of education and level of intelligence occurred for the Chinese (scatter range decreased as education and intelligence level increased) but not for the U.S. sample (scatter range increased as education and intelligence increased). The authors caution readers to understand that different exposure to educational approaches will lead to different performance patterns on cognitive tests. The ideal educational experience in the United States emphasizes creativity, individualism, and self-expression. Chinese teach students to value the collective society by practicing moderation and restraint, respecting authority and conforming to tradition. The obvious outcome is that as education increases for Chinese, there is more homogeneity in the WAIS-RC scatter and more heterogeneity for Americans (Ryan et al., 1992).

Personality Tests

Much cross-cultural research has reported differences in the personality structure of Asians as compared to Caucasians (Golden, 1978; Jones & Thorne, 1987; Cheung, Song, & Butcher, 1991; Christy, 1978; Song, 1991; Boey, 1985). Other research elucidates the specific moderating variables of social class, education, and so on, which play an important role in the differences (Greene, 1980, 1987, 1991). A few of the popular tests are discussed here.

The early studies of the Rorschach and TAT with Chinese and Japanese (Abel & Hsu, 1949; DeVos, 1955) pointed out specific patterns of rigidity, lack of creative responses, and "overstriving . . . blocking" interpreted as intrapsychic difficulties and inflexible orientation. In some instances the Chinese and Japanese were compared to depressed or catatonic patients. De Vos (1955) interpreted the inability to identify human forms on the inkblots as "lack of positive interpersonal relationships" (p. 245). Subsequent reports by many psychologists criticized the premise of using U.S. norms to judge other cultures as abnormal. Wang, Li, Burstein, and Loucks (1991) conducted a study of 53 Chinese adults in Changsha, Hunan, and 50 U.S. adults in San Antonio, Texas, who met specific criteria for the Rorschach test. They predicted and found differences between the two cultures. Lowered number of responses, lowered movement, color, and human emotion responses appeared in the responses of the Chinese. The study supports culture as a factor in personality development. When confronted with ambiguous materials such as "inkblots," many Asians generally react with anxiety and puzzlement because of their novelty, not because of an inability to free-associate. Color cards on the Rorschach symbolize affect. Asians may react to the red stimulus with a positive response because they believe red represents good luck, happiness, and prosperity. Texture and movement and other scores should also be interpreted with mindfulness to a culture's conception of vague stimuli.

The MMPI has been translated and revised for use with Chinese in Singapore, Hong Kong, and China and with many other Asian groups (Cheung, Song, & Butcher, 1991; Song, 1991, Boey, 1985; Ying, 1990). Discrepancies were noted when Asians were compared with the American norms: Some of the items were unanswerable, difficult, or awkward to answer (Song, 1991) or elevated on scale F (fake–good, fake–bad). The latter was explained as the tendency for Chinese to overendorse on items that are expected and valued by their culture. Cheung, Zhao, and Wu (1992) report 26 clinical studies with the Chinese and subsequently summed up the results of several in which the Chinese MMPI was administered to small samples of psychiatric patients in China. In a Chinese neurotic patient group, the MMPI results were compared with the Chinese norm, the U.S. original norm, and contemporary norm. When the U.S. norm was applied, many of the clinical scales were elevated: scales 2 Depression (D), 8 Schizophrenia (Sc), 7 Psychasthenia (Pt), 6 Paranoia (Pa), and 1 Hypochondriasis (Hs). On the Chinese MMPI, all psychiatric patients elevated on scales 2 (D) and 8 (Sc) consistently. When the criterion cutoff was lowered by using the Chinese norm, elevations on scales 8 (Sc) was eliminated and other clinical scales were only moderately elevated. These results did not show consistency when compared across different norms unless the criterion level was adjusted. Cheung et al. (1992) conducted a larger sample study with 1,112 Chinese neurotic outpatients from diverse age groups (16 to over 40), occupations, and regions in Eastern China. All were literate. Again they found that compared to the U.S. norms, the clinical T score elevations on the Chinese norm were much lower. Thus, they recommend that both the Chinese and American norms be used in the interpretation of the Chinese MMPI due to discrepancies in patterns of elevations. These studies point out more pathology with Chinese patients when using the American norm but, as the authors conclude, due more to cultural disparity than to cohort problems. Few studies of MMPI performances of Asian Americans have been conducted in the United States. Sue and Sue (1974) compared Chinese and Japanese students with white students on the MMPI at a student health psychiatric clinic in a university. Both Asian groups showed higher elevations than their white counterparts. Diagnoses of greater pathology for Asians again may be the ostensible conclusion.

The BDI has been translated into multiple languages for use in many countries. A Chinese version was developed and reported by Chan (1991). In the University of Hong Kong, 331 bilingual students were administered the English and Chinese versions of the BDI. They report that the scale has high internal consistency and both versions correlated significantly with each other. The predictive power of the test to assess psychiatric samples with mixed diagnoses was also relatively good. The BDI seems to have reliability with Chinese and can be used as a diagnostic tool in testing. An adaptation of the BDI for the Hmong examined the psychometric characteristics and the relationship between depression and demographic variables in 123 Hmong refugees ranging in age from 18 to 66 years old (Mouanoutoua, Brown, Cappelletty, & Levine, 1991). This measure was able to differentiate the depressed from nondepressed accurately and proved to be reliable. Interestingly, factors that helped to ameliorate depression appeared to be related to the quality and not quantity of social supports and years of education instead of length of stay in the United States.

ESTABLISHING RAPPORT

The clinic and testing culture can be alienating to many foreign-born Asians, as clinicians have reported. Starting with an initial interview is important to establish a history, lay groundwork, and develop rapport. It is also helpful for the examiner to be of the same race or ethnic background as the client. The tester's age, sex, and status can prevent initial rapport. In some situations, I have introduced myself as Ms. _____, compared dialects, and explained my role. Much of the time I describe myself as a PhD or "Doctor of Philosophy" to older people or males and other women who tend to respond with appropriate acceptance to a teacher/professor status, which is very respected in Asian society regardless of sex or age.

The examiner must respect adults of all ages by calling them Mr., Mrs., or Ms. until they become adjusted to therapy. Younger adults may ask the examiner to call them by their first name. If using a translator, it is best to ask or train a clinician who understands the interactional norms of that culture.

The examiner begins by giving his or her name in proper form and getting the client's name and asking what village, city, or region the client lived in. I have found that a quick bond is formed if the examiner's family happened to have originated from the same area. Examiners should empathize with the client's immigration process and apologize for the inconvenience of having to use a translator. Expressing respect for adults who do not speak English helps those adults to "save face" and to feel more comfortable and less apprehensive with the unfamiliar ambience of testing.

Next, examiners should explain in simple terms *what* the testing is like and *why*. Explaining the purpose of the test is important, especially that it is to help clients understand and orient to a new and sometimes threatening situation and to emphasize their current areas of strengths and difficulties that may be treated by medication or other appropriate means. These approaches will aid in developing the clients' motivation for testing.

For the history, examiners should begin with questions related to basic information and clients' practical experiences. The examiner should ask clients to talk about their immigration experiences, life in the United States, and previous life in their native country (family internetwork, births, deaths, losses, employment, health and healing practices, etc.). The examiner should have clients summarize their premorbid level of functioning (e.g., previous illnesses or hospitalization, any physical impairments, psychiatric symptoms, and overall quality of life). I find that this information may be obtained by administering a daily activities schedule and noting how clients describe their problems and daily adaptive functioning. This history taking provides a valuable tool in gathering information about clients' general flow and coherence of language and how they sequence past and present memory. The emotional quality of the presentation can also be ascertained.

It is difficult to obtain psychiatric, school, or medical information from other countries. For monolingual adults, I have found it useful to interview a family member or friend separately who knows the client best. If such a person is available, his or her version along with the client's, will help to corroborate and establish a premorbid level of functioning and cultural and environmental context. Establishing a premorbid level of functioning is especially valuable when records are missing or unavailable. It would be ideal if testing could provide a more accurate diagnosis, but without a method to estimate the accuracy of these clients' self-reports of multiple and complex symptoms, a conclusive or clear primary diagnosis may be missed or an incorrect diagnosis may be rendered. Without a solid initial understanding of a client's background, the validity of the specific cultural factors and the interpretation of testing is not complete. Only an estimate of a premorbid level of performance can be made.

Life history and background questions to ask both client and family include the following:

1. Education: Approximately how many years or levels of formal education in your native country did you complete (the number of years may not be equivalent to Western standards)?
2. Did you experience births, deaths, and loss of family and friends and when?
3. Were you in the midst of war and did you experience prolonged stress of images and sounds of gunfire, bombing, and the like?

4. How was the immigration process? Was it by sponsorship, escape, or another way?

5. Did the current symptoms emerge recently or a long time ago?

From these questions, clients have digressed into more private and precarious material, such as how they felt about the devastation of war and loss and other emotional aspects of their lives. When clients reach this delicate point, a domino effect may be set off, so the examiner must be careful about preventing or limiting their outpour and reminding them of the purpose of testing. Finally, the examiner should tender reassurance to offset clients' concerns and suspicions about who might see the results.

REASONS FOR REFERRAL

The reasons that a person is referred for psychological assessment in a community mental health outpatient or inpatient setting may vary, but the most common questions raised are the following:

1. What is the differential diagnosis? For example, does the person have schizophrenia or alcohol/drug psychosis, dementia or depression, bipolar or schizophrenic disorder, major psychiatric or organic disorder?

2. Is the person intellectually impaired?

3. What is the course predicted—progressive or acute?

4. Can the person be referred to rehabilitation and be capable of relearning to work?

5. What type of work is appropriate?

These are difficult questions to answer.

The particular Asian population entering community mental health clinics tends to manifest presenting symptoms in higher proportions of severity, intensity, acuteness, and or chronicity (Kinzie, 1981; Mollica, Caspi-Yavin, Bollini, Truong, et al., 1992; Nguyen, 1982; Sue & Morishima, 1982). Thus, the necessity for making a diagnostic differential is a crucial moving force to justify testing and to aid the clinician in assigning proper treatment for a client.

TEST SELECTION

Choosing which test to begin with depends on what the examiner is asked to diagnose. If the referral question is to determine a psychiatric or organic diagnosis, the general traditional battery (excluding neuropsychological tests) would include the Bender–Gestalt Visual–Motor Test, Goodenough–Harris Draw-A-Person Test (DAP; Goodenough, 1963), WAIS-R, TAT and Rorschach, Wechsler Memory Scale, and BVRT. Although the Leiter International Performance Scale and Raven's Progressive Matrices (Raven, 1960)—Standard or Colored have been used for the nonverbal or linguistically limited, they include increasingly complex items which are difficult and not applicable to this Asian group. The Stanford–Binet (Terman & Merrill, 1960, 1973), if translated, can be given to particular groups with lower levels of education and obvious signs of learning impairment. Some school-based psychologists have used the Hiske–Nebraska with children. Adults have also been tested with this measure because it is a nonverbal test for the hearing impaired and normed with non-hearing impaired. This measure has similarities to the Wechsler Intelligence Scale for Children—Revised (WISC-R) Performance section.

The test protocol can be approached by using a functional concept so strengths and weaknesses in behavior and thinking can be identified for survival in the social and environmental contexts. Intellectual functions can be divided into groups to be tested: receptive skills, expressive abilities, verbal and visual memory, attention and concentration and control functions; and how individuals start up, speed up, slow down, and stop; and how such individuals may regulate, modulate, and correct their behavior. Emotional functioning will follow in determining an individual's capacity and strength in ego functioning, how the individual may perceive the world, self-esteem, competence, sense of judgment, reality testing, interpersonal relating, defense mechanisms, affective responding, and personality integration. Some agencies that have the benefit of a multiple service center have used the System of Multicultural Pluralistic Assessment (SOMPA) developed by Mercer 1979 for ages 5 through 11. This test was used to counter misplacement of minority and other subcultural children by IQ test scores. Mercer believed social and cultural experiences contributed to observed differences. The SOMPA integrates medical, social and pluralistic assessments. Medical health, social, adaptive behaviors, and sociocultural background are combined and an estimated learning potential (ELP) is derived. The SOMPA can be applied to adults with an equivalent health profile, self and family information on social adaptiveness, and cultural environmental aspects in their lives. Finally, the familiarity approach can be used by starting with tests that can help the client acclimate to the testing situation. The following sections comprise a compendium of some tests used with monolingual Asians.

Test of Memory Functioning

The Wechsler Memory Scale (Wechsler, 1945) covers orientation and immediate, recent, associative, and visual motor memory. When trans-

lated for Asians, the test must include changes in information regarding history in the United States to items related to their specific country. Memory passages of stories must have similarity in content and number of words. Associations of paired words must also reflect the concept of simple to more complex vocabulary. Because vocabulary is based on a structurally different premise for Asians, a strict translation sometimes does not work. Associative memory can be measured in other ways.

Tests of Visuospatial Functioning

The DAP (Goodenough, 1963) has upper-age norms ending at age 15 but can be used with adults. This test can provide the client's developmental level in spatial and visual ability, but without the experience or opportunity to draw, the results may not mean much unless the examiner (1) understands that the strokes expected by Western standards may not be the same for Asians, (2) uses it as a projective task, and (3) can have the client practice with the instrument and retest to compare results of improvement.

The Bender–Gestalt Visual–Motor Test is the most popular test to use because of its easy and quick administration. It is both a projective test and a visual–spatial task (Bender, 1938). Recently, its use as a projective has been questioned. The directions are simple and an overview of the cutoff scores for brain impairment, psychopathology, and normals can be obtained (Hain, 1964). For Asians with specific drawing limitations, manual dexterity through practice can be learned and observed.

The BVRT (Benton, 1963, 1974) has age norms and estimated IQ available. When IQ is not available, the age norms provide an index of performance ability. This test, again, is a nonverbal task of immediate recall in reproducing geometric designs presented for 5, 10, or 20 seconds and removed. This test can be used in conjunction with the Wechsler Memory Scale to clarify visual motor memory. It is useful measure with certain Asian subgroups.

Tests of Intellectual Functioning

The WAIS or WAIS-R (Wechsler, 1955, 1981) with translated versions can be used for persons with higher educational level (high school level or 12 years). Specific functioning can be obtained within this test (e.g., overall cognitive level, attention and concentration, abstract and visual–motor functioning, and receptive, expressive, and planning abilities).

The Leiter International Performance Scale (Leiter, 1969a, 1969b) is an instrument devised for testing verbally handicapped and foreign language-speaking children. It is used for individuals from 2 to 18 years old. Mental age scores and ratio IQs are obtained. It has been used for adults in a neuropsychological battery, cross-culturally for Hawaiian and

African ethnic groups, and for Asian monolingual adolescents and adults. Although it is a nonverbal test, it is not well standardized for reliability or validity (Lezak, 1976, 1983) and can be very complex.

The Peabody Picture Vocabulary Test (PPVT; Dunn, 1959) has been considered for modification and translation as it was devised for testing verbally handicapped and foreign language-speaking children from 2½ to 18 years old. It has also been used for brain damaged adults in a neuropsychological battery (Lezak, 1976, 1983). Currently, the revised PPVT (PPVT-R) include adult norms obtained for ages 19 through 40. The PPVT-R has complex items and is not well standardized for reliability or validity. Sattler and Altes (1984) recommend that the PPVT-R not be used to estimate the intelligence level of bilingual and monolingual Hispanic children due to lowered scores not consistent with their normal intelligence. Anastasi (1988) feels that PPVT scores reflect the examinee's "degree of cultural assimilation and exposure to Standard American English" (p. 296).

Mood Checklists and Personality Profiles

Psychologists can use existing or newly developed symptom checklists to determine psychiatric diagnoses particular to Asian subgroups. The Hopkins Symptom Checklist (Mollica et al., 1986) can be used with Cambodian, Lao, and Vietnamese groups. A Vietnamese Language Depression Rating scale is validated for use encompassing items such as cognitive, affective and behavioral expressions (Kinzie, Manson, Vinh, et al., 1982).

The BDI (Beck, Ward, Mendelson, Mock, & Erbaugh, 1961) has English and Chinese versions. Test reliability and score equivalence were indicated from studies of bilingual Hong Kong University students.

The MMPI (Hathaway & McKinley, 1951; Dahlstrom, Welsh, & Dahlstrom, 1975) is a self-report inventory originally published by Hathaway and McKinley. The test has 550 true–false items. It can be used for individuals ages 16 and above with at least sixth-grade education. There are 10 clinical scales and three validity scales. Profile coding and interpretation help to objectify any pathological deviations. An MMPI Chinese version with different norms is available (National MMPI Coordinating Group, 1982). This version should be interpreted with both Chinese and American norms.

Tests of Emotional Functioning

The Rorschach tends to be a less familiar type of stimulus for Asians and results can be confusing or deleterious when interpreted, as previous research has indicated. However, the TAT is generally more applicable because it is structured and less ambiguous. Here a narrative account or story of the pictures can be more easily evoked and encapsulated into the

Asian cultural thinking style. Telling a narrative is a common way of expressing a culture group's constructs of meaning (Howard, 1991; Jones & Thorne, 1987) in rituals, morals, and values. Meaning can be conveyed through the storytelling of history, opera, Bhuddism and other religions, Confucian and Taoist philosophy, and societal and parental practices. Imagination and curiosity is not encouraged as much in Asian cultures as in American society. Many folk stories are told about how excessive curiosity can lead to a nasty outcome. Children are taught early through stories that taboo subjects such as sex, adult behavior, and so on. are not to be explored. Asian American psychologists have found the TAT to be less threatening for Asians because it is very much akin to their concept and practice of "culture tales" (Howard, 1991). Exceptions do occur; for example, a Chinese Vietnamese male whom I tested spoke both English and Cantonese well and responded to the "storytelling" as belittling his abilities "I'm not a child . . . children make up stories." I reassured him with explanations that people of all ages can utilize the concept of imagination and suggested he think of it as a way in which Asians have conducted the history of their culture through stories to their children. He then felt more comfortable and produced a rich TAT profile. Finally, when responses are terse or tentative on both cognitive and projective tests, the limits are tested to allow alternative or fuller responses. Again, it is a way of eliciting a more comprehensive and usable profile.

Tests of Social Adaptive Functioning and Social Competence

The Vineland Social Maturity Scale (Doll, 1965) assesses an individual's developmental level in daily practical needs and responsibilities in the mentally challenged. In 1984/1985 this scale was revised and the Vineland Adaptive Behavior Scales were produced. One scale is a report by the parent/caretaker, the second scale is used to prepare individualized educational or treatment programs, and the third scale is used in the classroom by a teacher. The original or revised caretaker scales can be useful for identifying social competence in adult Asian immigrants who are not literate in their own language or English, who have not attended school, and who are cognitively impaired.

Other measures can be developed to assess social adaptive behavior in adults with normal intelligence. A daily activities and social behavior checklist can be devised. Cultural adaptation scales and stress indices are in abundance to determine social competencies that can compensate for some of the intellectual language and environmental requirements of a new society. Cross-cultural studies have determined social competence to be a very important factor in coping under stress and in relational situations. Cooperation, empathy, sympathy, role adaptation and integration, and skills in social interaction all contribute to social smartness, which is required for survival and success.

THE TESTING PROCESS

Many barriers in testing exist, so a qualitative approach should be used during testing and in the interpretation. For example, examiners should test the limits and extend the inquiry. Many monolingual clients are not familiar with the testing process, so examiners should begin with the Information section of Wechsler Memory Scale because it is nonthreatening and covers a part of the client's mental status (orientation of time, place, and person). The remainder of the Memory test covers immediate, recent, remote, associative, and visual–motor memory. The translation for the memory passage of stories has to be similar in content and in the number of words. A common complaint of monolingual Asians is "I can't draw!" Asking a Chinese or Southeast Asian to draw may evoke embarrassment, anxiety, resistance, and hesitation to perform well, or even requests to terminate that section. Substituting the drawing tests with other more comfortable sections of the administration will decrease the anxiety. The drawing tests can be repeated with those who are able to draw. Encouragement and explanations are offered and examinees are reminded that it is not a skill of art and that they may draw as best they can. Many times, it is useful to have an initial session to observe the process of clients' learning to use new instruments and perform fine-motor tasks in drawing people and geometric shapes when they have been unable to do so because of lack of opportunity. A Laotian teenager examinee told me she had never used a pen or pencil. In the first session I had her write and draw with a pen and pencil and practice some sample drawings and printing of letters at home for a week. She then returned to the clinic to show me how she could use these instruments. In this fashion, I was testing her ability to learn from practice. Psychologists should use the test–teach–practice and retest format at the beginning to give the client an opportunity to learn and for them to measure the client's visual–motor memory and ability.

Both verbal and nonverbal intelligence are included in the WAIS-R; if the client is not literate, I would begin with the Performance section. Much of cognitive testing, specifically visual–motor tasks, is timed. If failure is due to speed, the examiner should test the limits to see if the client can succeed at a less rapid pace and note the client is only overtimed or just unable to grasp the concept.

INTERPRETATION OF RESULTS

Several points should be considered in the interpretation process:

1. Evaluate immigration and stress factors: (a) community of origin (rural, urban, indigenous peoples, etc.); (b) length of stay in the United

States; (c) quantity and quality of support system; (d) previous employment and current ability to work; (e) years of education; (f) language difficulties and literacy; (g) medical/physical problems; (h) premorbid history (psychiatric, political, and economic situations, etc.).

2. Consider educational level. If no education was achieved, premorbid intellectual capability cannot be compared to current results unless a reliable history is available.

3. Evaluate language. Does dialect match? How much is contaminated by the translation process?

4. Evaluate approach to testing and rapport. Is the client cooperative, embarrassed, angry, fearful, anxious, withdrawn? What are the subtle nonverbal behaviors? In some Asian cultures, when the person smiles, it may be a sign of anxiety and not confidence.

5. Confirm test validity. Does the test measure the same construct for Asians in terms of expectations and perceptions of stimuli (ambiguity in the Rorschach, depression, etc.)? Education is usually more cognitive and intellectual in nature; as such, spontaneous or free-flow responses to ambiguous situations are not advocated in the formal Asian educational context.

6. Ascertain familiarity with tests. (a) Forced choice "yes or no" items may compel Asians to endorse what's expected. (b) Conformity in learning may homogenize test results so that apparent deficiencies or pathology should be compared within the Asian norm. (c) Many Chinese and Southeast Asians were farmers, agricultural workers or fishermen; a bright Asian with farming and labor skills may fail on tasks that require writing, speaking, or drawing. The example of the Hmong, discussed earlier, highlights the problem of false scatter on test performance. (d) Awkward grip of pen for older Chinese and Asians occurs because of the specific learned habit of brushpen position in calligraphy, used throughout their education, which may inhibit a new pen-holding position.

7. Apply universal guidelines cautiously and describe the client's performance in the framework of adaptive versus nonadaptive functioning in their current life environment. Outline the strengths and deficiencies and offer compensatory suggestions.

8. Observe the chronology of events described so that all aspects of memory, attention, concentration, and mental status can be examined.

9. Interpret results in the context of the client's life experiences.

SUMMARY AND CONCLUSIONS

Concepts and perceptions are formulated and shaped by a culture's system of values and beliefs. Researchers are also bound by their own culture's colored glasses. Expecting similarities and differences to occur across cultures is recognized and accepted. However, judging another group unfavorably against one's own cultural standards is biased and unfair.

Psychological testing of monolingual Asians is a complex and time-consuming process. The large number of Asians and the lack of available bilingual psychologists add to the problem. The constraints and benefits of testing were weighed against using measures not relatively normed, language and translation, cultural dynamics and life, and educational experiences. Research highlighted these various barriers. The qualitative approach in the testing process and interpretation offset the shortcomings and provide a more effective profile. Conducting projectives with the concept of narrative tales enhanced the results. Other issues include the following:

1. Testing may be able to extrapolate the components and specifics of the primary emotional and cognitive diagnosis and point out strengths and weaknesses so that treatment can help to compensate for limitations in functioning and maximize competent skills.
2. Encouragement and testing of limits are highly recommended.
3. Attention must be paid to subtle nonverbal behavior and to nuances in performance.
4. Tests are basically white, middle-classed based and do not reflect the modes of thinking, expression, or problem solving for low-income monolingual or immigrant Asians. Thus, results must be interpreted with reference to both the standard norms and to Asian's own sociocultural norms.
5. An individual's effective functioning in his or her previous milieu is usually not transferrable to the United States in terms of occupation or other means of expected survival. Positive reinforcement of previous skills is advocated, but, realistically, immigrants need to be trained for the behaviors and employment necessary for survival.

RECOMMENDATIONS

1. More training of bilingual Asian psychologists in testing is needed. Currently few psychologists are experienced with test materials or in the assessment of monolingual Asians.
2. More support, in the form of adequate training and supervision, is needed from local resources in major communities, such as San Francisco where one of the largest population of Asian immigrants resides.

3. More research studies need to be conducted with monolingual Asians in the United States and other countries, which can be compared across cultures.

4. Adequate translations of current tests should continue. Translated versions should be standardized, normed, or modified with original measures and tested on a larger number of Asian subgroups.

5. Specific tests that are resistant to the effects of practice must be modified.

6. When particular difficulties are observed, methods should be recommended to augment strengths and to compensate for shortcomings. Psychologists should refer to local community resources.

7. Severe diagnoses or long-range predictions should not be hastily made and, as Sattler (1974) has suggested, performance differences should be accounted for by the context in which the client develops and expresses competence.

8. Developing culture-specific or cultures fair tests for separate groups should be determined by what the psychologist is measuring. Symptom clusters delineated in research for posttraumatic disorders have been critical in making accurate diagnoses with Chinese and Southeast Asians.

9. All psychologists who assess bilingual or monolingual clients should be sensitive to different cultural constructs of reality.

REFERENCES

Abel, T. M., & Hsu, F. L. (1949). Some aspects of personality of Chinese as revealed by the Rorschach test. *Rorschach Research Exchange* and *Journal of Projective Techniques, 13,* 285–301.

Anastasi, A. (1988). *Psychological testing* (6th ed.). New York: Macmillan.

Angoff, W. H. (1988). The nature–nurture debate, aptitudes and group differences. *American Psychologist, 43*(9), 713–720.

Beck, A. T., Ward, C. H., Mendelson, M., Mock, J., & Erbaugh, J. K. (1961). An inventory for measuring depression. *Archives of General Psychology, 4,* 561–571.

Bender, L. (1938). A visual motor gestalt test and its clinical use. *American Orthopsychiatric Association Research Monographs* (No. 3).

Benton, A. L. (1974). *The Revised Visual Retention Test.* New York: Psychological Corporation.

Benton, A. L. (1974). *The Revised Visual Retention Test* (4th ed.). New York: Psychological Corporation.

Boey, K. W. (1985). The MMPI response patter of Singapore Chinese. *Acta Psychologica Sinica, 17*(4), 377–383.

Brandt, M. E., & Boucher, J. D. (1986). Concepts of depression in emotion

lexicons of eight cultures. *International Journal of Intercultural Relations,*
10(3), 321–346.

Chan, A., Chan, H., Chen, M. Cheung, F., Chong, A., et al. (1977, 1979). *Wechsler*
Intelligence Scale, Manual, Cantonese translation. Workshop on Mental Testing
of the Hong Kong Psychological Society.

Chan, D. W. (1991). The Beck Depression Inventory: What difference does the
Chinese version make? *Psychological Assessment, 3*(4), 616–622.

Cheung, F. M., Song, W. Z., & Butcher, J. N. (1991). An infrequency scale for the
Chinese MMPI. *Psychological Assessment, 3*(4), 648–653.

Cheung, F. M., Zhao, J. C., & Wu, C. Y. (1992). Chinese MMPI profiles among
neurotic patients. *Psychological Assessment, 4*(2), 214–218.

Christy, L. C. (1978). Culture and control orientation: A study of internal–external
locus of control in Chinese and Chinese-American women. *Dissertation Abstracts*
International, 39, 2-A, 770.

Dahlstrom, W. G., Welsh, G. S., & Dahlstrom, C. E. (1975). *An MMPI handbook.*
Minneapolis: University of Minnesota Press.

Dao, M. (1991). Designing assessment procedures for educationally at-risk Southeast
Asian-American students. *Journal of Learning Disabilities, 24*(10), 594–601.

De Vos, G. (1955). A quantitative rorschach assessment of maladjustment and
rigidity in acculturating Japanese-Americans. *Genetic Psychology Monograph, 52,*
50–87.

Doll, E. A. (1965). *Vineland Social Maturity Scale: Manual of directions* (rev. ed.).
Minneapolis: American Guidance Service.

Dunn, L. M. (1959). *Peabody Picture Vocabulary Test.* Minneapolis: American Guidance Service.

Eysenck, H. J. (1991). Raising IQ through vitamin and mineral supplementation: An
introduction. *Personality and Individual Differences, 12,* 329–333.

Frydman, M., & Lynn, R. (1989). The intelligence of Korean children adopted in
Belgium. *Personality and Individual Differences, 10*(12), 1323–1325.

Golden, C. (1978). Cross-cultural second order factor structures of the 16 PF. *Journal*
of Personality Assessment, 42(2), 167–170.

Goleman, D. (1981, January). The new competency tests: Matching the right people
to the right jobs. *Psychology Today,* 35–46.

Gong, Y. X. (1982). *Manual for the Weschler Adult Intelligence Scale: Chinese revision.*
Changsha, Hunan China: Hunan Medical College.

Goodenough, H. (1963). *Children's drawings as measures of intellectual maturity.* New
York: Harcourt, Brace & World.

Gould, S. J. (1981). *The mismeasure of man.* New York: Norton.

Greene, R. L. (1980). *The MMPI: An interpretative manual.* Grune & Stratton.

Greene, R. L. (1987). Ethnicity and MMPI performance: A review. *Journal of*
Consulting and Clinical Psychology, 55(4), 497–512.

Greene, R. L. (1991). Specific groups: Adolescents, the aged blacks and other ethnic
groups. *MMPI-2/MMPI: An interpretative manual.* Boston: Allyn & Bacon.

Hain, J. D. (1964). The Bender–Gestalt Test: A scoring method for identifying brain
damage. *Journal of Consulting Psychology, 28,* 34–40.

Hathaway, S. R., & McKinley, J. C. (1951). *Minnesota Multiphasic Personality Inventory*
manual (rev. ed.). New York: Psychological Corporation.

Howard, G. S. (1991). Culture tales: A narrative approach to thinking—Cross-cultural psychology and psychotherapy. *American Psychologist, 46*(3), 187–197.

Jones, E., & Thorne, A. (1987). Rediscovery of the subject: Intercultural approaches to clinical assessment. *Journal of Counseling and Clinical Psychology, 55*(4), 488–495.

Kinzie, J. D. (1981). Evaluation and psychotherapy of Indochinese refugee patients. *American Journal of Psychotherapy, 35*(2), 251–261.

Kinzie, J. D., Fredrickson, R. H., Ben, R., Fleck, J., & Karls, W. (1984). Posttraumatic stress disorder among survivors of Cambodian concentration camps. *American Journal of Psychiatry, 141*(5), 645–650.

Kinzie, J. D., Manson, S. M., Ades, M., & Do, V. T. (1982). *The Vietnamese Depression Scale–Short form.* Portland, OR: Department of Psychiatry, Oregon Health Services, University and Mental Health Program, Indochinese Cultural and Service Center.

Kinzie, J. D., Manson, S. M., Vinh, D. T., Tolan, N. T., Anh, B., & Pho, T. N. (1982). Development and validation of a Vietnamese language depression rating scale. *American Journal of Psychiatry, 139*(10), 1276–1281.

Kokka, M., Lai, A., Nakagawa, K., Sue, D. W., Tinloy, M., & Wong, I. (1975). Issues in the testing of Asian Americans. *Newsletter of the Association of Asian American Psychologists, 2*(2), 14–15.

Leiter, R. G. (1969a). *Examiner's manual for the Leiter International Performance Scale.* Chicago: Stoelting.

Leiter R. G. (1969b). *General instructions for the Leiter International Performance Scale.* Chicago: Stoelting.

Lezak, M. D. (1976). *Neuropsychological assessment.* New York: Oxford University Press.

Lezak, M. D. (1983). *Neuropsychological assessment* (2nd ed.). New York: Oxford University Press.

Li-Repac, D. (1980). Cultural influences on clinical perception: A comparison between Caucasian and Chinese-American therapists. *Journal of Cross-Cultural Psychology, 11*(3), 327–342.

Lin, K. M., Masuda, M., & Tazuma, L. (1982). Adaptational problems of Vietnamese refugees: III. Case studies in clinic and field: Adaptive and maladaptive. *Psychiatric Journal of the University of Ottawa, 7*(3), 173–183.

Mann, E. M., Ikeda, Y., Mueller, C. W., Takahashi, A., Tao, K. T., Humris, E., Li, B. L., & Chin, D. (1991). Cross-cultural differences in rating hyperactive-disruptive behaviors in children. *Journal of Psychiatry.*

McClelland, D. C. (1973). Testing for competence rather than intelligence. *American Psychologist, 28,* 1–14.

Mercer, J. R. (1979). *System of Multicultural Pluralistic Assessment (SOMPA).* San Antonio, TX: Psychological Corporation.

Mercer, J. R., & Lewis, J. F. (1978). *System of Multicultural Pluralistic Assessment (SOMPA), Technical Manual.* San Antonio, TX: Psychological Corporation.

Mollica, R. F., Caspi-Yavin, Y., Bollini, P., Truong, T., et al. (1992). The Harvard Trauma Questionnaire: Validating a cross-cultural instrument for measuring torture, trauma and posttraumatic stress disorder in Indochinese refugees. *Journal of Nervous and Mental Disease, 180*(2), 111–116.

Mollica, R. F., Wyshak, G., Marneffe, D., Tu, B., Yang, T., Kuon, F., Coelho, R., &

Lavelle, J. (1986). *Hopkins Symptom Checklist–25. Indochinese versions (HSCL-25), Manual for use of Cambodian, Lao, and Vietnamese versions.* Funding by the U.S. Office of Refugee Resettlement. Developed by Indochinese Psychiatry Clinic; Brighton Marine Public Health Center; Department of Psychiatry, St. Elizabeth's Hospital; and the Harvard Program in Psychiatric Epidemiology, Brighton, MA.

Mouanoutoua, V. L., Brown, L. G., Cappelletty, G. G., & Levine, R. V. (1991). A Hmong adaptation of the Beck Depression Inventory. *Journal of Personality Assessment, 57*(2), 309–322.

National MMPI Coordinating Group. (1982). The revision, employment, and evaluation of MMPI on normal Chinese subjects. *Acta Psychologica Sinica, 17,* 346–355.

Nguyen, S. D. (1982). Psychiatric and psychosomatic problems among Southeast Asian refugees. *Psychiatric Journal of the University of Ottawa, 7*(3), 163–172.

Noh, S., Avison, W. R., & Kaspar, V. (1992). Depressive symptoms among Korean immigrants: Assessment of a translation of the Center for Epidemiological Studies–Depression Scale. *Psychological Assessment, 4*(1), 84–91.

Perez-Arce, P. (1992). *Lecture on neuropyschological testing of bilingual Hispanics.* Unpublished manuscript.

Raven, J. C. (1958). *Standard Progressive Matrices.* London: H. K. Lewis.

Raven, J. C. (1960). *Guide to the Standard Progressive Matrices.* New York: Psychological Corporation.

Rotter, J. B., & Rafferty, J. E. (1950). *Manual: The Rotter Incomplete Sentences Blank.* San Antonio, TX: Psychological Corporation.

Sattler, J. M. (1974). *Assessment of children's intelligence.* Philadelphia: Saunders.

Sattler, J. M., & Altes, L. M. (1984, June). Performance of bilingual and monolingual Hispanic children on the Peabody Picture Vocabulary Text–Revised and the McCarthy Perceptual Performance Scale. *Psychology in the Schools, 21,* 313–316.

Scarr, S., & Weinberg, R. A. (1978). The influence of "family background" on intellectual attainment. *American Sociological Review, 43,* 674–692.

Song, W. (1991). Use and evaluation of a modified MMPI in China. *International Journal of Mental Health, 20*(1), 81–93.

Sue, S., & Morishima, J. K. (1982). *The mental health of Asian Americans.* San Francisco: Jossey-Bass.

Terman, L. M., & Merrill, M. A. (1960). *Stanford–Binet Intelligence Scale: Manual for the Third Revision Form L-M.* Boston: Houghton Mifflin.

Terman, L. M., & Merrill, M. A. (1973). *Stanford–Binet Intelligence Scale: 1972 norms edition.* Boston: Houghton Mifflin.

Tuddenham, R. D. (1948). Soldier intelligence in World War I and II. *American Psychologist, 3,* 54–56.

Wang, M., Li, S., Burstein, A., & Loucks, S. (1991). *Culture and personality study based on a comparison of some Rorschach performance between Chinese and American normals.* Paper presented at the annual meeting of the American Psychological Association, San Francisco, CA.

Wechsler, D. (1945). A standardized memory scale for clinical use. *Journal of Psychology, 19,* 87–95.

Wechsler, D. (1955). *Wechsler Adult Intelligence Scale, Manual.* New York: Psychological Corporation.

Wechsler, D. (1981). *Wechsler Adult Intelligence Scale, Manual.* New York: Psychological Corporation.

Yee, J. (1983). *Parenting attitudes, acculturation and social competence in the Chinese American child.* Unpublished doctoral dissertation, Boston University, Boston, MA.

Ying, Y. W. (1990). Use of the CPI structural scales in Taiwan cultural graduates. *International Journal of Social Psychiatry, 36*(1), 49–57.

24

The Use of Psychotropic Medications in Working with Asian Patients

KEH-MING LIN
FREDA CHEUNG
MICHAEL SMITH
RUSSELL E. POLAND

Pharmacotherapy is an important and often indispensable component in the care of psychiatric patients, perhaps even more so in the case of patients with an Asian American background. Studies have indicated that Asian American psychiatric patients often significantly delay their help seeking (Lin, Tardiff, Douetz, & Goresky, 1978; Lin, Innui, Kleinman, & Womack, 1982). Those entering the mental health care system typically do so only after they have exhausted their own and their family's support and resources (Lin & Lin, 1981). Thus, most Asian patients enter treatment at a later stage, are likely to be more chronic, and are more severely afflicted than other ethnic groups (Lin, Kleinman, & Lin, 1981). Reflecting this tendency, a relatively larger proportion of Asian patients than other ethnic groups suffer from major psychiatric conditions (e.g., schizophrenia, major depression, and posttraumatic stress disorder) that require psychopharmacological intervention.

In addition, because of their belief in the unity rather than dichotomy of the psychological and somatic processes (Bond, 1986; Kleinman, 1976, 1982, 1988; Lin, 1981, 1996), most Asian American patients and their families expect and request treatment with medication when they interact with mental health professionals (Lin & Shen, 1991; Acosta, Yamamoto, & Evans, 1982). Such beliefs in the special curing power of medications . render psychopharmacotherapy a particularly important treatment modality in psychiatric care for this population.

Unfortunately, despite the significance of the issues involved, practitioners do not have a systematic understanding regarding the use of psychotropics with Asians. With few exceptions, practically all psychotropics have been developed in North America or Europe and tested predominantly with Caucasian populations. Ethnicity has rarely been examined in relation to the dosing range and profiles of the side effects of new drugs during their development. Notwithstanding, sporadic clinical reports over the past 30 years suggest that the database derived from Caucasian populations may not be readily applicable to Asian patients (Lin, Poland, Smith, Strickland, & Mendoza, 1991; Wood & Zhou, 1991). Some of these clinical observations have been confirmed by more rigorously designed studies conducted in the past decade (Lin et al., 1991). In addition, cultural factors also influence psychotropic responses through "nonbiological" mechanisms, including the perception and interpretation of symptoms and side effects, compliance, and placebo responses (Lin & Shen, 1991; Smith, Lin, & Mendoza, 1993). The following sections review these issues.

BIOLOGICALLY BASED DIFFERENCES IN PSYCHOTROPIC RESPONSES

Clinical observations and survey reports since the late 1960s suggest that Asians may be more sensitive to the effects of a large array of psychotropics (Lin, Poland, & Lesser, 1986; Lin & Poland, 1989; Rosenblat & Tang, 1987; Wood & Zhou, 1991), including neuroleptics, antidepressants, lithium, and benzodiazepines. More recent studies using state-of-the-art pharmacological research tools demonstrate that indeed biologically based mechanisms may be responsible for some of these clinically observed differences. This section briefly describes this issue. (For a more in-depth discussion, see Lin et al., 1986; Wood & Zhou, 1991; Lin, Poland, & Nakasaki, 1993.)

Neuroleptics

Several carefully designed studies of haloperidol have demonstrated that Asians and Caucasians differ significantly in terms of pharmacokinetics (the disposition and metabolism of drugs) and pharmacodynamics (brain receptor-coupled activities, or "sensitivity"). Asian normal volunteers (Lin, Lau, Smith, & Poland, 1988) and schizophrenic patients (Potkin et al., 1984) had approximately 50% higher plasma haloperidol concentrations than their Caucasian counterparts when given comparable doses of the medicine. These differences were not explained by ethnic variations in body weight or size and were most likely determined by the activities of drug-metabolizing enzymes. A series of recent studies (Chang, Chen, Lee, Hu, & Yeh, 1987; Chang et al., 1989, 1991; Jann et al., 1989; Jann, Lam, & Chang, 1993) indicated that Asians had a lower reduced haloperidol/haloperidol ratio, suggesting that a lower rate of reduction (a major metabolic pathway for haloperidol) in Asians may be responsible for a slower rate of metabolism and consequently for the more prominent effects when given equivalent doses.

In addition, a study with normal volunteers (Lin, Poland, Lau, & Rubin, 1988) demonstrated larger prolactin responses to haloperidol challenge in Asians as compared to Caucasians, which remained statistically significantly after controlling for differences in haloperidol concentrations, suggesting the existence of ethnic differences in brain receptor sensitivity. In a subsequent clinical treatment study (Lin et al., 1989), Asian schizophrenic patients responded optimally to significantly lower plasma haloperidol concentrations as compared to their Caucasian counterparts, again suggesting that pharmacodynamic factors contribute to ethnic differences in response to haloperidol.

To the extent the previously mentioned findings involving haloperidol are generalizable to other neuroleptics, they substantiate earlier clinical reports of lower dosage requirements (Lin & Finder, 1983; Yamamoto, Fung, Lo, & Reece, 1979) and higher risk for extrapyramidal side effects (Binder & Levy, 1981) in Asians. To what extent this is true, however, remains to be clarified.

Tricyclic Antidepressants

Survey findings (Yamashita & Asano, 1979; Rosenblat & Tang, 1987) and clinical studies (Kinzie & Manson, 1983; Kleinman, 1981; Yamamoto et al., 1979) reported that Asians require substantially lower doses of antidepressants for the treatment of depression. Results from three single-dose pharmacokinetic studies (Kishimoto & Hollister, 1984; Rudorfer, Lau, Chang, Zhang, & Potter, 1984; Schneider et al., 1991) revealed that Asians metabolize tricyclic antidepressants significantly more slowly than their Caucasian counterparts. Although other studies (Pi, Simpson, & Cooper, 1986; Pi et al., 1989) showed differences in the same direction, these differences did not reach statistical significance, particularly after controlling for body weight. Thus, at present it is unclear to what extent pharmacokinetic factors contribute to ethnic differences in response to tricyclics.

Pharmacodynamic factors have not been formally examined in studies comparing the use of antidepressants across ethnic groups. However, results from two clinical studies in Asia (Hu, Lee, Yang, & Tseng, 1983; Yamashita & Asano, 1979) reported that severely depressed hospitalized Asian patients responded clinically to lower combined concentrations of imipramine and desipramine (130 ng per ml) than had been previously reported in North American and European studies (180–200 ng per ml; American Psychiatric Association Task Force), thereby suggesting that differential brain receptor responsivity may also play a role in determining ethnic differences in tricyclic dosage requirement.

Lithium

Several recent cross-national comparison studies have replicated earlier reports from Japanese researchers regarding the need for lower doses of lithium as well as lower therapeutic lithium levels among Asians. Yang (1985) studied 101 Taiwanese bipolar patients treated over a 2-year period with clinically determined doses of lithium. He found that the plasma lithium level of the majority of good responders ranged between 0.5 and 0.79 mEq per liter. Lee (1992) reported that bipolar patients in Hong Kong were stabilized on an average lithium concentration of 0.63 mmol per liter. In two studies conducted separately in Shanghai and in Taipei, Chang, Pandey, Zhang, Ku, and Davis (1984) and Chang, Pandey, Yang, Yeh, and Davis (1985) reported remarkably similar pharmacokinetic profiles and therapeutic lithium concentrations for these two Chinese groups residing in drastically divergent socioeconomic environments. These Chinese patients did not differ from Caucasians in terms of pharmacokinetics. However, these patients responded optimally to mean lithium concentrations of 0.71 and 0.73 mEq per liter, respectively. These concentrations were significantly lower than the mean level of 0.98 mEq per liter for the matched Caucasian American patients, as well as the 0.8 to 1.2 mEq per liter therapeutic levels generally reported in Europe and North America. Thus, it appears that compared to their Caucasian counterparts, Asian bipolar patients may require lower doses of lithium because of pharmacodynamic reasons ("enhanced brain receptor responsivity").

Benzodiazepines

Confirming earlier clinical and survey reports, four studies (Ghoneim et al., 1981; Kumana, Lauder, Chan, Ko, & Lin, 1987; Lin et al., 1988; Zhang, Reviriego, Lou, Sjoqvist, & Bertilsson, 1990) involving Asians and Caucasians demonstrated significant pharmacokinetic differences between the two ethnic groups. Three of the studies used diazepam as the test drug, and one utilized alprazolam. These studies involved the administration of the test drugs either by oral or intravenous routes or both. Furthermore, they were conducted with Asians residing in diverse areas of the world, including Los Angeles, St. Louis, Hong Kong, and Beijing, China. Given the diversity of sites and research methodology, the consistency in these reports of a slower metabolism of benzodiazepines is quite remarkable, suggesting that perhaps genetic factors are more important than environmental factors in causing such a phenomenon.

Although prospective ethnic comparisons have yet to be conducted for patients treated with the benzodiazepines, the previously mentioned studies suggest that Asian patients indeed may require significantly smaller daily dosages to achieve similar steady-state levels and optimal clinical effects. In addition, because benzodiazepines are frequently prescribed on an as-needed basis, differences in single-dose pharmacokinetics may also have important clinical significance, especially in relation to their propensity to induce undesirable side effects, such as excessive sedation and anterograde amnesia.

SOCIOCULTURAL ISSUES

Pharmacological agents possess powerful symbolic and social meanings and implications in addition to their instrumental (biological) properties. These symbolic effects are without question strongly influenced by sociocultural forces (Moerman, 1979). The majority of Asians continue to be significantly influenced by traditional Oriental medical concepts and practices (Kleinman, 1980; Lin, 1981) despite the ready availability of modern Western medical services in most contemporary Asian societies. These culturally determined health beliefs and practices exert profound influences on the experiencing and reporting of symptoms and distress, the assessment of efficacy and toxicity of medication, placebo response, and compliance behavior. Further, the simultaneous use of traditional herbal medicine and psychotropics may also lead to drug–herb interactions. Although very little systematic research has been conducted on these issues, their importance in psychopharmacotherapy is without question and hence is discussed briefly here.

Cultural Influences on Symptom Manifestation and Assessment

Effective treatment relies on accuracy in assessment. Misdiagnosis often leads to poor treatment outcome. Because psychiatric nosological concepts and diagnostic systems have been developed in the context of Western culture, their applicability to non-Western culture settings, when performed in a simplistic and mechanistic manner, often leads to misdiagnosis and inappropriate patient care (Lin, 1996). For example, the strong "somatizing" tendency often observed among Asian psychiatric patients (Kleinman, 1980; Lin, 1990) may obscure potentially treatable conditions such as major depression from clinicians who are not familiar with such a phenomenon.

Interactions between Traditional Asian Herbal Medicine and Psychotropics

Despite the wide availability of Western-style medical services, the use of traditional herbal medicines continues to be popular and extensive in various Asian populations (Kleinman, 1980), including Asians residing in the United States (Chan & Chang, 1976). Some of these herbal drugs clearly have active pharmacological properties and may interact with psychotropic drugs in a number of ways (Egashira, Sudo, & Murayama, 1991; Jones & Runikis, 1987; Liu, 1991; Shader & Greenblatt, 1988). For example, the anticholinergic properties inherent in some of these drugs may cause atropine psychosis, particularly when ingested concomitantly with tricyclic antidepressants or low-potency neuroleptics. In a recent study, several Chinese herbs, including Fructus Schizandrae, Corydalis bungeane Diels, Kopsia officinallis, Clausena lansium, muscone, ginseng, and glycyrrhiza, have been found to have potent stimulating effects on enzymes responsible for the metabolism of psychotropics, and oleanolic acid contained in Sertia mileensis and Ligustrum lucidium Ait substantially inhibits the activities of these enzymes (Liu, 1991). Increased awareness and further clarification of these issues remain important as long as patients continue to rely on these traditional herbs along with pharmacotherapeutic agents.

The Assessment of Efficacy and Toxicity of Medication

Culturally ingrained health beliefs not only affect patients' decisions regarding the use of traditional Asian treatment methods but also determine how they expect "Western medicines" to work and what kind of side-effect profiles might occur. For example, a commonly held belief by Asians is that Western medicines are highly potent but often deal only with the "superficial" manifestations instead of the underlying conditions of the diseases. At the same time, they believe that Western medicines are more likely to cause serious untoward effects (Smith et al., 1993). These beliefs, probably passed down from earlier experiences with antipyretic and antibacterial agents, can be especially troublesome in the case of psychotropic agents. Unless it is carefully explained and emphasized, Asian patients often do not understand the need for maintenance therapy for most psychiatric conditions. The lack of immediate therapeutic effects for most psychotropics (especially tricyclic antidepressants) to exert their maximal effects are incongruent with the preconceptions of the patients toward Western medicines. Further, when side effects occur, they could easily be taken as proof that Western medicines were indeed too strong for the Asians. Therefore, looking into patients' indigenous health beliefs and eliciting their expectations about Western medicines are important when psychotropic agents are prescribed. Only through such inquiries can misunderstandings and mismatches in expectations be determined and minimized.

Issues of Compliance

Compliance is a significant problem in the treatment of chronic medical conditions (Sackett & Haynes, 1976). Because psychopharmacotherapies typically require long-term treatment, poor compliance can often be quite substantial. Indeed, several recent studies have found that compliance with psychotropics medication may be more problematic among non-Western populations (Smith et al., 1993). Discrepancies in the beliefs between patients and clinicians coupled with problems in communication have been regarded as the major reasons of such ethnic differences in compliance. Many Asians still are profoundly influenced by traditional Oriental medical beliefs. Unless clinicians routinely make an effort to elicit these indigenous beliefs and to provide medication education in an individualized and culturally congruent manner, noncompliance will continue to represent a major problem in the clinical settings.

Placebo Effects

Placebo effects are mediated through "symbolic" rather than "instrumental" mechanisms and are expected to be influenced a great deal by culture (Moerman, 1979). Paradoxically, at present there is very little specific information regarding how placebo responses might differ cross-culturally. Clinical lore has long suggested that Asians often express "excessive" concerns about the side effects of psychotropics (Lin & Shen, 1991), which may lead to placebo side effects and to subsequent discontinuation or lowering of the drug dosage. Cultural influences on the perception and expectation of drug effects are clearly demonstrated in a recent study of 57 Hong Kong Chinese psychiatric patients treated with lithium. In this study, Lee (1993; Lee, Wing, & Wong, 1992) found that in contrast to Western patients, Chinese rarely complained of "missing of highs," "loss of creativity," or weight gain and metallic taste. Although polydipsia and polyuria were present in the majority of these patients, these side effects were positively, not negatively, interpreted. Complaints such as lethargy, poor memory, and drowsiness appeared to be related to patients' fear of not being able to work and actually occurred at a similar frequency as age- and sex-matched normal controls. This study clearly demonstrates the importance of cultural beliefs in patients' interpretation and reporting of side effects.

CLINICAL IMPLICATIONS AND DIRECTIONS FOR FUTURE RESEARCH

As briefly reviewed earlier, responses to psychotropics are likely to differ significantly for Asian and non-Asian psychiatric patients for both pharmacological and nonpharmacological reasons. However, both the extent of and the mechanisms responsible for such differences remain largely unclarified. To further progress in such an admittedly complicated area, studies with diverse designs and strategies are needed. Future research should include (1) systematic surveys of prescription patterns, dosage, compliance, and side-effect profiles of patients receiving psychotropic medications and (2) longitudinal studies involving trials of specific regimens or therapeutic agents. Results and suggestions derived from these hypothesis-generating studies should then be tested further with research protocols utilizing more vigorous designs, including studies involving pharmacokinetic, pharmacogenetic, and pharmacodynamic measurements and double-blind testing for the treatment of specific conditions.

The need for future research notwithstanding, several important general clinical guidelines can be derived from this review.

1. Patients' beliefs and explanatory models of the cause(s) of their afflictions and help-seeking preferences should not be neglected. Complaints and expectations that do not fit the clinician's conceptualization should not be neglected. Rather, the meaning behind such complaints should be adequately explored. Treatment methods should be discussed in culturally appropriate and meaningful terms.

2. Inquiries should be made routinely regarding the use of traditional Asian medical practices (e.g., herbs). The possibility of drug–herb interactions should not be prematurely discounted.

3. Compliance issues should be discussed openly in a nonthreatening manner with patients and their family members. As an adjunct to ensure compliance, the measurement of serum or plasma drug concentrations might be of particular value in some situations.

4. Available research data indicate that compared to Caucasians, Asian patients may require substantially smaller doses of a number of psychotropics for comparable clinical results. However, at the same time, it should be kept in mind that huge (up to 40-fold) interindividual differences in the kinetics and dosage requirements exist within any ethnic group. In individual cases, such interindividual variations may override

cross-ethnic differences. If the patient has been compliant yet does not respond within a reasonable period of time or manifest significant side effects, the clinician should not hesitate to increase the dosage of a particular medication. Again, the determination of serum drug concentration might be useful in making this decision.

In conclusion, recent advances in research methodologies in both cross-cultural psychiatry and psychopharmacology have converged to enable researchers to conduct increasingly sophisticated research on issues relevant to the psychopharmacological care of patients with different ethnic and cultural backgrounds. In the coming decade, such clinical and research efforts should further clarify the mechanisms underlying such differences and render psychopharmacotherapy more culturally and ethnically specific for the rapidly expanding Asian American populations in different parts of the United States, as well as for Asians in many parts of the world.

ACKNOWLEDGMENTS

This work was supported in part by Research Center on the Psychobiology of Ethnicity MH47193 (Drs. Lin, Cheung, Smith, and Poland), National Research Center on Asian American Mental Health MH44331 (Dr. Lin), and NIMH Research Scientist Development Award MH00534 (Dr. Poland).

REFERENCES

Acosta, F. X., Yamamoto, J., & Evans, L. A. (1982). *Effective psychotherapy for low-income and minority patients.* New York: Plenum Press.

Binder, R. L., & Levy, R. (1981). Extrapyramidal reactions in Asians. *American Journal of Psychiatry, 138,* 1243–1244.

Bond, M. H. (1986). *The psychology of the Chinese people.* Hong Kong: Oxford University Press.

Chan, C. W., & Chang, J. K. (1976). The role of Chinese medicine in New York City's Chinatown. *American Journal of Chinese Medicine, 4,* 31–45, 129–146.

Chang, S. S., Pandey, G. N., Zhang, M. Y., Ku, N. F., & Davis, J. M. (1984). *Racial differences in plasma and RBC lithium levels.* Paper presented at the annual meeting of the American Psychiatric Continuing Medical Education Syllabus and Scientific Proceedings, Los Angeles, CA.

Chang, S. S., Pandey, G. N., Yang, Y.-Y., Yeh, E. K., & Davis, J. M. (1985, May 19–24). *Lithium pharmacokinetics: Inter-racial comparison.* Paper presented at the 138th Annual Meeting of the American Psychiatric Association, Dallas, TX.

Chang, W.-H., Chen, T.-Y., Lee, C.-F., Hu, W. H., & Yeh, E. K. (1987). Low plasma reduced haloperidol/haloperidol ratios in Chinese patients. *Biological Psychiatry, 22,* 1406–1408.

Chang, W.-H., Jann, W. M., Hwu, H.-G., Chen, T.-Y., Lin, S.-K., Wang, J.-M., Ereshefsky, L., Saklad, S. R., Richards, A., & Lam, Y. W. F. (1991). Ethnic comparison of haloperidol and reduced haloperidol plasma levels: Taiwan Chinese versus American non-Chinese. *Journal of the Formosan Medical Association, 90,* 572–578.

Chang, W.-H., Lin, S.-K., Jann, W. M., Lam, Y. W. F., Chen, T.-Y., Chen, C.-T., Hu, W.-H., & Yeh, E.-K. (1989). Pharmacodynamics and pharmacokinetics of haloperidol and reduced haloperidol in schizophrenic patients. *Biological Psychiatry, 26,* 239–249.

Egashira, T., Sudo, S., & Murayama, F. (1991). Effects of kamikihi-to, a Chinese traditional medicine, on various cholinergic biochemical markers in the brain of aged rats. *Folia Pharmacologica Japonica, 98,* 273–281.

Ghoneim, M. M., Korttila, K., Chiang, C. K., Jacobs, L., Schoenwald, R. D., Newaldt, S. P., & Lauaba, K. O. (1981). Diazepam effects and kinetics in Caucasians and Orientals. *Clinical Pharmacology and Therapeutics, 29,* 749–756.

Hu, W. H., Lee, C. F., & Yang, Y. Y., & Tseng, Y. T. (1983). Imipramine plasma levels and clinical response. *Bulletin of the Chinese Society of Neurology and Psychiatry, 9,* 40–49.

Jann, M. W., Chang, W. H., Davis, C. M., Chen, T. Y., Deng, H. C., Lung, F. W., Ereshefsky, L., Saklad, S. R., & Richards, A. (1989). Haloperidol and reduced haloperidol plasma levels in Chinese vs. non-Chinese psychiatric patients. *Psychiatry Research, 30,* 45–52.

Jann, M. W., Lam, Y. W. F., & Chang, W. H. (1993). Haloperidol and reduced haloperidol plasma concentrations in different ethnic populations and interindividual. Variabilities in haloperidol metabolism. In K. M. Lin, R. E. Poland, & G. Nakasaki (Eds.), *Psychopharmacology and psychobiology of ethnicity* (pp. 133–152). Washington, DC: American Psychiatric Press.

Jones, B. D., & Runikis, A. (1987). Interaction of ginseng with phenelzine. *Journal of Clinical Psychopharmacology, 7,* 201–202.

Kinzie, J. D., & Manson, S. (1983). Five years' experience with Indochinese refugee psychiatric patients. *Journal of Operational Psychiatry, 14,* 13–19.

Kishimoto, A., & Hollister, L. E. (1984). Nortriptyline kinetics in Japanese and Americans. *Journal of Clinical Psychopharmacology, 4,* 171–172.

Kleinman, A. (1976). Depression, somatization and the "new cross-cultural psychiatry." *Social Science and Medicine, 11,* 3–8.

Kleinman, A. (1980). *Patients and healers in the context of culture.* Berkeley: University of California Press.

Kleinman, A. (1981). Culture and patient care: Psychiatry among the Chinese. *Drug Therapy, 11,* 134–140.

Kleinman, A. (1982). Neurasthenia and depression. *Culture, Medicine and Psychiatry, 6,* 117–190.

Kleinman, A. (1988). *Rethinking psychiatry.* New York: Free Press.

Kumana, C. R., Lauder, I. J., Chan, M., Ko, W., & Lin, H. J. (1987). Differences in diazepam pharmacokinetics in Chinese and white caucasians—Relation to body lipid stores. *European Journal of Clinical Pharmacology, 32,* 211–215.

Lee, S. (1992). The first lithium clinic in Hong Kong: A Chinese profile. *Australian and New Zealand Journal of Psychiatry, 26,* 450–453.

Lee, S. (1993). Side effects of chronic lithium therapy in Hong Kong Chinese: An ethnopsychiatric perspective. *Culture, Medicine and Psychiatry, 17,* 301-320.

Lee, S., Wing, Y. K., Wong, K. C. (1992). Knowledge and compliance towards lithium therapy among Chinese psychiatric patients in Hong Kong. *Australian and New Zealand Journal of Psychiatry, 26,* 444–449.

Lin, K. M. (1981). Chinese medical beliefs and their relevance for mental illness and psychiatry. In A. Kleinman & T. Y. Lin (Eds.), *Normal and abnormal behavior in Chinese culture* (pp. 95–111). Dordrecht, The Netherlands: D. Reidel.

Lin, K. M. (1990). Assessment and diagnostic issues in the psychiatric care of refugee patients. In W. H. Holzman & T. H. Bornemann (Eds.), *Mental health of immigrants and refugees* (pp. 198–206). Austin, TX: Hogg Foundation for Mental Health, University of Texas.

Lin, K. M. (1996). Culture and DSM-IV: Asian-American perspectives. In H. Fabrega Jr. & D. Parron (Eds.), *Culture and psychiatric diagnosis* (pp. 35–38). Washington, DC: American Psychiatric Press.

Lin, K. M., & Finder, E. (1983). Neuroleptic dosage in Asians. *American Journal of Psychiatry, 140,* 490–491.

Lin, K. M., Innui, T. S., Kleinman, A., & Womack, W. (1982). Sociocultural determinants of the help-seeking behavior of patients with mental illness. *Journal of Nervous and Mental Disease, 170,* 78–85.

Lin, K. M., Kleinman, A., & Lin, T. Y. (1981). Overview of mental disorders in Chinese cultures: Review of epidemiological and clinical studies. In A. Kleinman & T. Y. Lin (Eds.), *Normal and abnormal behavior in Chinese culture* (pp. 237–272). Dordrecht, The Netherlands: D. Reidel.

Lin, K. M., Lau, J. K., Smith, R., & Poland, R. E. (1988). Comparison of alprazolam plasma levels and behavioral effects in normal Asian and Caucasian male volunteers. *Psychopharmacology, 96,* 365–369.

Lin, K. M., & Poland, R. E. (1989). Pharmacotherapy of Asian psychiatric patients. *Psychiatric Annals, 19,* 659–663.

Lin, K. M., Poland, R. E., Lau, J. K., & Rubin, R. (1988). Haloperidol and prolactin concentrations in Asians and Caucasians. *Journal of Clinical Psychopharmacology, 8,* 195–201.

Lin, K. M., Poland, R. E., & Lesser, I. M. (1986). Ethnicity and psychopharmacology. *Culture, Medicine and Psychiatry, 10,* 151–165.

Lin, K. M., Poland, R. E., & Nakasaki, G. (Eds.). (1993). *Psychopharmacology and psychobiology of ethnicity.* Washington, DC: American Psychiatric Press.

Lin, K. M., Poland, R. E., Nuccio, I., Matsuda, K., Hathuc, N., Su, T. P., & Fu, P. (1989). Longitudinal assessment of haloperidol dosage and serum concentration in Asian and Caucasian schizophrenic patients. *American Journal of Psychiatry, 146,* 1307–1311.

Lin, K. M., Poland, R. E., Smith, M. W., Strickland, T. L., & Mendoza, R. (1991). Pharmacokinetic and other related factors affecting psychotropic responses in Asians. *Psychopharmacology Bulletin, 27,* 427–439.

Lin, K. M., & Shen, W. W. (1991). Pharmacotherapy for Southeast Asian Psychiatric Patients. *Journal of Nervous and Mental Disease, 179,* 346–350.

Lin, T. Y., & Lin, M. C. (1981). Love, denial and rejection: Response of Chinese families to mental illness. In A. Kleinman & T. Y. Lin (Eds.), *Normal and abnormal behavior in Chinese culture.* Dordrecht, The Netherlands: D. Reidel.

Lin, T. Y., Tardiff, K., Douetz, G., & Goresky, W. (1978). Ethnicity and patterns of help-seeking. *Culture, Medicine and Psychiatry, 2,* 3–14.

Liu, G. T. (1991). Effects of some compounds isolated from Chinese medicinal herbs on hepatic microsomal cytochrome P-450 and their potential biological consequences. *Drug Metabolism Reviews, 23,* 439–465.

Moerman, D. E. (1979). Anthropology of symbolic healing. *Currents in Anthropology, 20,* 59–80.

Pi, E., Simpson, G. M., & Cooper, M. A. (1986). Pharmacokinetics of desipramine in Caucasian and Asian volunteers. *American Journal of Psychiatry, 143,* 1174–1176.

Pi, E. H., Tran-Johnson, T. K., Walker, N. R., Cooper, T. B., Suckow, R. F., Gray, G. E. (1989). Pharmacokinetics of desipramine in Asian and Caucasian Volunteers. *Psychopharmacology Bulletin, 25,* 483–487.

Potkin, S. G., Shen Y., Pardes, H., Phelps, B. H., Zhou, D., Shu, L., Korpi, E., & Wyatt, R. J. (1984). Haloperidol concentrations elevated in Chinese patients. *Psychiatry Research, 12,* 167–172.

Rosenblat, R., & Tang, S. W. (1987). Do Oriental psychiatric patients receive different dosages of psychotropic medication when compared with Occidentals? *Canadian Journal of Psychiatry, 32,* 270–274.

Rudorfer, M. V., Lan, E. A., Chang, W. H., Zhang, M. D., & Potter, W. Z. (1984). Desipramine pharmacokinetics in Chinese and Caucasian volunteers. *British Journal of Clinical Pharmacology, 17,* 433–440.

Sackett, D. L., & Haynes, R. B. (Eds.). (1976). *Compliance with therapeutic regimens.* Baltimore & London: Johns Hopkins University Press.

Schneider, L., Pawluczyk, S., Dopheide, J., Lyness, S. A., Suckow, R. F., & Cooper, T. B. (1991, May 11–16). *Ethnic difference in nortriptyline metabolism.* Paper presented at the 144th annual meeting of the American Psychiatric Association, New Orleans.

Shader, R. I., & Greenblatt, D. J. (1988). Bees, ginseng and MAOI's revisited. *Journal of Clinical Psychopharmacology, 8,* 325.

Smith, M., Lin, K. M., & Mendoza, R. (1993). "Non-biological" issues affecting psychopharmacotherapy: Cultural considerations. In K. M. Lin, R. E. Poland, & G. Nakasaki (Eds.), *Psychopharmacology and psychobiology of ethnicity* (pp. 37–58). Washington, DC: American Psychiatric Press.

Wood, A. J., & Zhou, H. H. (1991). Ethnic differences in drug disposition and responsiveness. *Clinical Pharmacokinetics, 20,* 1–24.

Yamamoto, J., Fung D., Lo, S., & Reece, S. (1979). Psychopharmacology for Asian Americans and Pacific Islanders. *Psychopharmacological Bulletin, 15,* 29–31.

Yamashita, I., & Asano, Y. (1979). Tricyclic antidepressants: Therapeutic plasma level. *Psychopharmacological Bulletin, 15,* 40–41.

Yang, Y. Y. (1985). Prophylactic efficacy of lithium and its effective plasma levels in Chinese bipolar patients. *Acta Psychiatrica Scandinavica, 71,* 171–175.

Zhang, Y., Reviriego, J., Lou, Y., Sjoqvist, F., & Bertilsson, L. (1990). Diazepam metabolism in native Chinese poor and extensive hydroxylators of S-mephenytoin: Interethnic differences in comparison with white subjects. *Clinical Pharmacology and Therapeutics, 48,* 496–502.

25

Clinical Case Management with Asian Americans

ALBERT ENG
EVELYN F. BALANCIO

For several decades, the vast majority of outpatient mental health services in this country have been provided to clients in an office-based, specialty clinic model. Mental health clinicians for the most part work in clinic offices, where they meet with clients referred to them for psychosocial assessment and/or psychotherapeutic treatment exclusively. This way of delivering mental health services is antithetical to important traditional Asian attitudes about seeking help for behavioral, interpersonal, and emotional difficulties. Recent models of clinical case management tend to be more culturally syntonic with these traditional Asian attitudes than has been the specialty clinic model in America. This chapter describes a further refinement of recent U.S. clinical case management models which has even greater potential for being culturally sensitive to the values and needs of many Asian Americans who may need or desire mental health services.

CASE MANAGEMENT AS A TREATMENT MODALITY

A development in the field of community mental health which holds promise of being effective with many Asian clients is the increasing number of case management services in the total array of services offered in a mental health program. Several models of case management have been proposed and implemented in recent years. One model combines the roles of therapist and case manager in the same individual (Lamb, 1980). A recent elaboration of this model identifies 13 types of activities: engagement, assessment, planning, linkage with community resources, consultation with families and other caregivers, maintenance and expansion of social networks, collaboration with physicians and hospitals, advocacy, intermittent individual psychotherapy, training in independent living skills, patient psychoeducation, crisis intervention, and monitoring (Kanter, 1989).

Clinical case management within this theoretical perspective is defined as a process of providing comprehensive treatment to individuals with severe mental illness (Surber, 1994). It is a treatment modality that integrates psychological treatment, medication, psychosocial rehabilitation, and provision of environmental supports (Kanter, 1989; Balancio, 1994). All interventions, including "concrete" help, are viewed from a treatment perspective and within the context of a therapeutic relationship. The major premises of clinical case management include an acknowledgment of the heterogeneity or diversity of clients and a broad definition of what is therapeutic. Its principles emphasize an individualized and flexible approach which takes into consideration the comprehensive needs of a client (medical, social service, vocational, education, spiritual, etc.). This approach underscores the importance of culture, which shapes an individual's world view and influences beliefs as to how an individual affects the environment and how the environment affects the individual. Likewise articulated in its principles are requirements for an effective client-centered therapeutic stance, namely, that clinical case managers have to be resourceful, accessible, tolerant, and culturally competent. The premises and principles of clinical case management allow for a treatment modality that is sensitive and responsive to clients of different cultures.

As mentioned earlier, important differences exist between Western and Asian belief systems regarding mental illness and its causes. A holistic model of health that is nondualistic in its concept of physical and mental/emotional/spiritual health has been the basis of traditional healing practices in much of Asia. In clinical case management, a comprehensive approach to treatment requires a responsiveness to all client needs. Clinical case management still approaches health and mental health as a dichotomy, but it acknowledges the dynamic interplay of multiple factors (including social and economic factors) that create or contribute to a client's distress. This comprehensive approach is more consonant to the Asian theory of holistic health, compared to other traditional mental health treatment approaches. A clinical case manager is not expected to be an expert in all a client's treatment and service needs, but by actively coordinating and consulting with other care providers, the clinical case manager is highly likely to address the multiple needs of a client.

As a treatment modality that integrates psychological treatment, biological treatment, psychosocial rehabilitation, and provision of environmental supports, the assessment of Asian clients using a clinical case management model takes into account the following areas:

Psychological factors

- Concept of self and its relationship to family and community
- Developmental stage, described in terms of culturally appropriate tasks and milestones
- Level of functioning prior to illness and prior to immigration
- Adaptive capacity in own culture and in new culture
- Immigration history
- Degree of impairment
- Precipitating event
- Individual's belief about cause of mental illness
- Individual's understanding of own illness
- Individual's reaction to own illness

Biological factors

- Use of traditional medications (e.g., herbs and tonics)
- Attitudes toward Western medication and their side effects
- Medical problems

Psychosocial rehabilitation variables

- Family structure
- Connection and degree of participation with community and other social supports
- Degree of acculturation
- Educational attainment and work history in country of origin
- English proficiency
- Experiences with racism

Environmental supports

- Knowledge of and attitudes about using Western social service institutions
- Financial situation
- Housing
- Transportation and mobility

In treating Asian American clients, it is important to remember that their concept of self is highly defined within the context of family. One's sense of identity is derived from one's role in a hierarchical family structure, and one's self-esteem depends on one's capacity to function and carry out the role. Family "obligation" is intertwined with one's very sense of being and thus is not questioned. It includes taking care of the older and younger members of the family in an interdependent relational context where its members share collective responsibility. The context of interdependent and collective responsibility is extended to the community. To this day, in many traditional communities or villages, families are able to trace some kind of far or extended kinship, by blood or social affinity, with their neighbors. Mutual help or assistance is part of community life, and individuals demonstrate a high level of awareness of the effect of their behavior on the social group. The group's acceptance or rejection of an individual reflects on the family, and it is an important factor which could determine individual and family honor or shame.

Much has been written about the effects of immigration on individuals and their families. Regardless of whether immigration was a choice (even a long-held dream) or a forced alternative (as in the case of refugees), separations, massive losses, and traumatic experiences are common issues that underlie affective and psychotic symptoms and manifestations of disorientation. Immigration affects the family structure, the defined functional roles of its members, and the balance of authority and power within. Well-functioning families become high risk for dysfunction and even chaos as they adapt to Western culture while dealing with their massive losses.

Beliefs about mental illness; differences in the concept of self, family, and community; and immigration history have profound implications for assessment and treatment approaches. Working with Asian clients requires a highly flexible, sensitive, and culturally competent treatment approach. Engaging Asian clients to receive mental health treatment and services presents a challenge which often cannot be met by traditional Western treatment models. Many Asian clients, particularly Asian refugees who escaped from civil wars and political persecution in Southeast Asia, maintain a guarded attitude toward strangers and governmental employees. It takes time for these potential Asian mental health clients to test mental health workers and to begin to trust them. Providing case management services is a good vehicle for this to take place.

CASE EXAMPLES

Case Example 1

In clinical case management, a broad definition of what is therapeutic, coupled with the principle of flexibility, allows for creative, "nontraditional" approaches and interventions. For example, a 36-year-old single

Asian female, an immigrant of 3 years, unemployed for 1 year, with no family and a small support system (Asian roommates), was referred to an outpatient clinic by a hospital after her third hospitalization within a year. She was diagnosed with a bipolar manic illness and was known to be noncompliant with treatment. She never followed through with previous outpatient referrals and stopped taking medications as soon as she left the hospital. The referring hospital also mentioned that she was in denial about her psychiatric condition and had many somatic complaints. The clinical case manager assigned to the case visited the client at the hospital before discharge to do an initial assessment and, especially, to start the engagement process. The client believed that her hospitalizations were a result of abnormalities in her menstrual cycle, became hostile when there was a slight suggestion that she had a psychiatric illness, and adamantly refused to come to a mental health clinic because she would be too ashamed to be seen in a "crazy" clinic. She was afraid she would be asked to leave her apartment by her Asian roommates. Her main concern was to find employment to support herself and be able to send money to her brother in Asia, whose education she was supporting. She refused mental health treatment but appreciated the case manager's offer to accompany her to a medical clinic with a strong focus on women's needs for the express purpose of addressing her concerns about her menstrual problems. She was also greatly relieved that the case manager would try to advocate for some public assistance when her unemployment benefits ran out and would refer her to a vocational training program at an appropriate time. The case manager did not insist on clinic visits at that time but offered to do regular home visits, to which the client agreed. The case manager referred the client to the women's clinic and made plans for the client to apply for public assistance. While addressing the client's identified needs, the case manager simultaneously discussed the meaning of mental health and mental illness in this country. The case manager provided psychoeducation without emphasizing psychiatric diagnosis. The client gradually started to acknowledge distressing experiences (i.e., symptoms) and became receptive to discussions about the role of Western medication. After approximately 2 months of home visits and brokerage of medical and social services by the clinical case manager, the client started to come to the outpatient clinic and agreed to try psychiatric medication. After 2 years of supportive treatment where the patient and therapist addressed issues of loss and family obligation, the client was able to find employment with the assistance of a vocational rehabilitation program.

Case Example 2

Differences between traditional Asian and contemporary U.S. concepts of family obligation can have a profound influence on treatment. The traditional Asian parent's beliefs and attitudes about the extent of parental responsibility often extend far beyond what is usually expected of parents in the United States. To work with a troubled Asian child, adolescent, or dependent adult, the clinician needs to recognize and address these attitudes in a concrete, supportive fashion. For example, a 17-year-old Asian male, whose family had immigrated to the United States 3 years earlier, was diagnosed with severe psychotic symptoms resulting from a progressive organic condition. He began to physically assault his father at home. These assaults often occurred when the father told the son not to leave the house or scolded the son for not attending to personal hygiene or appropriate dress. Despite these assaults, the father wanted the son to continue to live at home. When the son's psychotic symptoms and aggressive behavior first appeared shortly after the family arrived in the United States, the father refused to authorize the use of any Western psychiatric medications. He was suspicious of such medications and believed that their side effects were evidence of his son's worsening condition. During the previous year, the son was hospitalized three times in adolescent inpatient psychiatric wards and pediatric medical wards for acute episodes of acting-out behavior. The father harbored much anger toward the medical and psychiatric institutions for their failure to cure his son's condition. The father accused the hospital, medical clinic, and outpatient mental health therapists of not attending to his son's needs adequately, thereby causing his son's assaultive behavior. The father's frustration and anger were compounded by his inability to speak English and communicate directly with most line staff. Asian-language interpreters were present at treatment planning conferences and clinic appointments but not always available when he wanted to communicate with nursing staff who were attending to his son on the hospital wards. Furthermore, he complained that the interpreters did not take enough time with him and were doing a poor job. Almost all case managers, therapists, or other service providers who were assigned to work with the teenager felt helpless and frustrated. Moreover, they felt defeated by and were angry at the father. Although the father agreed that his son's behavior was out of control at home, he refused to participate in legal proceedings which would allow for placement of his son in a long-term, inpatient facility. Although the father acknowledged that he could not control his son's inappropriate behavior, he stated that nonetheless he could provide better care for his son than the acute care hospitals had done.

Prior to discharge from a recent medical hospital admission during which the teenager was medically and psychiatrically stabilized to a significant degree, the teenager was assigned to a bilingual Asian clinical case manager at an outpatient mental health clinic who could work with the family as intensively or frequently as required. Initially, the clinical case manager recognized that the father was not being "masochistic" by refusing to defend himself or refusing to call the police when his son assaulted him. Instead, the clinical case manager reframed this behavior as an understandable extension of the traditional Asian precept that parents should provide shelter for their dependent children. Second, instead of providing talk therapy to resolve the father's underlying psychological issues of loss and depression—he resisted all attempts to talk about his emotions—the clinical case manager provided active, concrete supportive services requested by the father, such as providing or arranging for transportation for the numerous outpatient medical clinic appointments. The clinical case manager spent long hours in medical clinics waiting with the father and son in order to be an interpreter when other interpreters could not be found. Over the course of 2 months, the father began to trust the clinical case manager. Despite the efforts of the case manager, the father, and the medical clinics, however, the son's condition deteriorated to the point that he needed to be hospitalized again for medical reasons. During the time the case manager had spent with the father, she learned that he wanted his son to be able to go to school. Furthermore, the son had a dream of going to school, something he had not done for 2 years. While the son was once again hospitalized, the clinical case manager continued to work with the family and began to educate the father about the concept of conservatorships and the possibility of out-of-home placement. After much discussion and negotiation with various parts of the mental health system during a series of clinical case planning meetings, an interagency treatment planning team decided that the client would be best served at a long-term, state hospital located some distance out of town. However, the parents, particularly the father, did not approve of the idea of keeping the son in a hospital indefinitely. Knowing that the state hospital had an on-site school, the case manager made an appointment with the intake staff at the state hospital, set aside an entire day for a visit, rented a car, and drove the parents there for an informational visit. On seeing that the hospital had adequate living quarters, a school, and extensive recreational facilities, as well as medical and psychiatric coverage, the parents enthusiastically embraced the idea of placing their son there. They surprised all the mental health workers who had attempted to work with them during the current hospitalization by demonstrating a spirit of cooperation, instead of vehement opposition, to the recommended placement plan. Key to this turnaround on the part of the parents was their belief that the clinical case manager actively supported their culturally determined parental obligation to care for their son in their home despite the tremendous emotional and physical costs in doing so. Only when they could see for themselves that the recommended placement met their own definition of adequate care (e.g., provision of schooling for their son) did they support the plan.

CONCLUSION

The two clinical vignettes discussed illustrate how traditional Asian cultures can shape Asian clients' world views in ways significantly different than U.S. culture does. Particularly, the attitudes of Asian clients or their caretakers regarding physical and mental health can be at odds with some of the basic values and principles underlying traditional outpatient U.S. mental health treatment. By using a clinical case management approach that is flexible and includes a broad definition of what is therapeutic, the treatment providers were able to design and implement comprehensive and effective intervention strategies that were affirming and respectful of their Asian clients' cultures.

REFERENCES

Balancio, E. (1994). Clinical case management. In R. W. Surber (Ed.), *Clinical case management: A guide to comprehensive treatment of serious mental illness* (pp. 21–41). Thousand Oaks, CA: Sage.

Kanter, J. (1989). Clinical case management: Definition, principles, components. *Hospital and Community Psychiatry, 40*(4), 361–368.

Lamb, H. R. (1980). Therapist-case managers: More than brokers of services. *Hospital and Community Psychiatry, 31*(11), 762–764.

Surber, R. W. (Ed.). (1994). *Clinical case management: A guide to comprehensive treatment of serious mental illness.* Thousand Oaks, CA: Sage.

Part V

Special Issues

26

Gay and Lesbian Asian Americans in Psychotherapy

BART K. AOKI

Gay and lesbian Asian Americans are entering psychotherapy in increasing numbers. Some seek therapy from openly identified gay or lesbian therapists, whereas others seek out Asian American or other ethnic minority psychotherapists. For others, the issue of sexuality and sexual identity arises in the course of an ongoing psychotherapy relationship. In each case, the psychotherapist is faced with understanding the relevant cultural context and influences affecting the Asian American client and the client's level of progress toward a constructive adaptation to his or her sexuality and, ultimately, with responding in affirmative and culturally specific ways to facilitate this process. This chapter addresses these three broad areas and ends with a brief discussion of clinical issues related to HIV/AIDS among Asians.

GAYS AND LESBIANS AND CULTURAL INFLUENCES

Self-identification as a gay or lesbian person requires the Asian American individual to face conflicting cultural values and expectations. Culturally based views regarding sexuality and, specifically, homosexuality influence the Asian American client to varying degrees depending on cultural identification and level of acculturation. Similarly, the emphasis on the family versus the individual's own wants and needs in traditional Asian cultures may pose particular difficulties for a gay or lesbian client. Traditional Asian cultural views of gender roles and responsibilities are also often critical issues as they relate to sexuality and familial responsibility. Finally, subcultural values and norms specific to the Asian American experience and contemporary gay and lesbian communities are particularly relevant to the process of adaptation and identity formation.

Sexuality, Homosexuality, and Asian Culture

The meaning and expression of sexuality have varied across cultures depending on such factors as historical time periods, class status, and the varying influences of external cultures (Adam, 1985). Variation in the expression and social context of homosexuality in Asian cultures, in particular, has been the subject of extensive study. These studies have included documentation of communities of homosexual women in Southern China (Sankar, 1986) and openly acknowledged male homosexual activity in contemporary Filipino and Indian cultures (Sechrest & Flores, 1969; Nanda, 1986) and feudal Japan (Ihara, 1972). However, Confucian values, emphasizing sexuality only as it perpetuates the family line, have predominated throughout much of Asian cultural history. These values have generally fostered attitudes that discourage the uninhibited expression of sexuality and homosexuality.

Related Asian Cultural Values

Given the priority of family relationships and the well-being of the family unit within traditional Asian cultures, an individual's personal needs and wants are secondary. Asian Americans who are gay or lesbian often experience the possibility of sexuality as a central organizer of identity as a conflict of opposing values. The Asian emphasis on the group and choices based on an essential understanding of the interrelatedness of individuals conflicts directly with choices made on the basis of personal sexuality.

As traditional Asian family structure includes clearly defined role responsibilities tied partially to gender, this factor also intensifies conflicts for gay and lesbian Asian Americans. Asian lesbians, for example, may experience overt pressure to fulfill traditional expectations regarding marriage and childbearing. Any behavior perceived as departing from traditionally prescribed heterosexual roles for women may bring subtle forms of disapproval and disengagement by family and friends (Chan, 1989). Similarly, gay Asian men, depending on birth order, may experience a specific sense of responsibility to bear children or to achieve or behave in ways that preserve or enhance the family's status.

Subcultural Values and Norms

In psychotherapy with Asian American gays or lesbians, it is critical for the therapist to understand the effects of immigration and minority status on cultural values, specifically those governing sexuality and homosexuality. Whereas Asian societies have changing mores regarding sexuality and homosexuality, immigrant groups bring with them values that are rooted in a specific time and are often class specific. These values are also shaped by the pressures and influence of immigration and minority status, often resulting in an increased rigidity and intensification of these values in the face of oppression and powerlessness. Thus, Asian American values and sanctions related to sexuality and homosexuality can also be understood as even more rigidified versions of cultural values perpetuated within minority families faced with threats to their cultural and familial integrity.

Similarly, values and norms specific to contemporary gay and lesbian communities are relevant to the Asian client's process of adaptation to his or her sexuality. When these norms overlap with Asian American norms, they are likely to ease the process of adaptation. Shared consciousness and identification around issues of oppression, power, and minority status can contribute to attaining stable levels of adaptation to sexuality. Cultural divergence or conflict, which often include standards of attractiveness and interpersonal behavior, may complicate the socialization and identity formation process for Asian American gays and lesbians. For many Asian American gay men, sexual objectification as "exotic" physical types or as "undesirable Orientals" may contribute significantly to periods of identity confusion and behavioral withdrawal, further slowing the process of identity formation.

PROCESS AND FORMATION OF POSITIVE IDENTITY

Gays and lesbians experience the formation of their sexual identity through specific developmental steps commonly referred to as "coming out." Each of these steps evokes psychological issues that may stimulate specific cultural issues and pose problems as well as afford an opportunity for growth. Garnets and Kimmel (1991) review the work that has been done to explicate the developmental tasks gays and lesbians face in the process of acquiring and affirming a gay or lesbian identity and to delineate common stages. These stages include (1) initial awareness, (2) exploration, and (3) integration of a positive identity.

Many gays and lesbians share a sense of being different early in life (Boxer & Cohler, 1989). Early awareness is also common among Asian Americans, but the family's emphasis on nonsocial aspects of development, particularly in the area of academics, may delay the person's own self-labeling of same-sex attraction. When combined with developmental tasks frequently complicated by ethnic minority status, persistent negative self-images often develop during adolescence. Social withdrawal, depression, suicide attempts, substance abuse, and avoidant and compulsive behaviors may arise as complications during this phase.

Behavioral exploration in the process of coming out usually involves both disclosure of being gay to others and first sexual experiences, which may in turn lead to further social and sexual experimentation. Once Asian Americans accept their same-sex attraction, disclosure to others often depends on a number of culturally based factors. In traditional families or social circles, where personal and/or sexual aspects of life are not discussed, the individual may proceed with behavioral exploration without any disclosure to others, particularly family members. A temporary or enduring duality may develop in which family and friends avoid direct discussion of the personal relationships of the gay or lesbian individual. Both the indirect nature of communication in traditional families and a cultural tolerance of duality and contradictions may contribute to and support this form of adaptation among Asians beyond that present in other groups.

Forms of initial sexual experience during this phase may follow this pattern of duality to varying degrees. In some individuals, this pattern manifests itself in sexual experiences restricted solely to secretive anonymous sexual contacts. Among other individuals, initial exploration in social settings raises issues of self-image as Asians in a predominantly white culture and also challenges culturally based interpersonal styles of initiating and developing relationships. If exploration is limited to anonymous sexual contacts, the process of identity development can be undermined by negative self-evaluations and ongoing guilt. Increased social exploration usually affords multiple opportunities to strengthen a biculturally based self-image. Clinical symptoms or complications are consequently much less likely during this phase.

Integration of a positive identity usually follows a substantial period of sexual and social exploration. In most groups, this integration is described ideally as involving a consolidated internal sexual identity as gay or lesbian corresponding with externally consistent behavior in multiple spheres (Troiden, 1988). For ethnic minority gays and lesbians, this process also includes an integration of ethnic identity as part of sexual identity (Morales, 1989). For Asian gays and lesbians, a culturally based model of this process of sexual identity formation may or may not involve an overtly apparent consistency across all spheres. It is as likely, for example, for a gay Asian man's family to have integrated his lifelong partner into family activities without ever having openly discussed the homosexual nature of their relationship. As important for Asian gays and lesbians is the ongoing process of recognizing and respecting often conflicting aspects of their ethnic and sexual identities and the continual exploration of mechanisms that affirm both.

AN AFFIRMATIVE CLINICAL APPROACH

Beginning with an assumption of gay and lesbian identities and lifestyles as equally valid, the clinician's primary task is to counteract the psychological effects of social oppression and to facilitate the process of identity formation. Such a gay affirmative approach is particularly appropriate with a culturally diverse clientele and uniquely suited for doubly oppressed subpopulations (Gock, 1986).

In engaging gay and lesbian Asians around the issues of sexuality, the clinician establishes an affirmative approach by actively defining and affirming both sexual and ethnic identity as valid issues and foci of the therapeutic process. Initially clinicians achieve this affirmative approach by their willingness to raise, explore, and provide relevant frameworks and information about sexual identity in the context of the client's own personal and cultural situation. Clinicians also demonstrate their affirmation of the importance of these issues by their willingness to seek further consultation or to explore with the client his or her interest in seeing a gay- or lesbian-identified psychotherapist at any particular point in the process.

As the client progresses through the process of identity exploration and formation, the clinician (1) seeks to bring to the surface both the gay and ethnic aspects in each of the primary issues raised by the client and (2) helps the client identify psychological or behavioral mechanisms by which he or she can address or resolve these issues.

For example, in the process of exploring disclosure to others, client and therapist examine motivations along culturally influenced lines in addition to the inherent press to further consolidate sexual identity. This press to consolidate might surface in the Asian client's felt need to belong or to be embraced by the family unit or in his or her fears of rejection and anger, which are closely related to feelings of marginality associated with ethnic minority status. Without therapeutic efforts focused specifically on these areas, the identity formation process is potentially distorted and the client risks further alienation from aspects of the self.

Once the clinician identifies such culturally based issues, he or she is then in a position to deepen clients' awareness of the complexity of their own ethnic identity as it relates to sexuality and to support perceptions and actions sensitive to these complexities. Felt pressure to come out, for example, once understood in the context of both Asian and mainstream gay cultural influences as well as potential manifestations of oppression-based anger, expands the alternatives for responding to this pressure. Gay

Asian clients in this situation may be assisted to explore further in the psychotherapy the sources and manifestations of anger, as well as to spend more time in the company of their family or to disclose their sexuality to an Asian friend. All potentially contribute to developing further a positive sexual and ethnic identity without negating each critical aspect of the self.

HIV/AIDS: CLINICAL ISSUES

Depending on their behavior, all individuals, whether gay or straight, are vulnerable to HIV infection. AIDS diagnoses among Asians in the United States have been increasing at a remarkable high rate over the last few years and include Asian women, children, and heterosexual men. In the late 1990s, however, Asian American men who have had high-risk sexual contact with other men are particularly affected.

An Asian American who is HIV positive is confronted by culturally specific issues that may have been dormant for a considerable amount of time. Parallel to and intersecting with these issues are additional concerns that are almost universal to those faced with becoming infected with HIV in the 1990s. These are (1) the need for information, quality health care, and services; (2) the need for social support; and (3) psychological issues and psychotherapeutic needs specific to HIV.

Provision of Information, Health Care, and Related Services

When confronted with being HIV infected, some are overwhelmed by the task of making sense of all the complicated and rapidly changing information about the nature and treatment of HIV illness. The clinician needs to assess the level of understanding and awareness of the implications of the disease in the context of the patient's culturally based health beliefs and practices. Clients may require specifically targeted informational materials in their own language and at their own reading level. Educating the client and the family involves detailed discussion of the implications of the serostatus itself as well as the risks of transmission. When the clinician uses interpreters in this process, he or she needs to identify specifically trained and HIV-sensitive interpreters so as to minimize the communication of misinformation, even indirectly.

An individual with AIDS also needs information and services related to finances, legal services, social services, housing, and access to specialized health care. The Asian client's willingness to seek and receive help in a variety of these areas when services may not be culturally comfortable is often an unspoken issue. Similarly, the client's relative comfort with his or her physician will affect overall adherence to any treatment or prophylactic regimen. A clinician sensitive to these issues will be prepared to raise them and to serve a facilitative or mediating role with these providers. This may be particularly necessary in relation to the client's physician, whose respected status may inhibit the more traditional Asian client's ability to communicate freely. Even the most behaviorally adaptive client's help-seeking patterns are likely to be taxed and potentially compromised by the frustration and depression often inherent to HIV illness.

Social Support

Social support beyond that provided in the clinical relationship is essential to the process of adapting to being HIV infected. For Asian Americans any forced disclosure of HIV status often challenges the normative communication processes of family/friends potentially creating intense conflict, anxiety, and fears of abandonment. Most frequently, social bonds are maintained and even strengthened when faced with the challenge of life-threatening illness. In other instances, profound issues of psychological loss and abandonment need to be processed as part of a client's experiences of rejection.

The need to turn to friends and family in such a vulnerable state often triggers other culturally based issues. Some patients' ability to seek and receive the necessary support from other Asians may be compromised. Moreover, what and who was supportive in the past may no longer be experienced as such, and clients may find themselves longing for forms of support experienced in childhood with its unique cultural flavor. If, as is sometimes the case with gay Asians, their social networks have previously excluded Asian friends or family members, the client may experience a vague sense of frustration and depression over these unmet needs.

Psychotherapeutic Issues and Needs

Psychotherapy with the HIV-infected client often addresses common themes that may take on specific forms in relation to an Asian American, including issues related to dependency, control, sustaining investment in life or hope, and the need to confront life-stage issues.

The reality of living with a potentially life-threatening illness understandably raises issues related to dependency in all its forms. An essential part of facilitating adaptation to the illness is an assessment of the client's personal and cultural feelings regarding this issue. Sometimes, culturally prescribed caregiving, especially among more traditional families, may prolong a natural regressive phase in the adaptation to the illness. While enhancing the sense of being cared for, efforts involving self-mastery, including seeking information and support from a variety of sources, also play an important part in enhancing an enduring sense of well-being among many Asian Americans.

As with issues of dependency, HIV also invariable triggers issues around control: the need to control and the ability to control in a specific way. Persons influenced by Eastern cultures have been described as gaining esteem through the control of processes (i.e., feelings) internal to the individual (Weisz, Rothbaum, & Blackburn, 1984). This pattern contrasts with that of many Westernized individuals who are more likely to gain esteem through activity aimed at exerting influence on external events and situations. When confronted with a seemingly uncontrollable situation such as AIDS, the Asian client may need to exert considerable control over his or her own feelings as a way to gain a sense of psychological stability. This pattern may also manifest itself periodically throughout the process of adaptation and may seem to come into direct conflict with alternative ways of "taking control" of the illness. Clinicians attuned to these issues are in a unique position to help clients explore fears regarding loss of control and to establish realistic mechanisms and activities that may be helpful in allaying some of these fears.

As for anyone with a potentially life-threatening illness, the HIV-infected Asian is faced with the task of sustaining hope. This process is often culturally based and may include ingrained but subconscious beliefs regarding destiny and fate. Even the most acculturated Asian may react to submerged but intense culturally determined beliefs about forces beyond his or her control. These beliefs need to be differentiated from a sense of powerlessness associated with any personal experiences of helplessness related to physical or sexual abuse, homophobia, and racial oppression. When the client is helped to experience these distinctions through recall within the therapy, psychological resources often become available for coping with the ongoing stress of the illness. Thus, while harboring a degree of fatalistic acceptance, many clients can be helped to act in ways that will effectively improve immediate health and psychological status.

When a person confronts life-threatening illness, his or her sense of personal mortality may foster a reprioritizing of activities and pursuits. Often, in an Asian American, much of this reprioritization centers around the need to become reinvolved with family members in an effort to heal previous rifts and wounds. Reprioritization is also balanced in the bicultural individual with desires to achieve certain personal goals. When facilitated by a clinician sensitive to cultural issues, the client can emphasize and appreciate the dual nature of what may seem like solely personal desires. For instance, further schooling is also an achievement to be shared with family members. Similarly, the increased importance of personal leisure may also free the client to participate more fully in selected family celebrations and activities, thus healing wounds and deepening these critically supportive relationships.

REFERENCES

Adam, B. D. (1985). Age, structure and sexuality: Reflections on the anthropological evidence on homosexual relations. *Journal of Homosexuality, 11*(3/4), 19–33.

Boxer, A., & Cohler, B. (1989). The life course of gay and lesbian youth: An immodest proposal for the study of lives. *Journal of Homosexuality, 17*(1–4), 317–335.

Chan, C. (1989). Issues of identity development among Asian American lesbians and gay men. *Journal of Counseling and Development, 68,* 16–20.

Garnets, L., & Kimmel, D. (1991). Lesbian and gay male dimensions in the psychological study of human diversity. In J. D. Goodchilds (Ed.), *Psychological perspectives on human diversity in America* (pp. 143–189). Washington, DC: American Psychological Association.

Gock, T. (1986, August). *Issues in gay affirmative psychotherapy with ethnically/culturally diverse populations.* Paper presented at the 94th Annual Convention of the American Psychological Association, Washington, DC.

Ihara, S. (1972). *Comrade loves of the Samurai.* Rutland, VT: Charles E. Tuttle.

Morales, E. S. (1989). Ethnic minority families and minority gays and lesbians. *Marriage and Family Review, 14,* 217–239.

Nanda, S. (1986). The Hijras of India: Cultural and Individual dimensions of an institutionalized third gender role. *Journal of Homosexuality, 11*(3/4), 35–54.

Sankar, A. (1986). Sisters and brothers, lovers and enemies: Marriage resistance in southern Kwantung. *Journal of Homosexuality, 11*(3/4), 69–82.

Sechrest, L., & Flores, L. (1969). Homosexuality in the Philippines and in the United States: The handwriting on the wall. *Journal of Social Psychiatry, 79,* 3–12.

Troiden, R. R. (1988). *Gay and lesbian identity: A sociological analysis.* New York: General Hall.

Weisz, J. R., Rothbaum, F. M., & Blackburn, T. C. (1984). Standing out and standing in: The psychology of control in America and Japan, *American Psychologist, 39,* 955–969.

27

Asian American Women

REIKO HOMMA-TRUE

HISTORICAL BACKGROUND

The term "Asian American women" refers to a diverse group representing as many as 35 ethnic–cultural groups, including Chinese, Filipinos, Japanese, Koreans, Indians, and various Southeast Asians. Their immigration to the United States began nearly 150 years ago with the entry of a small number of Chinese women, who accompanied their merchant husbands or were brought in as prostitutes (Kim & Otani, 1983). Their entry was soon blocked by the mounting anti-Chinese sentiment and enactment of a series of Chinese exclusion acts, and they were replaced by Japanese women, whose government actively encouraged the immigration of women as a way of preventing problems endemic to bachelor societies (e.g., prostitution, violence, and gambling) (Takaki, 1989).

Although Korean and Filipino women also immigrated during the early 1900s, their number was small at that time. It was after the liberalization of the immigration law in 1965 that a large number of Chinese, Filipino, and Korean women were permitted to immigrate with their families. They were followed by Southeast Asian women, who came with their families as refugees after the Vietnam War and settled in various parts of the country (Kim & Otani, 1983). For this reason, although women were far outnumbered by men in earlier years, they now constitute 51% of the Asian American population in the United States (U.S. Bureau of the Census, 1993).

Because of their diverse history of immigration, some Asian women, particularly Japanese and Chinese women, have been in the United States for several generations, but the majority are foreign-born (U.S. Bureau of the Census, 1993). The majority of adult women are married and live with their families. Although the traditional expectation for women in Asia has been that once they marry, they should stay home to take care of their families, 60.1% of them are working to supplement their husband's income, while the rate for all U.S. women is at 56.8% (U.S. Bureau of the Census, 1993). The aggregate educational achievement of Asian American women is high (32.7% with bachelor's degree or higher compared with 17.6% for all U.S. women), although there are significant subgroup differences ranging between 48.7% for Asian Indian women to 3.0% for Hmong women (U.S. Bureau of the Census, 1993). However, with the exception of a small number of professional and managerial women, most are employed at marginal, lower-level occupations and are earning considerably less than their white counterparts in a restricted labor market, such as the sweatshop garment industry, banking, insurance, hotels, telephone communications, and Silicon Valley factories (Wong & Hayashi, 1989; Villones, 1989).

PSYCHOSOCIAL STRESSES

Although they come from diverse cultural, ethnic, and socioeconomic backgrounds, certain common themes emerge in the stresses Asian American women encounter. For a large number of immigrant women, coping with the many stresses of adjusting to a new culture, learning a new language, working in marginal occupations, and securing basic survival needs for themselves and families are major sources of frustration and stress. While their stress level increases significantly, their difficulties are compounded by the fact they can no longer rely on the help they had from their extended families in the old country. They often have to work to help their husbands, who are unable to find work or can get only marginal jobs. When the husband's role as a breadwinner for his family is thus eroded, it often leads to changes in marital roles, power balance, and strains in their relationship. In extreme situations, it leads to domestic abuse, in which victims are invariably wives who often do not know how to seek help. Another source of stress for Asian immigrant women is the changing relationship with their children, who can usually adapt more rapidly to the new culture and begin to question the old-world values and challenge parental authority (Bradshaw, 1994; Homma-True, 1990).

Among the immigrant groups, there is general agreement that the Southeast Asian refugees face the greatest stresses in adjusting to the life in the new country. Many suffered traumatic experiences and major losses of close family members prior to their immigration. Often coming from rural backgrounds without the necessary language capability, education, or job skills, they were ill prepared to cope with the life in a modern, industrialized country. Their strains are frequently manifested through psychiatric and somatic symptoms, such as depression, anxiety attacks, headaches, and, in extreme cases, functional blindness (Chung, 1991; Rozee & Van Boemel, 1989).

Native-born Asian American women born in the United States, and others who are freer of the basic survival needs faced by immigrant women, face different types of stresses. Within their own Asian families and communities, many are still discriminated against because they are considered inferior to men (Kingston, 1976). Although most older women, particularly those who are foreign-born and who have had limited exposure to the Western ideologies of a woman's role and status, are more accepting of this traditional cultural expectations, others are unhappy with them and are increasingly challenging the old order to define new roles for themselves (Kim & Otani, 1983).

When they interact with larger communities, Asian American women often encounter a double dose of racism and sexism despite recent efforts to eliminate gender and racial discriminations in the United States. Many blame the fact that Asian women in this country are still perceived with negative stereotypes perpetuated in movies and literature (sex object, subservient, passive, helpless person or, if somewhat aggressive, a bitchy dragon lady) (Homma-True, 1990). Because of these stereotypes, Asian women are often exploited at their workplace or in their interpersonal relationships. An added factor that creates additional difficulty is the fact that Asian American women are often socialized by their families to uphold the traditional virtues, to be modest and reserved, and to be helpful to others, putting aside their own personal needs. These personal traits are in stark contrast to the traits encouraged by the dominant culture (e.g., assertiveness, competitiveness, and individualism) and put them at a disadvantage in competing with others in work and social situations, which in turn often leads to frustration and self-doubt.

Another source of strain for Asian American women arises from an increasing trend for them to marry outside their ethnic communities (Kikumura & Kitano, 1973). Although interracial marriages were strongly discouraged earlier, not only by Asian families but by most U.S. communities as well, they are now viewed with less stigma and the number of interracial marriages is likely to continue to increase. When couples are in love, they usually do not realize that there are a number of potential relationship problems in a union of people with divergent cultural backgrounds. Unless the couple recognizes these strains and conflicts early and deals with them, they will eventually destroy the relationship. This is particularly true for couples with widely divergent backgrounds (e.g., the so-called war brides and other foreign-born Asian women and their partners) (Kim & Otani, 1983). Although the U.S.-born Asian American women who outmarry are much better prepared culturally than the foreign-born women, many of them are still struggling with a variety of conflicts rooted in their cultural differences and experiences of racism and discrimination (Bradshaw, 1994). The challenges faced by biracial or multiracial Asian women who are the offspring of these marriages are also complex and could lead to additional strains (Root, 1994).

CLINICAL CONSIDERATIONS

Partly because of cultural stigma attached to seeking professional psychological help and partly because of the lack of linguistic and culturally appropriate services, the utilization of mental health services by Asian American women is significantly lower than that of the general population of women in the United States. Although a review of the utilization rate of Asian men and women at a public mental health system did not indicate significant differences between them (Homma-True, 1989), there were differences in the types of problems they sought help on—that is, the men had more serious psychotic illnesses while the women had more problems related to depression and other affective disorders. A similar pattern of Asian women with depressive conditions was also found in a health clinic in Boston (Yu & Wong, 1987). This pattern also parallels the pattern of depression among women in many parts of the world (Weissman & Olfson, 1995).

Some of the reasons that drive Asian women to seek help include the strains of coping and surviving in the new country, difficulty within their marriage and families, and dealing with the separation from or losses of loved ones. The information about the treatment approaches used by therapists who see Asian American women is limited, but it appears that many of them try to be eclectic and adapt the existing theoretical framework and treatment strategies by incorporating the client's specific cultural environment (Bradshaw, 1994; Homma-True, 1990; Sue & Morishima, 1982).

When attempting to conduct an assessment for Asian American women, it is important to keep in mind that the standardized diagnostic instruments may be inappropriate because they do not include culturally sensitive items or have not been validated for the Asian American population. For this reason, it is critical to conduct a thorough intake interviews with careful attention to the client's social, cultural, generational, and historical background (Lee, 1982). Based on the assessment, the treatment strategies will need to be adapted to the individual's needs, problems, and receptivity to psychological interventions. These interventions could include an active or a directive approach with concrete assistance around survival issues for those in crisis and with limited psychological sophistication; behavior therapy or short-term psychotherapy focusing on a specific problem area; longer-term psychotherapy for those with psychological receptivity to deal with more extensive and long-standing difficulties; family therapy when problems are enmeshed within the family structure; selective use of psychotropic medication or traditional herbal medicine; and a combination of psychotherapy and other adjunctive therapy such as acupuncture or meditation.

Therapists need to be particularly sensitive about the struggle many Asian American woman face between their wish to be autonomous and assert their personal needs, like other U.S. women, and their deep-rooted bond and loyalty to their families. They must understand the degree to which certain cultural values need to be respected, including those relating to sex-role issues, and balance them with other competing interests. Therapists can help their clients see the traditional values not in absolute terms but with a different perspective that allows them some flexibility and modification. When conflicts are too pathological and seriously crippling to a client's well-being (e.g., conflicts that involve domestic abuse, in extreme cases), clients should be given support and assistance in making appropriate changes, including creating psychological or interpersonal distances from their families. Therapists need to help clients understand that it is generally not realistic to try to challenge or change the traditional belief system of one's family, but it is possible to confront and change their own internalized expectations if these expectations are seriously interfering with their personal growth.

Strategies advocated by feminist therapists are often viewed with skepticism by Asian American therapists as potentially more harmful to Asian American women in their relationship to their partners and families. However, if used with sensitive concerns, some feminist approaches can be beneficial (Gilbert, 1980; Mays & Comas-Díaz, 1988). For example, assertiveness training can be effective for those who are being exploited at work if it focuses on the specific situation and careful attention is given to separate and maintain an acceptable pattern of behavior within the context of the Asian American community (Yanagida, 1979). Therapists, particularly Asian American female therapists, can also serve as a role model for successfully balancing these conflicting demands both within and outside their own families and community.

CASE EXAMPLE

The following clinical vignette illustrates some of the issues faced by Asian women who seek psychotherapeutic assistance. To protect the confidentiality of the individuals involved, their names have been altered.

Mary was a 33-year-old, second-generation Chinese American, who was seriously depressed and feeling suicidal. She was working as a legal secretary and was having frequent marital difficulties with Sam, her 40-year-old Chinese American businessman husband. Sam came from an affluent mercantile family in Hong Kong, immigrated to the United States as a student, and started his own business. Sam had a series of extramarital affairs but expected Mary to accept his behavior, insisting that a successful Asian man must have his freedom. He was critical about Mary's working-class background and often was verbally abusive to her for not being a supportive wife. Mary's parents were not sympathetic to her unhappiness, pointing out that Sam was not physically abusive and that as long as the husband provides for his family, a good Asian wife needs to forgive his occasional dalliances. In fact, both Sam's and Mary's mothers had husbands who committed similar indiscretions, but tolerated these indiscretions as part of the cultural tradition and to keep peace in the family.

As Sam refused to become involved in a couple therapy, the therapist saw Mary in individual sessions and helped her to recognize how her deep sense of anger and hurt toward her husband was internalized against herself and manifested in the form of depression and suicidality. By illustrating how women's status and roles have undergone many changes, not only in the United States, but in China and in other parts of Asia as well, the therapist was able to help Mary understand her family's expectations as a reflection of the social mores of the earlier times in China which might no longer be as valid for contemporary Asian American women and in Mary's situation.

The therapist helped Mary to understand the importance of maintaining a respectful relationship with her parents and not trying to change their inflexible, traditional values and ideas but to begin to cultivate other sources of support and reference point for herself outside her family. Mary was encouraged to join an Asian American women's organization, cultivate friendship with other Asian American women, read literature on the struggles of other Asian and Asian American women, and develop plans for personal growth. Eventually Mary decided to leave her husband. She survived a stressful divorce process and went back to school to pursue a career in law. Despite their original disapproval, Mary's family gradually became more supportive of her effort and ultimately became proud of her achievements.

SUMMARY

There are significant degrees of psychosocial stresses among a diverse group of Asian American women. Although immigrants and refugees are particularly vulnerable to the stresses of adjustment, U.S.-born women are also exposed to a variety of stresses, including those stemming from their exposure to the racism and sexism around them. Despite their reluctance to seek outside help, there are indications that integrating the existing treatment approaches with culturally sensitive approaches can be useful in resolving the psychosocial conflicts Asian American women face, both within their own families and with their relationships outside their communities. If therapists use such approaches sensitively, they can be effective in helping to clarify the balance between traditional Asian sexism and cultural values and those of the surrounding community's cultural values. While respecting the old order, therapists should help their clients develop newer, more complementary male/female relationships and create stronger, more positive roles for Asian American women.

REFERENCES

Bradshaw, C. K. (1994). Asian and Asian American women: Hisotorical and political consideration in psychotherapy. In L. Comas-Díaz & B. Greene (Eds.), *Women of color: Integrating ethnic and gender identities in psychotherapy* (pp. 72–113). New York: Guilford Press.

Chung, R. C. (1991, August). *Predictors of distress among Southeast Asian refugees: Group and gender differences.* Paper presented at Asian American Psychological Association Conference, San Francisco.

Gilbert, L. A. (1980). Feminist therapy. In A. M. Brodsky & R. Hare-Mustin (Eds.), *Women and psychotherapy: An assessment of research and practice* (pp. 245–265). New York: Guilford Press.

Homma-True, R. (1989). *Mental health service utilization by Asian American women in San Francisco.* Paper presented at the Annual Convention of the Asian American Psychological Association, New York.

Homma-True, R. (1990). Psychotherapeutic issues with Asian American women. *Sex Roles, 22,* 477–486.

Kikumura, A., & Kitano, H. (1973). Interracial marriage: A picture of the Japanese Americans. *Journal of Social Issues, 29,* 67–81.

Kim, E. H., & Otani, J. (1983). Asian women in America. In E. H. Kim (Ed.), *With silk wings: Asian American women at work* (pp. 120–135). San Francisco: Asian Women United.

Kingston, M. H. (1976). *The women warrior.* New York: Knopf.

Lee, E. (1982). A social system approach to assessment and treatment for Chinese American families. In M. McGodrick, J. K. Pearce, & J. Giordano (Eds.), *Ethnicity and family therapy* (pp. 527–551). New York: Guilford Press.

Mays, V., & Comas-Díaz, L. (1988). Feminist therapy with ethnic minority populations: A closer look at blacks and Hispanics. In M. A. Dutton-Douglas & L. D. Walker (Eds.), *Feminist psychotherapies: Integration of therapeutic and feminist systems* (pp. 228–251). Norwood, NJ: Ablex.

Root, M. P. P. (1994). Mixed-race women. In L. Comas-Díaz & B. Greene (Eds.),

Women of color: Integrating ethnic and gender identities in psychotherapy (pp. 455–478). New York: Guilford Press.

Rozee, P. D., & Van Boemel, G. (1989). The psychological effects of war trauma and abuse on older Cambodian refugee women. *Women and Therapy, 8*(4), 23–49.

Sue, S., & Morishima, J. K. (1982). *The mental health of Asian Americans.* San Francisco: Jossey-Bass.

Takaki, R. (1989). *Strangers from a different shore: History of Asian Americans.* Boston: Little, Brown.

U.S. Bureau of the Census. (1993). *We, the American . . . Asians.* Washington, DC: U.S. Department of Commerce.

Villones, R. (1989). Women in the Silicon Valley. In Asian Women United of California (Ed.), *Making waves: An anthology of writings by and about Asian American women* (pp. 172–175). Boston: Beacon.

Weissman, M. M., & Olfson, M. (1995). Depression in women: Implications for health care research. *Science, 269,* 799–801.

Wong, D., & Hayashi, D. (1989). Behind the unmarked doors: Developments in the garment industry. In Asian Women United of California (Ed.), *Making waves: An anthology of writings by and about Asian American women* (pp. 159–171). Boston: Beacon.

Yanagida, E. H. (1979). Cross-cultural considerations in the application of assertive training. *Psychology of Women Quarterly, 3,* 400–402.

Yu, E. S. H., Liu, W. T., & Wong, S. C. (1987). Measurement of depression in a Chinatown health clinic. In W. T. Liu (Ed.), *A decade review of mental health research, training, and services* Chicago: Pacific/Asian American Mental Health Research Center, University of Illinois at Chicago.

28

Asian Intermarriage: Love versus Tradition

JOEL CROHN

In the last 30 years, the once unthinkable possibility of interracial marriage has become a commonplace reality in many Asian American communities. A majority of third-generation Japanese Americans, the Sansei, are choosing non-Japanese and non-Asian partners, most often Caucasians. Although Chinese and members of other Asian American groups are not marrying out as frequently as Japanese Americans, their rates of intermarriage continue to climb. This explosion of intermarriage in communities in which societal racism, as well as strong internal familial, communal, and psychological forces, had long made interracial marriage a rarity has had a tremendous impact on Asian American families and communities.

The new demographics of love in the United States are a result of several interrelated factors: the high educational achievement and rapid upward economic mobility of almost all Asian groups, gradually lowering barriers of discrimination, and the image that has evolved in recent years of Asians as the "model minority."

CULTURAL CONTRASTS

The contrasts between Western and Asian values can form the basis of both the attraction and the conflict in interracial marriages involving Asian Americans and non-Asians. The values of the hyperindividualistic white American Protestant culture, which elevates the separate, bounded, and autonomous self, stand in sharp contrast to the collective and communal values of Asian cultures in which individual and group identity are tightly intertwined. Although Asian Americans have absorbed more of the individualistic American culture than their Asian-born relatives, even second- and third-generation Asian Americans retain strong if conflicted attachments to traditional cultural and family values.

In many ways these contrasts in Asian and Anglo-American values lead to basic assumptions about relationships that are mirror images of one another. In Asian cultures, the roles of men and women are more clearly, but rigidly, differentiated. In modern American culture, with men and women from many different backgrounds interacting and a public ideology of equal opportunity, sex roles are increasingly blurred. Although Asians tend to be most comfortable with hierarchical social structures that emphasize cooperation and clear lines of power and authority, American myths repeatedly idealize the common man who singlehandedly triumphs over adversity and challenges the status quo. If Americans praise their children for "expressing their feelings," Asian cultures tend to praise children who are "quiet and obedient."

The bonds of loyalty and obligation in Asian cultures are tremendously strong and extend back through the generations. In middle-class Anglo-American culture, the present and future are stressed, and in a fantastically mobile society, it is expected and accepted that one generation may be geographically and emotionally isolated from the next. In Asian cultures, marriage exists in the context of extended family and long-term interfamily relationships. Americans expect to make new sets of friends several times in their lives and are quite expert at building new, if sometimes superficial, relationships.

As Asian Americans increasingly come into close contact with non-Asians in work, academic, and neighborhood settings, cultural assumptions that were secure and stable for generations are challenged, and sometimes, uprooted. People living under the communal and hierarchical values of Asian cultures who are exposed to the relative freedom of Western values suddenly find themselves feeling constricted by a social system that until now always seemed inevitable and necessary. And when non-Asian Americans who have prided themselves on their independence and freedom from the constraints of tradition are exposed to the unity, support, and structured sex roles that Asian cultures offer, they suddenly find themselves increasingly aware of the isolation, alienation, and confusion that are often the price of their freedom.

THE SEARCH FOR SYNTHESIS

Marriage, at its best, is motivated by a search for synthesis, a wish for completion and wholeness. In cross-cultural relationships, both persons look to their partner, and the values of the partner's culture, to open possibilities they feel are lacking in their own family and culture.

Cross-cultural couples face a paradox that is inherent in their attraction to each other: the cultural style and sense of identity that one partner finds so attractive may be precisely what the other is trying to escape from. It is as if two people traveling in opposite directions meet one another as their paths cross.

This dynamic was quite clear in the relationship of an interracial couple who came to me for psychotherapy.

Susan was 12 when she immigrated with her family to the United States from mainland China after spending a year in Hong Kong. She attended high school in California and went on to study business at the university while continuing to live with her parents.

She felt that her marriage to Alan, who was a rising star in the firm at which she went to work after her graduation, would allow her a personal and professional freedom that she believed would be very difficult to find in a marriage to an Asian man from a similar cultural background. She characterized Asian American men as domineering and controlling.

> "Asian men are used to seeing women as possessions, to be bought, sold, used or abused. And while it obviously isn't so overt anymore, Chinese men, even American-born Chinese men of traditional families whose parents were born overseas, still expect a whole lot of male prerogatives. I'm not going to put up with it. I haven't come this far to be someone's slave or possession."

Alan was from a middle-class white Protestant background and Susan believed that he valued her because she was an "independent woman who thought for herself." She also recognized that her marriage to Alan would help her achieve a greater separation from her family, which she had found very difficult to accomplish. She complained that even though she was 25 and self-supporting, her mother felt free to constantly criticize her independence as "selfishness." She also repeatedly resisted her mother's offers of helping her find an appropriate young Chinese man for a husband.

Alan's unspoken expectations of his relationship with Susan were in many ways the opposite of hers. Although he valued her intelligence, his attraction was not so much to Susan's independence but to how well she fit into his fantasy of the exotic, beautiful Asian woman who would ultimately defer her needs for his. His own relationships with American women led him to conclude that they were "too pushy and demanding and always thinking about themselves." He saw Susan as someone who would think about him first.

Not surprisingly, they had not clarified their fantasies or their expectations before they married. They also tended to minimize their cultural differences. It was not until they moved in together and began arguing over the division of household labor that the contradictions in their unarticulated fantasies about each other came to light. Each of them felt betrayed by the other.

As Susan and Alan began the process of negotiating their differences, they realized that they had never spelled out their expectations of married life. Choosing one another over the opposition of their families led to an idealization of their relationship. Angered by their families' lack of support, they ignored their normal ambivalence about their own relationship. Like a nation threatened by enemies from without, they closed ranks and forgot, until time reminded them, of their own differences.

RECLAIMING CULTURAL HISTORIES

Unacknowledged contrasts in the meaning and intensity of each partner's cultural identity can also lead to conflict in Asian/non-Asian intermarriages. Because of their rapid assimilation, Japanese Americans are particularly prone to a kind of cultural amnesia. Ron and Julie's story illustrates how life cycle transitions can reveal denied or minimized aspects of identity in disturbing ways.

Until the birth of their child, Ron, who is Japanese American, and Julie, who is from a white, Protestant family, always felt proud of their transcendence of the limiting identities of their birth cultures. They often quoted John Lennon's song "Imagine," which looks forward to a better time when people have left behind the racial, cultural, and religious attachments that seem to be the cause of so much conflict in the world. Even after Julie got pregnant, they never felt that it was necessary to talk about how they would shape the cultural identity of their biracial child.

When Julie went into preterm labor, she called Ron, who was at a conference in a nearby city. He quickly left the meeting to join her at the hospital, but their new son arrived before his father. As Ron ran into the delivery room, the first words that burst out of his mouth were, "What shape are his eyes?" Julie looked up at him in shock and confusion. Several hours after the baby's birth, Ron told Julie for the first time about his wish to name their child after his grandfather. In spite of their shared ideology emphasizing the universal, Ron found himself obsessed with the particular. Ron and Julie finally had to deal with old and deep cultural loyalties which do not simply disappear.

Talking openly about their cultural contrasts had always seemed dangerous rather than potentially enriching. They both feared that the past might highlight their differences and pull them apart. Underlying the bond of their common values, they each had very different feelings about their pasts. They both sensed that dealing directly with these issues might open old wounds from their own complicated and conflicted histories.

Ron and Julie's therapy focused on helping them share the experiences that had shaped their cultural identities in their families of origin. As they explored their cultural pasts, they began to understand their differences better. Although Ron felt both burdened and enriched by his hidden, intense history, Julie hungered for a sense of belonging and cultural identity she had never experienced.

Julie sounded a bit apologetic as she spoke about her cultural history:

> "In a lot of ways I feel like my cultural heritage is of being a nothing. I mean, I guess I would be considered a white Protestant, but really, I don't feel like I'm anything. I have always felt kind of pale and empty. I'm a 'wannabe.' I always wanted to be something distinct. I remember as a little girl visiting my Italian friend's family. They seemed lively, close, and at times combative. I wanted what they seemed to have, and when I was at their house, I used to pretend that I was a member of their family and their culture. But then it would be time to leave, and I would feel like Cinderella at the stroke of midnight. I had to go back to being the ordinary me, the nothing."

Ron's story was very different. His parents were Nisei, the first American-born generation. They were raised in Hawaii by their immigrant families who had moved there from Japan after World War I. Ron grew up as a Sansei, a grandchild of the immigrant generation.

His mother and father invested their life savings in a small shop in Los Angeles, involved themselves in a thriving Japanese American community, and were already doing better than they had expected when a day came that changed their lives forever—December 7, 1941. The Japanese attack on Pearl Harbor resulted in the internment of thousands of West Coast Japanese Americans, the majority of whom, like Ron's parents, were U.S. citizens and guilty of nothing but their Japanese ancestry. His family was forced to sell their store at a fraction of its worth. Then they were transported to a desolate outpost in central California. They were devastated.

After they were released, they moved back to Hawaii to live with their parents. Ron was born in Honolulu in 1950. Ron was able to use the therapeutic setting to talk with Julie for the first time of the difficulties of his move to the mainland.

> "When I was eight, we moved from a totally Japanese American world in Honolulu to a neighborhood outside of San Francisco where we were the only non-Caucasians. It was a tremendous shock. Some of the older white kids taunted me, and one of my classmates threw a rock at me and called me a dirty Jap. My mother waited at the bus stop with me every day for fear of leaving me alone."

Although Ron's parents continued to stress the importance of associating only with Japanese, there were no other Japanese with whom to associate. Even though they lived just a few miles from San Francisco, they made little effort to interact with the vital Japanese community up the road. They might as well have moved to a cornfield in Iowa. The disparity between their words and their actions was confusing and disturbing. But because it was against the rules to question elders, Ron and his brother and sister could not challenge their parents' mixed messages. They suffered in silence, condemned to a joyless social isolation.

His parents were so successful at adapting and fitting into American life after the wartime betrayal by their own country that it almost seemed as if the internment had never happened. Their children were faced with the task of digesting an enormous history that they were not even allowed to taste. His parents often used the expression *shogamai,* which roughly translates to "you can't do anything about it," to deal with difficult realities. Ron now realized that their attempts to make the past invisible were consistent with the passive fatalism revealed by the way they used *shogamai.*

Julie and Ron now began to understand the problem with their agreement "to leave the past behind." By reviewing their cultural histories, they learned that Julie actually longed for a sense of closeness and connection that she felt lacking in her own family. Ron revealed that his disinterest in his history was designed to conceal a confusing and painful legacy with which he needed to come to terms. For the first time they could clearly see the connection between their failure to deal with the past and their current crisis over naming their child.

With some encouragement, they approached Ron's parents with questions about their past. After several months of brief and awkward conversations, they agreed to "tell a few stories." Their talks gradually evolved into a series of deep, quietly intense, and very personal revelations about their wartime experiences in the camps. These conversations brought them all closer than they ever imagined they could be. After talking late into the evening one night, Ron's mother said to Julie, "I never thought that someone who didn't go through it could possibly understand. But you do." Ron and Julie's patience and persistence had paid off.

The crisis brought on by the birth of their child revealed the very different cultural roots they always feared acknowledging. As their little unnamed infant pushed open the doors that hid their pasts, their fears seemed confirmed because of the pain and conflict they experienced. But as they became less anxious talking about their backgrounds with each other and their families, they began to realize that by facing the difficulties of the past, they could enrich their future together.

PRINCIPLES OF WORKING WITH INTERRACIAL COUPLES

Culture shapes every aspect of how a person views the world and what he or she considers "normal" and "abnormal." It molds attitudes toward time, family, sex monogamy, and identity. Cultural rules govern how anger and affection are expressed, the ways that children are disciplined and rewarded, how strangers and friends are greeted, and the roles of men and women. Behavior that one culture defines as neighborly, another may label as seductive; what one defines as friendly disagreement, the other may see as a threat.

In intermarriages, partners may not be aware of the different cultural value systems that shape their perceptions of reality. When one partner says he visits his parents "often," he may mean twice a year, but to the other, "seldom" might mean twice a week. Partners in mixed matches raised in different countries may have very different cultural definitions of normal. Just imagine the potential value conflicts in an intermarriage between a Japanese man from a culture where men average 11 minutes of housework a day and a woman from the United States where men average 108 minutes ("The Reluctant Princess," 1993). Expectations of what is normal may not easily mesh.

The following principles are useful in working with interracial couples when one is an Asian American partner. Although many of these methods echo established therapeutic practice in treating any couple, they especially emphasize the cultural component of working with cross-cultural couples and families.

Be Aware of "Cultural Countertransference"

There is no such thing as cultural "neutrality," and to help couples bridge the differences in their cultural values, therapists must recognize their own.

Kleinman (1988) reported on a Chinese psychiatrist treating a patient who was depressed and anxious about a family obligation to support an ungrateful mother-in-law. He quotes the therapist as saying: "She is your family member. It is your responsibility to care for an old mother-in-law. You must contain your anger. You know the old adage: 'Be deaf and dumb! Swallow the seeds of the bitter melon! Don't speak out.' "

Contrast the Chinese psychiatrist's advice with the core values of U.S. culture distilled in the "Gestalt Prayer" by Fritz Perls (1969). Its individualistic assumptions are echoed in many American and Western forms of psychotherapy:

> I do my thing, and you do your thing.
> I am not in this world to live up to your expectations.
> And you are not in this world to live up to mine.
> You are you and I am I,
> And if by chance we find each other, it's beautiful.
> If not, it can't be helped.

The therapist who can recognize his or her own values about culture, family, and community and who can also appreciate the validity of a wide range of cultural perspectives is in the best position to work with cross-cultural families. Separation and individuation are relative values, not absolute.

Confront Cultural Amnesia

The therapist should not collude with a couple in defining cultural differences as irrelevant. Especially when the Asian partner is U.S.-born and highly assimilated, the couple may assume that their cultural differences are minimal and may object when the therapist places their conflicts in a cultural framework. Taking a cultural history of each partner with the other present can help clarify differences in cultural expectations and identity. Conflict can sometimes be depolarized by exploring each partner's ambivalence about certain aspects of his or her own cultural identity.

Clarify Differences in Cultural Codes

The therapist must help partners see how contrasts in their expectations of each other and of their children's behavior are rooted in the cultural framework of their own childhoods. When parents can acknowledge the culturally influenced behavioral contrasts in their backgrounds, they are more able to depathologize their discomfort with their partner's beliefs. Therapists should see themselves as a simultaneous translator for two people who think they are speaking the same language but are not.

Clarify Differences between Culture and Religion

Intermarried couples often find negotiating the identity of their family complicated by each partner's confusion about religious and cultural identity. Although they traditionally overlap, culture and religion are not the same.

Religious faith offers a language for the soul and brings order out of the chaos of human life by creating moral codes that regulate the relationships between husbands and wives, parents and children, workers and employers, and even friends and enemies. Its rituals comfort people through times of loss and sanctify and give meaning to the life cycle transitions of birth, marriage, and death.

Culture is more particular. Although each religion includes many cultures, cultural identity is an affirmation of a distinctive sense of peoplehood. Whether mythical or literal, cultural identity honors common ancestors and is reinforced by food, festivals, folkways, language, and ritual. It is rooted in the remembrances of a shared past and the expectation of a common fate in the years to come.

Help Parents Help Their Children Build a Positive Identity

The therapist should challenge parents of interracial children to find ways to enable their children to have positive attachments to both of their cultural heritages. Although the culture of one parent may be emphasized for a variety of reasons, obliterating the culture of the other, even in families separated by divorce, is seldom helpful to children who literally embody both cultures. Often parents have to be helped to acknowledge their own confusion about their own cultural identities before they can help their children clarify theirs.

Do Not Overemphasize Cultural Explanations

Although a cultural perspective is important, therapists should not overemphasize cultural differences to the point of ignoring the universal. No framework explains everything and every marital conflict cannot be explained by exploring differences in cultural backgrounds. Some partners in cross-cultural relationships create conflict in all their relationships, whether or not they are cross-cultural.

Be Aware of the Social Context of Intermarriage

The therapist should help intermarried couples understand and deal with the social context of their marriage. Interracial marriage in Hawaii, where it is the norm, has a very different social meaning than in a small town in Alabama, where an interracial couple may experience various forms of racism or social isolation that puts strains on their relationship. Paradoxically, it may be the couple in the more tolerant milieu that has difficulty recognizing that their cultural differences are part of any conflict in their relationship, whereas the couple in the more parochial setting may have difficulty realizing that not all their difficulties are created by community intolerance.

Help Couples Attempt to Rebuild Family Relationships

For too many intermarried couples, the failure to reconnect with family members who have expressed disapproval of their relationships results from a failure to try. While some couples try for too long to negotiate with family and others who clearly will never accept their relationship, more often, couples retreat in hurt and anger before the situation is truly hopeless.

CONCLUSION

History has always involved dramatic shifts, but the accelerating rate of change has never approached that of today's world. In the past, change was measured in generations, and the distant horizon was more likely to be the next village than an alien land halfway around the world. Throughout most of history the practice of religion was inseparable from the life of a community. Because they were so intertwined, it was not necessary or even possible to separate family loyalty, cultural identity, and religious belief. Each reinforced the other, and all were integral in giving each person a clear sense of belonging and identity. The family was part of a community that was rooted in a culture that was linked to a religion.

Although people living in more stable, traditional cultures might face many hardships, they were sustained by a clear knowledge of who they were, where they belonged, and what they believed in. Everyone in a community understood the link between themselves and their ancestors and between their religious faith and their actions. Yesterday and today were as inseparably bound as heaven and earth.

Today the bonds connecting the three cornerstones that have always formed the foundation of identity—family, culture, and religion—are weakened by the pace of change and the new world disorder. As a result, our clients are constantly confronted with crises of definition and find themselves asking questions that most of their great-grandparents could not even have imagined. *What is the nature of my allegiance to my family, my tribe, my nation, and my God? Are they of different intensities? Could they come into conflict with one another?* Religious and cultural identities are no longer just accidents of birth. Today each person must pick from among shattered remnants of the past to create answers to the question, Who am I? Along with these questions comes the more mundane ones of defining the rules that govern behavior in daily life. When intermarried partners learn to identify and negotiate the cultural differences that influence their relationships, they are more able to successfully deal with the problems and possibilities of cross-cultural family life.

ACKNOWLEDGMENT

Parts of this chapter are from Crohn (1995). Copyright 1995 by Random House, Inc. Adapted by permission.

REFERENCES

Crohn, J. (1995). *Mixed matches: How to create successful interracial, interethnic, and interfaith relationships.* New York: Fawcett/Ballantine.
Kleinman, A. (1988). *Rethinking psychiatry: From cultural category to personal experience.* New York: Free Press.
Perls, F. (1969). *Gestalt therapy verbatim.* Lafayette, CA: Real People Press.
The reluctant princess. (1993, May 24). *Newsweek*, p. 34.

29

Domestic Violence in the Asian Community

BECKIE MASAKI
LORENA WONG

Sue (not her real name) came to the Asian Women's Shelter in San Francisco when she was 5 months' pregnant. She was encouraged by her doctor to call the shelter. Less than a year ago, she had suffered a miscarriage because of the beatings. The beatings continued, and she wants to deliver a healthy baby this time. Sue has a 3-year-old son as well, and she worries about how she will give birth and care for her son without the help of her husband and in-laws. Her own family is in China. The in-laws and husband want Sue to return, but Sue is frightened for her safety and especially that of her son and unborn baby.

Sue is not alone.

Domestic violence is a social problem of epidemic proportions. It is the single greatest cause of injury to women: In one year alone, almost four million American women are physically abused by their intimate partners (The Commonwealth Fund, 1993); 42% of murdered women are killed by their intimate male partners (Center for the Study and Prevention of Child Abuse, 1991); One in three Americans has directly witnessed an incident of domestic violence (Family Violence Prevention Fund, 1993).

There is a pervasive myth that domestic violence does not exist in the Asian community. In fact, domestic violence exists in every segment of our society—it crosses all racial, class, and religious lines. Domestic violence is a pattern of coercive control that one person exercises over another in a relationship. Domestic violence comprises of several forms of violence that batterers use as ways to dominate their partners and get their way: physical battering, emotional abuse, verbal abuse, sexual abuse, property and economic abuse.

Often the batterer, the victim, and the community want to minimize how severe domestic violence is, but in fact 25% of all female homicide victims were murdered by their husbands or partners. Studies show that in domestic violence relationships, the abuse increases in both severity and frequency over time.

Domestic violence has a devastating impact on children. One-quarter of batterers who abuse their partners abuse their children as well. Even if children are not directly abused, they suffer the serious psychological affects of living in fear, not feeling protected by their mothers, and being surrounded by an unpredictable, explosive, and uncontrollable environment. Some 80% of the boys who see their fathers beat their mothers grow up to become batterers (Strauss, Gelles, & Steinmetz, 1980).

Many people believe domestic violence is caused by alcohol, gambling, immigrant stresses, and so on. These things often feed into the problem but are not the cause. The cause of domestic violence is embedded in how societies define and value power and control: the way we are raised. Boys are taught that being powerful means having power over someone else, and being in control means controlling others. Girls are taught that responsibility means putting everyone else's needs before theirs, that nurturing and caring means sacrificing themselves for their families and giving power, not taking it. The unequal position of women and men in our societies, the deep patterns and values we were raised with, and the promotion of violence as a solution on every level of our society all create the seeds from which domestic violence grows.

DOMESTIC VIOLENCE IN THE ASIAN COMMUNITY

The basic dynamics and root causes of domestic violence are the same as in any community. There are some differences, however, because culture and background affect every aspect of who we are and what we do, including domestic violence relationships.

Asian Battered Women

All battered women face isolation, low self-esteem, lack of resources, and self-blame. For the Asian battered women, these factors are often magnified:

1. *Extreme isolation.* Many Asian battered women do not have family or friends in this country. They may not speak English and may not know the laws and their rights.

2. *Immigration.* Many Asian battered women depend on their batterers for sponsorship in the United States. The batterers use this as another means of control.

3. *Reinforced powerlessness from society.* For Asian battered women and other battered women of color, the ability to break out of a domestic violence relationship is compounded by barriers of racism, undocumented status, no resources, no place to go, no one who speaks their language, no marketable job skills, and unfamiliarity with systems.

4. *Traditional views regarding family and community.* Most Asian cultures deeply value putting one's family before oneself; community before the individual. Asian families emphasize extended family relations versus the nuclear family alone. The extended family and close community are strong supports and resources for survival for Asians in the United States, but when domestic violence exists, the close ties and deep commitment to family and community can be an additional barrier (both physically and emotionally) to escaping from the violence.

5. *Lack of resources.* All battered women lack resources, but few services are designed to address the needs of Asian battered women. In the United States, only four shelter programs exist that specifically address the language and cultural needs of Asian battered women. Economically, a woman often depends on the batterer, and when she leaves, she may have no job skills, no family or friends to turn to, no education in this country, and no access to government assistance.

The Batterers

Non-Asian batterers who abuse Asian women use their privileged position as a further means to control their partners (immigration status; knowledge of systems and law; access to resources; everyone believes batterer, no one believes or understands woman).

Asian batterers blame their violence on racism, "immigrant stresses," and their status in the United States. They believe that they have right to beat their partners because it is part of their culture and tradition. They do not have access to resources designed specifically for Asian batterers.

The Asian community, as many other communities, often reinforces domestic violence by minimizing the problem. The Asian community may not want the larger society to use this as yet another negative attribute and the community may also believe that domestic violence is acceptable because it is "traditional."

The Asian community can be a strong force against domestic violence, especially because many Asian communities have highly organized leadership and promote a sense of belonging and interdependence. Asian community members at large could effectively change the prevalence of domestic violence by actively speaking up against domestic violence, supporting battered women and their children in breaking the cycle of violence, and passing on traditions without passing on violence.

The Non-Asian Community

The larger society reinforces domestic violence in the Asian community by not acknowledging the existence of the problem. The larger society perpetuates the model minority myth about Asians and often believes Asians have no societal problems. If members of the larger society acknowledge that Asians have this problem, they often choose to ignore it because "they take care of their own" or "it is accepted in their culture." The invisibility of the issue of domestic violence in the Asian community by the larger society is particularly insidious because it affects funding and the availability of services, perpetuates racism, and oversimplifies cultural values.

CULTURAL CONSIDERATIONS IN COUNSELING DOMESTIC VIOLENCE SURVIVORS

Culture

To have a better understanding of domestic violence in the Asian communities, it is necessary to understand and appreciate the interplay between the individual and cultural dynamics. The term "Asian" in the United States has come to represent hundreds of nationalities of people, all with diverse cultural backgrounds. In addition, the immigration history of Asian groups to the United States ranges widely from those whose ancestors immigrated more than 100 years ago to those who recently arrived. Add to this the changing values with regard to the status of women, both in the United States and in countries of ancestry, and it becomes clear that any attempt to describe "cultural considerations" is a dynamic process prone to oversimplification or overgeneralization. We encourage readers to view the following points about culture as a background guide, focused primarily on enhancing our understanding of domestic violence in the Asian communities.

Perception of the Individual

The individual in Asian culture is defined as a part of a larger group: one's family before oneself; community before the individual. Individual behavior has great bearing on the family and community. Although shame and guilt are experienced in Western culture, they are much more magnified in Asian culture as the whole family is affected by the actions of any one family member.

Because domestic violence is generally viewed as shameful to the family, there is often pressure to keep it secret or even to deny that the violence exists. It is common for an Asian woman to live with her husband and his family. She is isolated from her own family members, who are often back in her home country. When domestic violence exists, she is sometimes scapegoated by her husband's whole family. If the husband's family does empathize with her, they often plead with her to stay with the batterer "to change him" or "give him another chance."

The difference between Western and Asian perceptions of the individual have significant implications for work with Asian battered women. Empowerment has been viewed as central to enabling battered women to rebuild self-esteem and confidence and to overcome the learned helplessness endured in a battering relationship. Empowerment in Western society often reflects the Western values of independence and individualism: "I can make it on my own," "I'm strong, I don't need anyone." Empowerment for Asian battered women often reflects more interdependence rather than individualism: "My group of friends is like the extended family that I no longer have. We help each other out."

Patriarchy

Rule and domination by men continue to be the prevailing social order in most societies, although this is being challenged on many levels and in many countries, including Asian countries. Even though the status of women throughout the world is changing, many men still see domestic violence as their male and husbandly right—to control the woman he feels he possesses. Other men believe it is their responsibility as head of the household to "discipline" the wife if she is not performing the way he thinks she should be. That discipline may take the form of battering, but he believes that is the way to teach her how to do things "correctly." Batterers use every means available to them to control and assert power over their partners. Male dominance and the abuse of male privilege are major factors used by batterers.

Immigrant Asian batterers often resent abuse laws in the United States: "How dare the U.S. government interfere with the way I discipline my wife. How dare they get involved in private matters!" In addition, the Asian community as well as the larger U.S. society often reinforces the myth that domestic violence is acceptable in Asian culture. This type of thinking reflects a common misconception that domestic violence is "cultural." The fact is, domestic violence crosses all lines of race, culture, class, religion, and sexual orientation.

Fatalism and Karma

Fatalism and some aspects of Confucian philosophy have commonly been interpreted to condone domestic violence. Such is the case around suffering. Suffering is the path to maturity. The one who endures suffering will develop a stronger and better character. A woman is expected to have patience and tolerate difficult situations, to accept bitterness. The woman can rest her hopes on a Chinese saying: "When all the bitterness ends, sweetness will come." She can also resign herself to fate—this is how her life was meant to be; he was born this way; I am doing penance for past wrongs.

Although some women believe it is their karmic fate to endure the violent relationship, others interpret fate in more empowering ways. One woman attributed her husband's violence to his fate for having killed so many people in the war. "He killed so many, he is haunted by their spirits and cannot free himself from his killing ways. We cannot help him, we must leave so that my children and I can survive in peace."

Immigration Status

Another issue that many Asian women must deal with is immigration status and its consequences. Many Asian battered women depend on their batterers for sponsorship in the United States. The batterers use this as another means of control: "If you ever try to leave me, I'll get you deported!" When an immigrant woman first marries a man living in the United States, he sponsors her for residency by filing an initial petition with the Immigration and Naturalization Service. After this first process, she is issued conditional permanent residency for at least 2 years. After the 2-year period the couple goes through a joint interview before she is granted permanent residency status. In a domestic violence relationship, the batterer wields the power of his sponsorship over the woman. He could file for a divorce, claiming fraudulent marriage, thereby leaving the woman to face possible deportation. This is a serious problem for the woman, especially if she was denoted as the bridge by which other family members would eventually come to the United States. When her marriage fails, sometimes an immigrant woman chooses not to return home rather than face shame in letting her family down.

A battered woman's waiver to the Marriage Fraud Act was established in 1990 to address the danger that women face when they are trapped in violent relationships for the 2-year period before the joint interview. Now those who can document their situation as battered women are eligible to go to the second interview without their husbands to receive their permanent resident status. Women in this situation should consult an immigration attorney.

Marriage and Divorce

The concept of marriage in Asian culture is another factor in the domestic violence situation. Marriages are purposeful—to continue the family line or to fulfill some prearranged contract. Marriages unite not only the individuals but their families as well. Arranged marriages, which are still common, are sometimes viewed as business contracts, to be honored and adhered to, lest the extended family lose face. Because women are generally not as valued as men in Asian cultures, their happiness is often considered less than their worth in bargaining for things the family can benefit from (i.e., caretaking, citizenship, and money). Many arranged marriages take place sight unseen until the day of the ceremony or after only a few weeks of meeting each other. Clearly, in such situations a solid foundation for marriage is not established and the man commonly assumes control immediately. Frequently the woman may leave her own relatives and home country to live with her husband and in-laws. When the husband is abusive and controlling, he often does not allow his wife to have contact with the world outside the home, does not allow her to learn English, and keeps her isolated from her own relatives and friends.

Although divorce is more generally accepted in the United States, most Asian cultures do not find divorce acceptable. Strong religious and cultural values oppose divorce, even in violent relationships. In addition, the legal procedures for divorce in this country are extremely foreign to many Asian sensibilities. Views toward divorce are changing, however, especially for Asian women who see no other option in ending the violence in their lives. As the issue of domestic violence in the Asian communities becomes more visible, religious and community leaders are also changing their views.

Other Factors

Violence is compounded when the batterer is dealing with exacerbating conditions such as gambling, financial insecurity, social/cultural adjustment, alcoholism, and so on. The degree of violence may also be more intense with a male who has experienced the violence and aftermath of war.

Assessment

Because the battered Asian woman will be looking toward the treatment provider as not only a counselor but also a liaison to myriad other needed services, the treatment provider must make a comprehensive assessment of both psychological and social needs. There are several factors to consider in assessing the woman's situation.

Safety

This is the most immediate need. To survive in a violent, unpredictable environment, many women minimize and deny the danger: "He points the gun at me and threatens me, but I know he won't pull the trigger." As she begins to acknowledge the degree of danger she and her children are in, it is important to gradually help her break through that denial while immediately addressing current safety. Does her partner know her whereabouts? Has he followed her? Does she have access to a safe place to stay for the immediate future or can the therapist help her with such a task? Therapists should impress on their clients the need for their whereabouts to be secret from their partner or those who might have contact with him during the crisis. The decision to leave a battering relationship is extremely difficult. It is the most dangerous time because the batterer's power has been threatened. If a woman chooses to stay, however, statistics show that the violence will continue, increasing in frequency and severity over time.

Culture-Specific Values of Sex Roles

Although most Asian cultures are paternalistic, the degree of accepted male dominance and rights in relation to women varies. It is important to understand how the woman views her role in relation to the man based on her cultural and family upbringing. It is also important to learn how the woman and her family view physical aggression in a marriage.

Geography and Generation

Where a person is from and his or her cultural roots have bearing on how the person experiences him- or herself. For example, a Chinese woman from China will have a different cultural and self experience than the Chinese woman from Taiwan or Hong Kong or the Chinese American woman. The generation and the degree of traditionalism versus Western exposure affect the woman's expectations of sex roles as well as her ideas of sexuality. Whether a woman lives in a rural or an urban area also determines differences.

Self-Esteem and Power

Most battered women struggle with issues of self-esteem. Low self-esteem and powerlessness are reinforced by the external world, which frequently does not provide adequate support and resources to help the woman gain control of herself and her situation. Her psychological and emotional world is further negatively influenced by the batterer. It is important to help the client recognize and identify some of her strengths, even in the initial assessment. These identifications become part of the building blocks of her treatment.

Internal and External Resources

The therapist should assess the woman's strengths that she draws on in times of crises, as well as during noncrisis periods. What have been her past and current coping skills? What options has she previously explored and tried? How does she care for herself and her children? How does she deal with frustration and stress? Outside of marriage, is she able to foster positive, nurturing relationships? External resources are important to consider especially in times of crisis. Does the woman have people to whom she can turn for support and possible refuge? What were her relationships with friends and family like?

Language Skills

When possible, language compatibility with the treatment provider is preferable. If not possible, a trustworthy third party may serve as an interpreter. Understanding the woman's situation to the fullest degree and having her be able to understand and communicate her needs are essential. She will need to learn about her rights and the various resources available to her. It is important that she understand and present any questions she may have in regard to the legal system and the social services system.

Finance

Many battered women do not have access to expendable funds and may not have been allowed to work. Assessing a woman's financial situation helps in planning of her recovery. How much money is available to her immediately and how long will it last? Does she need governmental financial help? Will she have lost wages if she is employed and unable to return to work for a period of time? Would she lose her job?

Legal Concerns

Exploring legal concerns and directing the woman to appropriate legal counsel can be a great relief and help to her. Is she knowledgeable about restraining orders? If not a U.S. citizen, how might her immigration status be affected should she decide to leave her husband? What legal recourse is there for her situation? How will her children be affected (*Domestic Violence in Immigrant and Refugee Communities*, 1991; Kanuha, 1990)?

Physical Health

When working with a battered woman, one of the most immediate concerns is her physical health. Immediate medical care may be necessary.

To survive the violence, many battered women have learned to minimize and deny the abuse. Sometimes women go to a shelter or to counseling without realizing they have broken ribs, wrist, concussions, and other physical injuries. It is useful to take Polaroid photos of a woman's injuries. The photos can help document the abuse for legal matters the woman may want to pursue and also help her realize what she has endured. If no immediate care is needed, other health concerns may need follow-up. For example, a woman may have had to leave her home abruptly and may have left her medications behind.

Belief System/Philosophy of Life/Religion

The underpinnings of an individual's motivation or survival and life are often found in the individual's belief system—a combination of his or her philosophical, religious, and cultural values. Understanding the woman's belief system and working with her within that framework will be most helpful from the assessment stage through termination of the work.

Children's Needs

The therapist cannot assess the needs of a mother without also assessing the needs of her children. Many of the children have experienced abuse and neglect themselves, and all have experienced the emotional effects of living in a violent home. Children who witness abuse may develop learning, developmental, language, speech, and stress-related problems; they may blame themselves or feel unprotected. Can counseling be made available to the children? What are their special needs now? Women may need support in parenting skills, helping their children to feel protected, and adjusting to single parenting if they choose to leave the batterer. If a woman is escaping from the batterer, are the school and child care still safe? Although disruptive, it is often safer to change schools and child care for the safety of the children as well as the mother.

Suicidality and Self-Mutilation

The potential for suicide is assessed in any mental status exam, but it is important to make a special note of the need for assessment in battering situations. Violence toward oneself and toward another is often a blur. Some battered women, having internalized the violence, blame, and humiliation heaped on them, become self-destructive. The lack of alternatives to escape or stop the violence and lack of avenues to deal with her feelings make the risk of suicide and self-mutilation especially high.

General Mental Status

An assessment of general mental status includes information on mood and affect, orientation, recent and remote memory, any hallucinations (audio and visual) or thought disorder, cognitive functioning and intelligence, bodily posture, any vegetative signs, organicity, suicidal or violent ideation, and so on, as well as any past or current substance abuse, eating disorder, and emotional, physical, or sexual abuse.

Reliving Past Traumas

Posttraumatic stress is a common experience for battered women. Their current trauma may also trigger memories and responses to past traumas that occurred during wartime, in their families, and in their immigration experiences.

Treatment

Treatment in the domestic violence situation requires the treatment provider to wear several hats. The treatment provider must be willing to assume more than a therapist role to help with the complexities of the woman's situation. Besides being a counselor (a term more acceptable than "therapist" to many Asian clients), the treatment provider sometimes needs to serve as a liaison and advocate to various social services and legal resources.

Social Services

A woman trying to free herself from a violent relationship may need immediate access to money, clothing, food, translation, housing, medical care, schooling, and child care for her children.

Legal Resources

The battered woman may need legal assistance and information on obtaining a restraining order, how her immigration status may be affected, the criminal justice system, and such family court matters as custody, legal separation, and divorce.

Advocacy/Case Management

If the treatment provider is unable to assist the women as an advocate/case manager, it is important to connect her to another resource for assistance (preferably someone who speaks her primary language).

Counseling

As in other counseling situations involving Asian clients, a task-oriented approach in the beginning of treatment is important to reassure the client that she is getting something tangible and useful from treatment. This is particularly true when the woman enters treatment in crisis, under tremendous fear, and facing many barriers. Counselors should provide some structure and guidance and let the client know their expertise to help instill confidence in their ability to help her. Education about domestic violence and the dynamics in the relationship are important issues to address with the client early on, as well as communicating the resources available to her. Helping the client understand her options while always keeping the power of choice with her is an important part of counseling. Many Asian women have not learned the concept of choice because of the oppression in their relationship and their socialization. It is common for the client to look to the treatment provider for decisions, but it is imperative that the client be allowed to make her own decisions. The counselor can assist the client in understanding possible consequences of each option. Because Asians frequently experience emotional stress through physical symptoms, elucidating this response is important. Explaining and teaching the language of feelings, which to most Asians is a new concept, will help in the empowerment process. The counselor should also educate the client on the relationship between physical and emotional health. Many women experience physical symptoms in response to posttraumatic stress. The counselor should help the client gradually to break through the denial that is common among abused persons. If a support group in the woman's language is available, the counselor should offer that as an adjunct to individual work. The woman needs to build a community and support as she is trying to free herself from a violent situation.

Individual counseling is important for batterers to own responsibility for the violence in the relationship and to find alternatives to coercion, controlling behavior, and violence. Individual counseling is important to assist the battered woman in focusing on her safety, needs, and feelings; addressing her fears; and dispelling the victim blaming.

Couple work in domestic violence relationships is controversial because of the power imbalance within the relationship and the degree to which the batterer owns responsibility for the violence. *If couple work is done before the batterer is ready to own responsibility for the violence, the risk of danger to the woman is greatly exacerbated.* A woman may feel encouraged to express her feelings in the presence of the counselor, only to face retaliation from the batterer at home. She may not express her true feelings in the sessions because of threats and fear of retaliation. Treatment providers need to carefully assess the violence existing in the relationship and the benefits or detriment in couple work. Otherwise couple work can place the woman at serious risk or set up a false image of the battering dynamic as mutual fighting and conflict.

CONCLUSION: BREAKING THE CYCLE OF VIOLENCE

Individuals in battering relationships face the challenge of breaking the cycle of violence, and because domestic violence is not just an individual's problem but a societal one, each of us in the community has that responsibility as well. That means that survivors of domestic violence work to find their power and build their determination and hope, batterers confront their abusive behavior and seek treatment, and all of us support survivors, create resources to help end domestic violence, refuse to accept abuse and violence, and help change values to overcome violence in all forms. Asian communities have rich cultures and many traditions. Domestic violence does not have to be a tradition we pass on to our children.

ACKNOWLEDGMENTS

We gratefully acknowledge Mary Tam Ma, LCSW, Victims Services Coordinator, Center for Special Problems, San Francisco, CA; Violet Ng, LCSW, Group Facilitator for Asian Male Batterers, Center for Special Problems, San Francisco, CA; Mayseng Saetern, Women's Advocate, Asian Women's Shelter, San Francisco, CA; and Tina Shum, Battered Asian Women's Program, Cameron House, San Francisco, CA.

REFERENCES

Center for the Study and Prevention of Violence. (1991). *1988–1991, analysis of the Uniform Crime Reports, FBI*. Boulder, CO: University of Colorado.

The Commonwealth Fund. (1993). *First comprehensive national health survey of American women*.

Domestic violence in immigrant and refugee communities: Asserting the rights of battered women. (1991). San Francisco: Family Violence Prevention Fund, Coalition for Immigrant and Refugee Rights and Services.

Family Violence Prevention Fund. (1993). *Men beating women: Ending domestic violence, a qualitative and quantitative study of public attitudes on violence against women*. New York: EDK Associates.

Kanuha, V. (1990). Compounding the triple jeopardy: Battering in lesbian of color relationships. In L. S. Brown & M. P. P. Root (Eds.), *Diversity and complexity in feminist therapy* (pp. 169–184). New York: Haworth Press.

Strauss, M., Gelles, R., & Steinmetz, S. (1980). *Behind closed doors: Violence in the American family*. Garden City, NY: Anchor Press.

30

Chinese Buddhism:
Its Implications for Counseling

WING H. YEUNG
EVELYN LEE

The Buddha once said: "There are two kinds of illnesses. What are those two? Physical illness and mental illness. There seem to be people who enjoy freedom from physical illness even for a year or two. . . . But, rare in this world are those who enjoy freedom from mental illness even for one moment" (Rahula, 1978). When one's mind is healthy, physical illness will diminish. If all the illnesses of one's mind are cured, one is "liberated."

Curing the human mind and producing a state of perfect mental health, equilibrium, and tranquillity are major aims in Buddhism. The extensive scriptures containing Buddha's teachings outline the methods and means to eliminate sufferings and bring happiness to all beings. The aim of this chapter is to summarize several important principles of Buddhism and discuss how these can be applied in therapy.

THE BUDDHA

The founder of Buddhism was Sakyamuni, who lived in Northern India in the sixth century B.C. Though a crown prince in the Kingdom of the

Sakayas (in modern Nepal), he felt unfulfilled, even though he seemed to have everything—lots of riches, a wife, and a son (Dhammananda, 1982). One day, while visiting the city, he saw the "Four Passing Sights," namely, an old man, a sick man, a dead man, and a holy recluse (Smith, 1986). These sights, which he had never seen inside the palace before, made a dramatic impact on him. He then realized that life is susceptible to age, death, and suffering.

Sakyamuni wanted to find a "cure," not only for himself, but for all mankind. So he left the palace as a monk, to search for enlightenment. With 6 years of ascetic practices under different religious teachers, he realized that would not lead him to liberation. Thus, he went on his own way. One night, seated under a tree, he attained enlightenment at the age of 35. He then became known as the Buddha, meaning "The Awakened" or "The Enlightened One." The teachings of the Buddha are known as *dharma*. This word literally means "law," meaning the universal laws that represent things as they really are. The Buddha went on to teach all men and women, without distinction regarding their social class, occupation, or ethnic origin. At the age of 80, the Buddha passed away at Kusinara (Rahula, 1978; Narada, 1982).

Among the founders of the major religions on earth, Buddha was the only teacher who did not claim to be other than a human being. He attributed all his realization, attainments, and achievements to human endeavor and human intelligence. Every person has within himself or herself the potential of becoming a Buddha. The Buddha taught and encouraged each person to develop him- or herself and to work out his or her emancipation, for each human has the power to escape all bondage through his or her own personal efforts and intelligence.

BUDDHA'S TEACHINGS

The doctrines of Buddha's teachings (Dhammananda, 1982; Narada, 1982; Niwano, 1990; Rahula, 1978) explain very clearly the causes of human suffering, how we can fundamentally solve the problem of the suffering and distress that we face with in our daily lives, and how we can achieve a mental state of peace and quietude. The following is a brief summary of the basic principles in Buddhism.

Four Noble Truths

According to Buddha's teachings, the problem of existence and its solution are precisely expressed in the Four Noble Truths. The First Truth *diagnoses* the symptom of an illness and the Second determines its *cause*. The Third Truth describes the final *cure* of the disease once the cause has been eliminated, and the Fourth prescribes the medicine or *treatment* that will bring about the cure. Following are the chief characteristics of the Four Noble Truths:

1. All existence entails suffering.
2. Suffering is caused by ignorance, which leads to craving and illusion.
3. There is an end to suffering, and this state of nonsuffering is *nirvana.*
4. *Nirvana* is attained through the practice of the *bodhisattva way.*

The first of the Four Noble Truths is the *Truth of Suffering.* Buddha explained the eight causes of suffering. The human condition has always entailed countless sufferings, as exemplified by the eight types enumerated by the Buddha. The first four sufferings are birth, old age, sickness, and death. The second four sufferings are separation from loved ones, association with unpleasant persons and conditions, not getting what one desires or due to unfulfilled wishes, and finally, suffering due to the raging *skandas.* The five *skandas* are form, feeling, perception, volition, and consciousness. This is the suffering of the body and the mind. Our physical bodies are subject to birth, old age, disease, death, hunger, thirst, heat, cold, and weariness. Our minds, on the other hand, are afflicted by anger, worry, love, hate, and other emotions. The word "suffering" here does not represent a pessimistic view of life but rather presents a realistic view of life and the world.

The *Truth of Cause* means that we must reflect on what causes have produced these sufferings, and we must investigate them and understand them clearly. The Buddha found that the fundamental cause of suffering is ignorance. Ignorance, in turn, leads to the rise of self-centered desire. Ignorance and desire combine to blind us and preclude any possibility of realizing our inherent spiritual nature. Because of ignorance, living beings create *karma.*

The *Truth of Extinction* is the state of absolute quietude wherein all the sufferings in human life are extinguished. This is a state attained only by awakening to the three great truths that Buddha has taught us: "All things are impermanent," "Nothing has an ego," and "*Nirvana* is quiescence."

Ordinary people cannot easily realize these three great truths. However, the *Truth of the Path* shows the way how people can practice the *bodhisattva way* with their mind, body, and actions. This means that they must devote themselves to the practice of the doctrines of the Eightfold Path and the Six Perfections (Tables 30.1 and 30.2). The Eightfold Path consists of right view, right thinking, right speech, right action, right living, right endeavor, right memory, and right meditation. The Six

TABLE 30.1. The Eightfold Path (Niwano, 1976)

Right view	To see all things rightly, based on the Buddha's wisdom, which discerns and understands the principle of the Reality of All Existence.
Right thinking	To think rightly, avoiding the three evils of the mind
Right speech	To speak right words, avoiding the four evils of the mouth
Right action	To act rightly, avoiding the three evils of the body
Right living	To gain food, clothing, shelter, and other daily necessities in a right way
Right endeavor	Never to do evil and always to do good
Right memory	To have a continuous right mind toward both oneself and others
Right meditation	To strive constantly for the true Law and to be fixed and settled in it

Perfections teaches us the six kinds of practice: donation, keeping the precepts, perseverance, assiduity, meditation, and wisdom.

In summary, the Four Noble Truths teach us to face the reality of human suffering, to grasp its real cause, to practice daily the *bodhisattva way* to help ourselves and others and thereby to extinguish various sufferings.

TABLE 30.2. The Six Perfections (Niwano, 1976)

Donation	"Makes a miserly one raise the mind of donation": to serve sincerely the community and other people
Keeping the precepts	"Makes an arrogant one raise the mind of keeping the commandments": to remove the mind of arrogance and to admonish and discipline oneself
Perseverance	"Makes an irascible one raise the mind of perseverance": to remove anger and to endure
Assiduity	"Makes an indolent one raise the mind of assiduity": to endeavor constantly
Meditation	"Makes a distracted one raise the mind of meditation": to calm one's mind and not be agitated
Wisdom	"Makes an ignorant one raise the mind of wisdom": to remove prejudice and evil thinking through correct judgment

Karma

Karma means "deed" or "action." Whenever there is action, there will be consequences. This is the concept of *cause and effect.* All the things *we do* in body, speech, and thought are causes. And all the *things that happen* to us are results. All that we are at the present moment is the result of the *karma* that we have produced in the past. *Karma* is complex and serious. Our deeds, however trivial, leave traces—physically, mentally, and environmentally. The traces left in our minds include memory, knowledge, habit, intelligence, and character. They are produced by the accumulation of our experiences and deeds over a long period of time (Niwano, 1976).

The *"karma* of a previous existence" that Buddhism teaches is more profound, as it include the *karma* that our own life has produced through the repetition of birth and death from the infinite past to the present (Niwano, 1976). However, this is not a fatalistic view that everything is predestined, because in between the cause (seed) and effect (fruit), there are many variable conditions (new sets of *karma*) which can be changed. Thus they can affect the outcome. The idea of *karma* teaches us clearly that we will reap the fruits of what we have sown. *People should take total individual responsibility of their own actions.*

Reincarnation

According to Buddhist teaching, reincarnation is part of life. Buddhists believe there are at least five planes of life: the Heavenly Beings, Human, Ghosts, Animals, and Hells. All beings in these classes continue in the cycle of rebirth and death until they can be liberated. They also can "transmigrate" from one class to another, from one life to another. Death is part of the endless life cycle.

Four Virtues

Buddha teaches four virtues for laymen to pursuit happiness:

1. One should have faith and confidence in moral, spiritual, and intellectual values.
2. One should abstain from destroying and harming life, stealing and cheating, adultery, falsehood, and intoxicating drinks.
3. One should practice charity and generosity, without attachment and craving for one's wealth.
4. One should develop wisdom which leads to the complete destruction of suffering, to the realization of *nirvana.*

In addition to the four virtues, Buddha also teaches "noble discipline." Six family and social groups should be treated as sacred and worthy of respect and worship. They are parents; teachers; spouse and children; friends, relatives and neighbors; servants, workers, and employees; and religious men. Budda provides a practical guide in how to deal with these family and social relationships in our daily lives.

Compassion and Wisdom

According to Buddhism, for a man to be perfect, he should develop two qualities equally: compassion on one side and wisdom on the other. Here, compassion represents love, charity, kindness, tolerance, and such noble qualities on the emotional side, or qualities of the heart. Wisdom would stand for the intellectual side, or qualities of the mind. If one develops only the emotional, neglecting the intellectual, one may become a good-hearted fool. To develop only the intellectual side and neglect the emotional may turn one into a hardhearted intellect without feelings for others. Therefore, to be perfect, one has to develop both compassion and wisdom equally (Rahula, 1978).

APPLICATIONS OF BUDDHISM IN COUNSELING

Recently, an increasing number of clinicians have begun to explore the possibilities of employing Buddhist principles and techniques in therapeutics contexts. This trend is important, in view of the increasing number of Asian clients who are Buddhists and non-Asian clients who are interested in alternative healing methods. This respect for clients' religious and spiritual backgrounds is vital, in view of the fact that religious and spiritual beliefs affect how these clients identify and present their problems, explain the causes of the problems, and seek health care.

Many possible approaches to counseling exist that use Buddhist teachings. Here, we discuss only three such approaches.

Conceptual Therapy

This is a cognitive approach of therapy based on the Buddhist concepts that "all of existence is a creation of the mind." People can gradually learn and understand these Buddhist concepts and change their way of thinking, feeling, and acting. Thus, they can change their "negative" behavior to "positive" behavior and attain the therapeutic goal of mental harmony. Following are some case examples of applying Buddhism principles in counseling.

The Concepts of Eight Sufferings and Impermanence

A 50-year-old Chinese woman came for counseling because of depression. Mrs. L took a disability leave from her job as a computer programmer. The bank where she worked was recently "taken over" by other institutions. Consequently, Mrs. L was reassigned to a different department and was under the supervision of a much younger boss who was very demanding and showed no respect for her contribution to the company over the past 20 years. In addition, her mother had passed away recently after suffering from cancer for 3 years. Mrs. L's husband, who used to be quite supportive of his wife, appeared to be less caring because he was preoccupied with his own job security, as his company was planning on "downsizing." Mrs. L's only daughter had just finished graduate school and moved far away to take a new job.

In the beginning phase of counseling, Mrs. L spent most of her time complaining of her "misfortune" and "bad luck." She felt life was unfair to her after years of hard work at business and at home. She asked "why" about her suffering. As a Buddhist, she was encouraged to examine her misfortunes from the Buddhist teachings of eight sufferings, impermanence, and the concept of *karma*. She realized that the sufferings in her life, such as disease, death, old age, separation from loved ones, unfulfilled wishes, and work with someone whom she hated, were part of human condition. Company mergers or downsizing was part of change and impermanence. This understanding helped her to let go of her grief and anger. She gradually accepted responsibility for taking care of herself. She accepted the situations she was not able to change and focused her energy on those areas in which she was able to make positive changes.

The Concept of Reincarnation

A 48-year-old woman, became angry and depressed after she was told by her husband that he had been seeing another woman for the past 4 years. She had thought that she was happy and lucky to have a wonderful marriage and three nice children. Now, all seemed to be an illusion. With therapy, she was able to understand that in her past lives, she also had different people as spouses, and so did her present husband. In their future lives, they are likely to have different people as spouses too. The only change that led to her present misery was her finding out what her husband had done in the past 4 years. Realizing that we are like travelers meeting and separating in time and space, she was determined not to be bothered by the entanglements from past lives and the uncertainties about future lives. She took responsibility for turning her anger into caring so she would not continue her entanglements with her husband. She learned new communication skills to improve the marital relationship and be a better mother. She was able to regain her confidence and happiness. Her husband was so impressed by her positive changes that he decided to end his extramarital affair.

Treatment providers should note that belief in reincarnation is one of the biggest cultural differences between Western and Eastern thought. However, the concept of reincarnation is being explored in mass media today because more and more people are receptive to this idea (Yeung, 1995). There are also many case studies and reports on reincarnation by mental health professionals. Studies on reincarnation vary from reports on individual clinical treatment under hypnosis (Weiss, 1988, 1992), long-term case studies of people who could remember their past-life events (Stevenson, 1977; Story, 1975), and life-before-birth experiences revealed under hypnosis (Wambach, 1979). Books on past-life therapy break through the barriers of conventional psychotherapy to present an innovative and effective treatment approach (Weiss, 1988, 1992).

The Concept of Birth and Death

A 68-year-old woman who used to enjoy life with enthusiasm became despondent and worrisome after a fortune teller told her that she would die at age 70. She became preoccupied with the fear of dying and was frightened about the uncertainties before and after death. She started to worry about missing her four children and grandchildren. As a Chinese Buddhist in beginning practice, she was encouraged to explore the Buddhist concepts of death, cause and effect, and reincarnation. She also studied the *Heart Sutra* to understand the concept of "no self" and illusion. Gradually, she overcame her fear of dying and death by believing that death is not an end but the beginning of life. Knowing that she has done a lot of good in this life, she felt confident that she would come back as a human being and may meet with her loved ones again. She suffered a major heart attack at the age of 72 and has made a remarkable recovery. She is still alive at age 77.

The Concept of Compassion

A 60-year-old depressed man had lost his business and become utterly bitter and isolated after he was humiliated by a young man whom he had helped to build a successful business enterprise. The young man refused to reciprocate. Prior to this loss, he had been sympathetic and helpful to others and was now quite disappointed that his friends did not offer help when he was in need of assistance. In the beginning of therapy, he was resistant to any help and spent most of the counseling sessions expressing his anger toward his ungrateful friends. One day, he picked up a booklet in temple about the concept of compassion in Buddhism. He tried to apply it to deal with his personal crisis. One day, he said, "I was compassionate before and I was very happy. I should not assume the role of a victim after I had setbacks. There is not much time to waste in life. Unable to forgive, I was full of grudges which actually hurt myself. I am going to resume being compassionate and forgiving again." He gradually regained his physical and mental health and eventually his business.

The Concept of Interdependence

A 16-year-old boy was very arrogant and selfish. Even though he was the best student in class, he had no friends and was isolated. At home, he bullied his younger sisters, and because he was the only son, he was favored by his grandparents. He became depressed after he lost the number-one position in class after being hospitalized for a few weeks because of a viral infection. In therapy, the boy and the counselor discussed the concept of interdependence. The counselor used various analogies. For example, to highlight the concept the counselor used the analogy of a car needing the proper combination of the engine, the tires, and even a small screw to run smoothly. The boy started to realize that many family members, teachers, and friends had contributed to his academic success in the past and he should not be so arrogant. Gradually, he was able to appreciate the importance of mutual respect and the equal contributions of other people in life. He eventually regained his number-one position in class but shed his arrogance and selfishness. He became a happier person and made many friends.

Practical Therapy

This is a behavioral approach of therapy that teaches people to do something to achieve mental harmony and stability. It emphasizes the need to persevere and practice every day.

Meditation

Meditation is the principal practice used to develop one's mind along the path to the end of suffering. The goal is to calm the scattered and unbalanced mind. In Buddhism, meditation does not mean "hard thinking." It means calming the body and thought processes and then observing all that goes on inside oneself. The most general and widely practiced meditative technique is breathing meditation, which consists of focusing one's attention on the breath and then observing the consequent bodily and mental processes. Counting numbers and walking can also be used as preliminary meditation techniques. Its primary contribution to mental development is in the establishment of the calm that arises when one banishes all enmity and ill will from one's mind. While we practice conscious breathing, our thinking slows down and we can give ourselves a real rest. Most of the time, we think too much, and mindful breathing helps us to be calm, relaxed, and peaceful. It helps us stop thinking so much and stop being possessed by sorrows of the past and worries about the future. It enables us to be in touch with life, which is wonderful in the present moment (Hanh, 1992). Meditation is generally helpful for most people with or without emotional stress. However, people who have such psychotic symptoms as hallucinations should not meditate without close supervision (some people may experience hallucination during meditation).

Buddhist masters developed many different meditation techniques. For example, mindfulness and walking meditation are very useful in dealing with negative emotions (Hanh, 1992). Many mental health professionals also apply meditation in conjunction with psychotherapy. For example, Epstein (1995) explains the unique psychological contributions of the teaching of Buddhism, and also describes the path of meditation in contemporary psychological language and lays groundwork for a meditation-inspired psychotherapy.

Chanting

When we are worried or emotionally disturbed, we can concentrate on chanting the Buddha's name to feel connected to and protected by the Buddha. This also helps to remind us about the Buddha's virtues of perfect compassion and wisdom. Chanting is also used in certain life conditions. For example, for the Mahayana Pure Land Sect, when a person is dying, family members and friends gather around and chant the name of the Amitabha Buddha. This is to stabilize the mind of the dying person and to help him or her chant. Members of this sect believe that if the dying person chants the name of the Amitabha Buddha with absolute sincerity, it is enough to bring him or her into the most connection with the Buddha (Yeung, 1995)

Practicing the Buddha's Teachings

As mentioned in the previous section, Buddha's teachings offer a profound analysis of the problem of suffering while providing both an alternate vision free of suffering and the actual methods we need to realize that awakening. The Buddha established the *Five Moral Precepts* as basic virtues for human life and the very essence of spiritual cultivation. They are as follows: Do not kill, do not steal, do not engage in sexual misconduct, do not speak falsely, and do not take intoxicants. The moral precepts are rooted in self-respect and respect for others. The path that leads to the cessation of suffering is to practice the *bodhisattva way*. This means that an individual should devote him- or herself to the practice of the doctrines of The Eightfold Path (Table 30.1) and The Six Perfections (Table 30.2).

Applying Buddhist Stories in Therapy

Storytelling can be used effectively to enhance the client's understanding of a certain situation. Many Buddhist stories can be used in counseling sessions. Following are three examples:

"Are you still carrying her?" This story can be used to illustrate the concept of "letting go" and not hanging on to the past. A young monk went on a trip with his master. On their way, they met a young woman who was hesitating near a small stream. To cross the stream would mean that she would get her dress wet. The old master offered to carry her across. After some thought and with a certain embarrassment, she agreed. After they had crossed the stream, they parted and went on their separate ways. However, the incident bothered the young monk. That night after they were settled, he said to the old monk that monks were not supposed to be near women, let alone carry them. To which the old monk replied: "I left the woman at the bank of the stream. Are you still carrying her?" (Cheng & Lo, 1991).

"Can you save my son?" This story helps a client accept certain realities in life, such as dying. A woman lost her only infant, and she became extremely distraught. She carried her dead son's body to the Buddha. She wanted him to revive her son. She was beyond reason. Seeing the woman in such overwhelming grief, the Buddha agreed to help if she would bring back some mustard seeds. She was very happy to hear that. However, the Buddha told her that the seeds had to be from a household where no one had died. Without hesitation, she set forth to look for the seeds from village to village. After a long and exhaustive search, she found no such seeds but discovered the nature of life (Narada, 1982). When she went back to see the Buddha, she was calm and peaceful.

"Can you help me find enlightenment?" This story helps a client become less arrogant and become more open to learning new skills. One day, a proud young man went to a *Ch'an* (Zen) master for advice on how to become enlightened. The master looked at the young man for a few minutes, not saying anything. He then invited the young man to have tea with him. He poured the hot tea until it overflowed. The young man was stunned; he asked why the master did not stop pouring. The master answered: "If your mind is like this cup—already full—there is no hope you'll ever learn anything new."

CONCLUSIONS

Buddhism and psychotherapy share common goals: to alleviate human suffering and achieve inner peace. While Western psychology has contributed much to the understanding of the biological and social aspects of human behavior, Buddhism has also provided a clear understanding of human spirit and the nature of the mind. In a systematic way, it identifies and diagnoses the symptoms of human suffering, determines its cause, describes cures for illnesses, and prescribes treatments that will bring happiness and lasting contentment. The timeless message of Buddhist *dharma* may have been the best counseling repository in the past 2,500 years. The Buddha, as a healer with compassion and wisdom, can serve as an excellent teacher and role model. The practical Buddhist teachings of love, understanding, tolerance, and impermanence are all applicable to modern life.

REFERENCES

Cheng, L. Y., & Lo, H-T. (1991). On the advantages of cross-culture psychotherapy: The minority therapist/mainstream patient dyad. *Psychiatry, 54,* 386–396.

The Dalai Lama. (1994). *The way to freedom.* New York: HarperCollins.

Dhammananda, K. K. (1982). *What the Buddhists believe.* Kuala Lumpur, Malaysia: Buddhist Missionary Society.

Epstein, M. (1995). *Thoughts without a thinker: Psychotherapy from a Buddhist perspective.* New York: Basic Books.

Hanh, T. N. (1992). *Peace is every step.* New York: Bantam Books.

Narada, M. T. (1982). *The Buddha and his teachings.* Singapore: Buddhist Meditation Center.

Niwano, N. (1976). *Buddhism for today.* Tokyo: Kosei.

Rahula, W. P. (1978). *What the Buddha taught.* London: Gordon Fraser.

Smith, H. (1986). *The religions of man.* New York: Harper & Row.

Stevenson, I. (1977). The explanatory value of the idea of reincarnation. *Journal of Nervous and Mental Disease, 5,* 305–326.

Story, F. (1975). *Rebirth as doctrine and experience.* Sri Lanka: Buddhist Publication Society.

Wambach, H. (1979). *Life before life.* New York: Bantam Books.

Weiss, B. L. (1988). *Many lives, many masters.* New York: Simon & Schuster.

Weiss, B. L. (1992). *Through time into healing.* New York: Simon & Schuster.

Yeung, W. H. (1995). Buddhism, death, and dying. In J. K. Parry & A. Shen Ryan (Eds.), *A cross-cultural look at death, dying, and religion.* Chicago: Nelson-Hall.

31

Mental Health Care Delivery to Asian Americans: Review of the Literature

PHILLIP D. AKUTSU

Prior to the 1970s, little research attention was given to the mental health needs of Asian Americans. However, in the past two decades, mental health providers and researchers have tried to increase and expand their findings to clinical practice with Asian Americans. Because of such efforts, a growing number of clinical studies focusing on counseling and psychotherapy issues with Asian Americans have begun to appear in the literature.

To date, six bibliographies of this expanding body of Asian American mental health research have been published (Doi, Lin, & Vohra-Sahu, 1981; Morishima, Sue, Teng, Zane, & Cram, 1979; Silver & Chui, 1985; Vohra-Sahu, 1983; Williams, 1987; Yu, Murata, & Lin, 1982). Also, a significant number of books and journal articles have made major contributions to a greater awareness and understanding of the special issues involved in working with Asian American clients (e.g., Leong, 1986; Mokuau, 1991; Owan, 1985; Sue & Sue, 1990; Sue & Morishima, 1982). More recently, two other reviews of the mental health literature on Asian Americans have been published: a bibliography of the books, book chapters, journal articles, and dissertations on Asian Americans in the PsychINFO database dating from 1967 to 1991 (Leong & Whitfield, 1992) and a book of the counseling and psychology research on personality, ethnic identity, and mental health issues with Asian Americans (Uba, 1994).

This chapter provides a brief update of recent findings in the mental health literature on Asian Americans. Because no single chapter can provide an exhaustive review of this literature, this chapter focuses on specific topics that are particularly salient to current discussions of mental health care delivery to Asian American populations.

SOMATIZATION

Both psychotherapists and researchers alike have focused special attention on the concept of somatization or the reporting of physical complaints as a possible substitute for emotional or psychological distress by Asian Americans. Previous reviews have shown that many of the more established Asian American groups, including the Chinese, Japanese, Filipinos, and Koreans, report a higher frequency of somatic complaints than European Americans (Kleinman & Good, 1985; Sue & Morishima, 1982). Similar reports of a relatively higher incidence of somatic problems were found among such Southeast Asian groups as the Cambodians and Laotians (Foulks, Merkel, & Boehnlein, 1992; Mattson, 1993), Hmong (Westermeyer, 1989), Iu-Mien (Moore & Boehlein, 1991), Vietnamese (Foulks et al., 1992; Matkin, Nickles, Demos, & Demos, 1996; Niem, 1989), and Vietnamese–Chinese (Nishimoto, 1988). Despite this growing consensus, a few studies have failed to report a significant difference in the rate of somatic complaints between Asian and European Americans (Lai & Linden, 1993; Raskin, Chien, & Lin, 1992).

Why is there a higher rate of somatization among Asian American groups? First, Asian Americans may be socialized to express their symptoms of emotional distress in ways that are appropriate or acceptable to others in their same culture yet are viewed by Western practitioners as somatization (Brislin, 1993). In general, these types of culture-bound symptoms and syndromes are commonly found in Asian and non-Asian cultures (Blue & Gaines, 1992; Carr & Vitaliano, 1985; Yamamoto, 1992). Second, by reporting somatic problems to nurses or physicians, Asian clients may be able to receive access to mental health services at medical facilities without having to face the stigma or shame that is often associated with reporting psychological problems (Jun-mian, 1987; Uba, 1994). Third, this somatic process may indicate the more holistic view of the mind and body that is common to many Asian cultures (Nishio & Bilmes, 1987; Cheung & Lau, 1982). For example, more traditional Chinese and Southeast Asians may be surprised that different therapists are needed for treating the physical and emotional symptoms of what they believe is the same underlying disorder (Flaskerud & Anh, 1988; Uba, 1994). Finally, less acculturated Southeast Asians report a higher rate of somatization than more acculturated Southeast Asians (Westermeyer, Bouafuely, Neider, & Callies, 1989). Because of problems with language proficiency as well as a limited knowledge of Western concepts of psychotherapy, it is not surprising that more recent immigrants and refugees turn to familiar forms of folk medicine or traditional medical facilities to deal with their emotional or psychological trauma (Brislin, 1993; Sue & Morishima, 1982; Ying & Miller, 1992).

Given these considerations, mental health providers must be cautious in their interpretations of the somatic complaints of Asian Americans. It could be that Asian Americans who present physical symptoms may be suffering from genuine medical problems and are not simply denying psychological distress (Uba, 1994). Also, although Southeast Asians may initially present somatic complaints, research has shown that these clients are capable of discussing their personal problems in psychological terms (Akutsu & Vuong, 1996; Chung & Okazaki, 1991). Therefore, there is still some controversy about whether or not Asian Americans actually somatize their psychological problems to a greater degree than European Americans.

SERVICE UTILIZATION

Another area undergoing much scrutiny by mental health providers and researchers focuses on patterns of help seeking and utilization of mental health services by Asian Americans. Previous reviews based on clinical admissions and treated cases at mental health settings have shown that Asian Americans are usually underrepresented as clients and have higher dropout rates and shorter stays in treatment than do European Americans (e.g., Leong, 1986; Sue & Morishima, 1982). In a review of the mental health literature, Uba (1994) reported that this service underuse occurred for "a variety of Asian American groups (Chinese, Japanese, and a mix of Asian Americans), with both students and adults, in both inpatient and outpatient facilities, at numerous mental health facilities (Loo, Tong, & True, 1989; Sue & Morishima, 1982) and over decades" (p. 196).

Recent studies, however, have been somewhat mixed in their conclusions about service utilization among Asian Americans. Some of these studies have shown that Asian Americans continue to underutilize both inpatient (Hu, Snowden, Jerrell, & Nguyen, 1991; Snowden & Cheung, 1990) and outpatient (Bui & Takeuchi, 1992; Loo et al., 1989) mental health services. For example, although Asian Americans represent about 9 percent of the population in Los Angeles County, they make up only 3% of the client population in the mental health system (Sue, Fujino, Hu,

Takeuchi, & Zane, 1991). In contrast to these findings, other studies report that Asian Americans use comparable or even higher rates of mental health services than do European Americans (Hu et al., 1991; O'Sullivan, Peterson, Cox, & Kirkeby, 1989). Several mental health experts speculate that service improvements may be a result of the introduction of culturally responsive programs to heavily populated Asian American communities.

How can this discrepancy in the reported rates of service utilization be explained? Several factors may contribute to a low rate of help seeking and service utilization for Asian American groups. First, Asian Americans are less likely initially to seek out mental health services for psychological problems because of the stigma and shame that are identified with having a mental illness. For example, Chinese (Mau & Jepsen, 1990; Ying, 1990) and Japanese (Narikiyo & Kameoka, 1992; Suan & Tyler, 1990) subjects who view their personal problems as psychologically based are more likely to turn to themselves, family, or friends for support and assistance rather than professional counseling. Second, even when they recognized a clearly identified need for counseling, Asian Americans delayed much longer in seeking mental health treatment than did other ethnic groups (Cheung, 1987; Lin, Inui, Kleinman, & Womack, 1982). Third, the level of acculturation plays a significant role in determining help-seeking behaviors for Asian Americans (Leong, Wagner, & Tata, 1995; Solberg, Choi, Ritsma, & Jolly, 1994). For Chinese, Japanese, and Korean subjects, those who were most acculturated were most able to recognize a need for psychological help, most tolerant of the stigma and shame associated with counseling services, and most open to discussing their personal problems with a psychologist (Atkinson & Gim, 1989; Ying & Miller, 1992).

Several factors, however, may also facilitate a greater rate of service utilization for Asian American groups. First, Asian Americans were found to make better use of mental health services when they had access to ethnically similar therapists (Kim, 1978; Wu & Windle, 1980). Recently, Asian Americans were found to remain in treatment longer and were less likely to drop out of treatment if they were matched with ethnically similar therapists (Sue et al., 1991; Wu & Windle, 1980) or therapists who spoke their primary language (Flaskerud, 1986; Flaskerud & Liu, 1990, 1991; Leong, 1986). Second, rates of service utilization also increased substantially when Asian Americans were able to participate in ethnic-specific or parallel programs in their own communities (e.g., Hatanaka, Watanabe, & Ono, 1975; Sue & McKinney, 1975). In comparison to more traditional programs, Asian clients were also found to have lower dropout rates and stayed in treatment longer at these ethnic-specific programs even when the significant effect of client–therapist ethnic matching was controlled for (Takeuchi, Mokuau, & Chun, 1992; Takeuchi, Sue, & Yeh, 1995; Yeh, Takeuchi, & Sue, 1994; Zane, Hatanaka, Park, & Akutsu, 1994).

Given these results, it would appear that improvements in service utilization by Asian Americans may be significantly influenced by the introduction of culturally responsive programs to their communities. However, this initial conclusion must be considered preliminary and tentative until more empirical studies have been completed in regard to the significant impact of client–therapist ethnic and language matching and participation in ethnic-specific programs.

DIRECTIVE THERAPY

In the past decade, a growing number of mental health providers have described the importance of using a structured or directive counseling approach with Asian American groups. Recent studies have shown that Asian Americans report a preference for therapists with a directive rather than a nondirective counseling style in therapy (Sue & Sue, 1990; Uba, 1994). For example, in analogue studies, both Chinese (Exum & Lau, 1988) and Korean (Foley & Fuqua, 1988) subjects rate therapists with a directive approach as more attractive and effective than therapists with a nondirective approach. Previous literature suggests that Asian Americans may view counseling as a more directive, paternalistic, and autocratic process, which is in contrast to European Americans who may view counseling as a more explorative and democratic process (Sue & Morishima, 1982; Waxer, 1989). In general, a directive approach, which entails providing the client with advice, explanations, and a recommended course of action, meets the expectations that many of the more traditional Asian Americans have about counseling and psychotherapy (Uba, 1994). Moreover, if therapists are not directive in their initial therapy session, the client may misinterpret this approach as indicating incompetence or disinterest (Fugita, Ito, Abe, & Takeuchi, 1991).

Although Asian Americans express a preference for a directive approach, they may still benefit from a nondirective counseling approach that focuses on emotions or feelings. For example, Okamura and Agbay-ani (1991) suggest that nondirective therapy may not be appropriate for foreign-born Filipinos, but such an approach may be appropriate for American-born Filipinos. Also, although Asian American therapists are more likely to use assertive, directive, structured, and formal approaches with traditional Asian clients, they tend to use more assertive, confrontational, and interpretive methods with acculturated Asian clients (Matsushima & Tashima, 1982). Interestingly enough, Merta, Ponterotto, and Brown (1992) found that high-acculturated Asian foreign students rated authoritative counselors higher in overall effectiveness, but low-acculturated students rated colloborative counselors higher. Despite this latter finding, it would appear that directive therapy strategies may prove to be productive with most Asian American clients. However, these particular techniques will not ensure that Asian clients will perceive their counselors as credible or trustworthy (Akutsu, Lin, & Zane, 1990). Invariably, it may be that achieving counselor credibility in the eyes of the Asian client may be more important than the use of such specific therapeutic techniques as structuring or directiveness (Sue & Zane, 1987).

Much research in this area is still needed as past studies have not adequately compared the efficacy of different types of therapy with Asian clients and intraethnic differences in responsivity to nondirective therapies as a function of presenting problem, generation, acculturation level, personality characteristics, education level, and so on (Uba, 1994). Similarly, these initial claims that directive approaches in therapy are more effective with Asian Americans are based primarily on clinical experiences or analogue studies rather than controlled clinical studies.

PSYCHOPHARMACOLOGY

Another phenomenon that has gained a great deal of attention concerns possible ethnic differences in physiological reactivity to prescribed medications. Recent studies have shown that physiological responses to pharmacological drugs, both psychiatric (e.g., Lin & Poland, 1989) and nonpsychiatric (e.g., Zhou, Koshakji, Silberstein, Wilkinson, & Wood, 1989), may be somewhat different for Asian Americans in comparison to European Americans. For example, pharmacokinetic differences have been reported for psychotropic medications such as haloperidol and some benzodiazepines (e.g., Lin, Poland, Lau, & Rubin, 1988; Lin et al., 1989), although the results from other studies on tricyclic antidepressants have been inconclusive (e.g., Lin, Poland, Smith, Strickland, & Mendoza, 1991). If these reported differences in responsivity to psychiatric medications hold true, these preliminary findings may have a significant influence on side-effect profiles and dosage requirements.

Beyond the pharmacokinetic properties of prescribed medications, other problems have also arisen as a result of cultural differences in expectations about drug effects and in medical compliance (Lin & Shen, 1991). For example, Southeast Asian groups have a high rate of noncompliance in taking prescribed medications (Kinzie, Leung, Boehlein, & Fleck, 1987). Although compliance rates improved for Vietnamese and Cambodians after patient education and a discussion of the problems and benefits of medicine, the Iu-Mien remained noncompliant to the prescribed medication regime. Thus, certain Asian immigrants and refugees who may be at risk for developing major depressive disorder and post-traumatic stress disorder may not reap the benefits from modern advances in psychopharmacology due to these high rates of noncompliance (Kroll et al., 1990; Lin & Shen, 1991).

Invariably, most of these studies reporting possible differences in physiological responses and patient compliance to psychiatric medications were completed in the past 10 years. As such, there has not been enough time to replicate these preliminary findings concerning dosage requirements and prescribed maintenance treatments. Also, it is not clear whether physical reactivity to certain dosages of medications, both psychiatric and nonpsychiatric, is specific to certain Asian American groups and not to others. In summary, these results support the great importance of conducting cross-racial studies to evaluate drug effects and physiological reactivity to these drugs, particularly when treating Asian Americans (Lin, Poland, & Nakasaki, 1993; Pi, Wang, & Gray, 1993; Zhou et al., 1989). Also, to prevent possible misuse of medications with Asian American groups, psychopharmacology should be included in the curriculum for psychiatric professionals and further research should be conducted to assess the physiological effects of psychiatric medications not only for Asian Americans but also for other ethnic minority groups (Tien, 1984).

CONCLUSIONS

In reviewing the mental health literature, it becomes apparent that there is a growing knowledge base on Asian Americans which is steadily moving beyond mere descriptive studies. As the Asian population continues to become more culturally diverse in the United States, particularly with the large influx of Southeast Asians and Pacific Islanders, there will be new challenges for mental health providers to develop culturally appropriate and accessible services for this ethnically diverse group.

Invariably, clinical studies conducted in the past may not be as applicable or generalizable to this new group of Asian Americans. For example, concepts of acculturation and its effect on ethnic identity formation as well as intra- and intergroup relations and conflicts will become more complex. In this age of changing international relations and pressures in our society, we cannot assume that the past experiences of Asian immigrants in the late 1800s will be similar to that of current immigrants and refugees who are now entering the United States (Sue & Sue, 1990).

We have just begun to identify some of the general clinical issues in working with Asian Americans; what we now need is to determine "what services work with which Asian groups under what conditions?" In other words, treatment providers must recognize that Asian Americans in the United States represent a largely heterogeneous group. For example, although there is a considerable movement among mental health professionals to develop culturally appropriate intervention strategies for treating Asian Americans as a whole, it will be just as important to determine whether Asian subgroup specificity is warranted. Although it might be helpful to point out how traditional counseling practices may act as barriers to effective cross-cultural help, a greater emphasis on culture-specific methods is likely to occur (Sue & Sue, 1990). Likewise, increasing concern should be given to specific issues and problems in the Asian American community that have plagued the general population, such as alcoholism and substance abuse (e.g., Ja & Aoki, 1993; Zane & Sasao, 1992), child or elder neglect and abuse (e.g., Ima & Hohm, 1991; Tomita, 1994), domestic violence (e.g., Nah, 1993; Song-Kim, 1992), and juvenile delinquency (e.g., Covey, Menard, & Franzese, 1992; Nagata, 1989).

REFERENCES

Akutsu, P. D., Lin, C. H., & Zane, N. (1990). Predictors of utilization intent of counseling among Chinese and Caucasian American students: A test of the proximal–distal model. *Journal of Counseling Psychology, 37,* 445–452.

Akutsu, P. D., & Vuong, T. (1996, November). *Symptomatology reports of Southeast Asian refugee groups.* Paper presented at the annual meeting of the Association for Advancement of Behavior Therapy, New York.

Atkinson, D. R., & Gim, R. H. (1989). Asian-American cultural identity and attitudes toward mental health services. *Journal of Counseling Psychology, 36*(2), 209–212.

Blue, A. V., & Gaines, A. D. (1992). The ethnopsychiatric repertoire: A review and overview of ethnopsychiatric studies. In A. D. Gaines (Ed.), *Ethnopsychiatry: The cultural construction of professional and folk psychiatries* (pp. 397–484). Albany: State University of New York Press.

Brislin, R. (1993). *Understanding culture's influence on behavior.* Fort Worth, TX: Harcourt Brace Jovanovich.

Bui, K. T., & Takeuchi, D. T. (1992). Ethnic minority adolescents and the use of community mental health care services. *American Journal of Community Psychology, 20*(4), 403–417.

Carr, J. E., & Vitaliano, P. P. (1985). The theoretical implications of converging research on depression and the culture-bound syndromes. In A. Kleinman & B. Good (Eds.), *Culture and depression* (pp. 244–266). Berkeley: University of California Press.

Cheung, F. M. (1987). Conceptualization of psychiatric illness and help-seeking behavior among Chinese. *Culture, Medicine, and Psychiatry, 11*(1), 97–106.

Cheung, F. M., & Lau, B. W. (1982). Situational variations of help-seeking behavior among Chinese patients. *Comprehensive Psychiatry, 23*(3), 252–262.

Chung, R., & Okazaki, S. (1991). Counseling Americans of Southeast Asian descent: The impact of the refugee experience. In C. C. Lee & B. L. Richardson (Eds.), *Multicultural issues in counseling: New approaches to diversity* (pp. 107–126). Alexandria, VA: American Association for Counseling and Development.

Covey, H. C., Menard, S. W., & Franzese, R. J. (1992). *Juvenile gangs.* Springfield, IL: Charles C Thomas.

Doi, M. L., Lin, C., & Vohra-Sahu, I. (1981). *Pacific/Asian American research: An annotated bibliography* (Bibliography Series No. 1). Chicago: Pacific/Asian American Mental Health Research Center.

Exum, H. A., & Lau, E. Y. (1988). Counseling style preference of Chinese college students. *Journal of Multicultural Counseling and Development, 16*(2), 84–92.

Flaskerud, J. H. (1986). The effects of culture-compatible intervention on the utilization of mental health services by minority clients. *Community Mental Health Journal, 22*(2), 127–141.

Flaskerud, J. H., & Anh, N. T. (1988). Mental health needs of Vietnamese refugees. *Hospital and Community Psychiatry, 39,* 435–437.

Flaskerud, J. H., & Liu, P. Y. (1990). Influence of therapist ethnicity and language on therapy outcomes of Southeast Asian clients. *International Journal of Social Psychiatry, 36,* 18–29.

Flaskerud, J. H., & Liu, P. Y. (1991). Effects of an Asian client–therapist language, ethnicity, and gender match on client outcomes. *Community Mental Health Journal, 27,* 31–42.

Foley, J. B., & Fuqua, D. R. (1988). The effects of status configuration and counseling style on Korean perspectives of counseling. *Journal of Cross-Cultural Psychology, 19*(4), 465–480.

Foulks, E. F., Merkel, L., & Boehnlein, J. K. (1992). Symptoms in nonpatient Southeast Asian refugees. *Journal of Nervous and Mental Disease, 180*(7), 466–468.

Fugita, S., Ito, K., Abe, J., & Takeuchi, D. (1991). Japanese Americans. In N. Mokuau (Ed.), *Handbook of social services for Asian and Pacific Islanders* (pp. 61–77). New York: Greenwood Press.

Hatanaka, H. K., Watanabe, W. Y., & Ono, S. (1975). The utilization of mental health services by Asian Americans in Los Angeles. In W. H. Ishikawa & N. H. Archer (Eds.), *Delivery of services in Pan Asian communities* (pp. 33–39). San Diego: San Diego Pacific Asian Coalition Mental Health Training Center, San Diego State University.

Hu, T., Snowden, L. R., Jerrell, J. M., & Nguyen, T. D. (1991). Ethnic populations in public mental health: Services choice and level of use. *American Journal of Public Health, 81*(11), 1429–1434.

Ima, K., & Hohm, C. F. (1991). Child maltreatment among Asians and Pacific Islander refugees and immigrants: The San Diego case. *Journal of Interpersonal Violence, 6*(3), 267–285.

Ja, D. Y., & Aoki, B. (1993). Substance abuse treatment: Cultural barriers in the Asian-American community. *Journal of Psychoactive Drugs, 25*(1), 61–71.

Jun-mian, X. (1987). Some issues in the diagnosis of depression in China. *Canadian Journal of Psychiatry, 32*(5), 368–370.

Kim, B. L. (1978). *The Asian Americans: Changing patterns, changing needs.* Montclair, NJ: Association of Korean Christian Scholars in North America.

Kinzie, J. D., Leung, P., Boehlein, J. K., & Fleck, J. (1987). Antidepressant blood levels in Southeast Asians: Clinical and cultural implications. *Journal of Nervous and Mental Disease, 175*(8), 480–485.

Kleinman, A., & Good, B. (1985). *Culture and depression.* Berkeley: University of California Press.

Kroll, J., Linde, P., Habenicht, M., Chan, S., Yang, M., Vang, T., Souvannasoth, L., Nguyen, T., Ly, M., Nguyen, H., & Vang, Y. (1990). Medication compliance, antidepressant blood levels, and side effects in Southeast Asian patients. *Journal of Clinical Psychopharmacology, 10*(4), 279–283.

Lai, J., & Linden, W. (1993). The smile of Asia: Acculturation effects on symptom reporting. *Canadian Journal of Behavioural Science, 25*(2), 303–313.

Leong, F. T. L. (1986). Counseling and psychotherapy with Asian-Americans: Review of the literature. *Journal of Counseling Psychology, 33,* 196–206.

Leong, F. T. L., Wagner, N. S., & Tata, S. P. (1995). Racial and ethnic variations in help-seeking attitudes. In J. G. Ponterotto, J. M. Casas, L. A. Suzuki, & C. M. Alexander (Eds.), *Handbook of multicultural counseling* (pp. 415–438). Thousand Oaks, CA: Sage.

Leong, F. T. L., & Whitfield, J. R. (1992). *Asians in the United States: Abstracts of the psychological and behavioral literature, 1967–1991* (Bibliographies in Psychology, No. 11). Washington, DC: American Psychological Association.

Lin, K. M., Inui, T. S., Kleinman, A. M., & Womack, W. M. (1982). Sociocultural determinants of the help-seeking behavior of patients with mental illness. *Journal of Nervous and Mental Disease, 170*(2), 78–85.

Lin, K. M., & Poland, R. E. (1989). Pharmacotherapy of Asian psychiatric patients. *Psychiatric Annals, 19*(12), 659–663.

Lin, K. M., Poland, R. E., Lau, J. K., & Rubin, R. T. (1988). Haloperidol and prolactin concentrations in Asians and Caucasians. *Journal of Clinical Psychopharmacology, 8*(3), 195–201.

Lin, K. M., Poland, R. E., & Nakasaki, G. (1993). *Psychopharmacology and psychobiology of ethnicity.* Washington, DC: American Psychiatric Press.

Lin, K. M., Poland, R. E., Nuccio, I., Matsuda, K., Hathuc, N., Su, T. P., & Fu, P. (1989). A longitudinal assessment of haloperidol doses and serum concentrations in Asian and Caucasian schizophrenic patients. *American Journal of Psychiatry, 146*(10), 1307–1311.

Lin, K. M., Poland, R. E., Smith, M. W., Strickland, T. L., & Mendoza, R. (1991). Pharmacokinetic and other related factors affecting psychotropic responses in Asians. *Psychopharmacology Bulletin, 27*(4), 427–439.

Lin, K. M., & Shen, W. W. (1991). Pharmacotherapy for Southeast Asian psychiatric patients. *Journal of Nervous and Mental Disease, 179*(6), 346–350.

Loo, C., Tong, B., & True, R. (1989). A bitter bean: Mental health status and attitudes in Chinatown. *Journal of Community Psychology, 17*(4), 283–296.

Matkin, R. E., Nickles, L. E., Demos, R. C., & Demos, G. D. (1996). Cultural effects on symptom expression among Southeast Asians diagnosed with posttraumatic stress disorder. *Journal of Mental Health Counseling, 18*(1), 64–79.

Matsushima, N. M., & Tashima, N. (1982). *Mental health treatment modalities of Pacific/Asian-American practitioners.* San Francisco: Pacific Asian Mental Health Research Project.

Mattson, S. (1993). Mental health of Southeast Asian refugee women: An overview. *Health Care for Women International, 14*(2), 155–165.

Mau, W., & Jepsen, D. A. (1990). Help-seeking perceptions and behaviors: A comparison of Chinese and American graduate students. *Journal of Multicultural Counseling and Development, 18*(2), 94–104.

Merta, R. J., Ponterotto, J. G., & Brown, R. D. (1992). Comparing the effectiveness of two directive styles in the academic counseling of foreign students. *Journal of Counseling Psychology, 39,* 214–218.

Mokuau, N. (1991). *Handbook of social services for Asian and Pacific Islanders.* New York: Greenwood Press.

Moore, L. J., & Boehnlein, J. K. (1991). Posttraumatic stress disorder, depression, and somatic symptoms in U.S. Mien patients. *Journal of Nervous and Mental Disease, 179*(12), 728–733.

Morishima, J. K., Sue, S., Teng, L. N., Zane, N. W. S., & Cram, J. R. (1979). *Handbook of Asian/Pacific Islander mental health* (Vol. 1) (DHHS Publication No. ADM 80-754). Rockville, MD: National Institute of Mental Health.

Nagata, D. (1989). Japanese American children and adolescents. In J. T. Gibbs & L. H. Huang (Eds.), *Children of color: Psychological interventions with minority youth* (pp. 67–113). San Francisco: Jossey-Bass.

Nah, K. (1993). Perceived problems and service delivery for Korean immigrants. *Social Work, 38*(3), 289–296.

Narikiyo, T. A., & Kameoka, V. A. (1992). Attributions of mental illness and judgments about help seeking among Japanese-American and White American students. *Journal of Counseling Psychology, 39*(3), 363–369.

Niem, T. T. (1989). Treating Oriental patients with western psychiatry: A 12-year experience with Vietnamese refugee psychiatric patients. *Psychiatric Annals, 19*(12), 648–652.

Nishimoto, R. (1988). A cross-cultural analysis of psychiatric symptom expression using Langer's twenty-two item index. *Journal of Sociology and Social Welfare, 15*(4), 45–62.

Nishio, K., & Bilmes, M. (1987). Psychotherapy with Southeast Asian American clients. *Professional Psychology: Research and Practice, 18*(4), 342–346.

Okamura, J., & Agbayani, A. (1991). Filipino Americans. In N. Mokuau (Ed.), *Handbook of social services for Asian and Pacific Islanders* (pp. 97–115). New York: Greenwood Press.

O'Sullivan, M. J., Peterson, P. D., Cox, G. B., & Kirkeby, J. (1989). Ethnic populations: Community mental health services ten years later. *American Journal of Community Psychology, 17*(1), 17–30.

Owan, T. C. (1985). *Southeast Asian mental health treatment, prevention services, training, and research.* Washington, DC: National Institute of Mental Health.

Pi, E. H., Wang, A. L., & Gray, G. E. (1993). Asian/non-Asian transcultural tricyclic antidepressant psychopharmacology: A review. *Progress in Neuro-Psychopharmacology and Biological Psychiatry, 17*(5), 691–702.

Raskin, A., Chien, C. P., & Lin, K. M. (1992). Elderly Chinese- and Caucasian-Americans compared on measures of psychic distress, somatic complaints, and social competence. *International Journal of Geriatric Psychiatry, 7*(3), 191–198.

Silver, B. J., & Chui, J. (1985). *Mental health issues: Indo-Chinese refugees. An annotated bibliography* (DHHS Publication No. ADM 85-1404). Rockville, MD: National Institute of Mental Health.

Snowden, L. R., & Cheung, F. K. (1990). Use of inpatient mental health services by members of ethnic minority groups. *American Psychologist, 45*(3), 347–355.

Solberg, V. S., Choi, K-H., Ritsma, S., & Jolly, A. (1994). Asian-American college students: It is time to reach out. *Journal of College Student Development, 35*(4), 296–301.

Song-Kim, Y. I. (1992). Battered Korean women in urban United States. In S. M. Furuto, R. Biswas, D. K. Chung, K. Murase, & F. Ross-Sheriff (Eds.), *Social work practice with Asian Americans* (pp. 213–226). Newbury Park, CA: Sage.

Suan, L. V., & Tyler, J. D. (1990). Mental health values and preference for mental health resources of Japanese-American and Caucasian-American students. *Professional Psychology: Research and Practice, 21*(4), 291–296.

Sue, D. W., & Sue, D. (1990). *Counseling the culturally different: Theory and practice* (2nd ed.). New York: Wiley.

Sue, S., Fujino, D. C., Hu, L. T., Takeuchi, D., & Zane, N. (1991). Community mental health services for ethnic minority groups: A test of the cultural responsiveness hypothesis. *Journal of Consulting and Clinical Psychology, 59*(4), 533–540.

Sue, S., & McKinney, H. (1975). Asian Americans in the community mental health care system. *American Journal of Orthopsychiatry, 45,* 111–118.

Sue, S., & Morishima, J. (1982). *The mental health of Asian Americans.* San Francisco: Jossey-Bass.

Sue, S., & Zane, N. (1987). The role of culture and cultural techniques in psychotherapy: A critique and reformulation. *American Psychologist, 42*(1), 37–45.

Takeuchi, D. T., Mokuau, N., & Chun, C. A. (1992). Mental health services for Asian Americans and Pacific Islanders. *Journal of Mental Health Administration, 19*(3), 237–245.

Takeuchi, D. T., Sue, S., & Yeh, M. (1995). Return rates and outcomes from ethnicity-specific mental health programs in Los Angeles. *American Journal of Public Health, 85,* 638–643.

Tien, J. L. (1984). Do Asians need less medication? *Journal of Psychosocial Nursing and Mental Health Services, 22*(12), 19–22.

Tomita, S. K. (1994). The consideration of cultural factors in the research of elder mistreatment with an in-depth look at the Japanese. *Journal of Cross-Cultural Gerontology, 9*(1), 39–52.

Uba, L. (1994). *Asian Americans: Personality patterns, identity, and mental health.* New York: Guilford Press.

Vohra-Sahu, I. (1983). *The Pacific/Asian Americans: A selected and annotated bibliography of recent materials* (Bibliography Series No. 4). Chicago: Pacific/Asian American Mental Health Research Center.

Waxer, P. H. (1989). Cantonese versus Canadian evaluation of directive and non-directive therapy. *Canadian Journal of Counselling, 23*(3), 263–272.

Westermeyer, J. (1989). Dr. Westermeyer replies. *American Journal of Psychiatry, 146*(3), 411.

Westermeyer, J., Bouafuely, M., Neider, J., & Callies, A. (1989). Somatization among refugees: An epidemiologic study. *Psychosomatics, 30*(1), 34–43.

Williams, C. L. (1987). *An annotated bibliography on refugee mental health* (DHHS Publication No. ADM 87-1517). Rockville, MD: National Institute of Mental Health.

Wu, I., & Windle, C. (1980). Ethnic specificity in the relative minority use and staffing of community mental health centers. *Community Mental Health Journal, 16,* 156–168.

Yamamoto, J. (1992). Psychiatric diagnoses and neurasthenia. *Psychiatric Annals, 22*(4), 171–172.

Yeh, M., Takeuchi, D. T., & Sue, S. (1994). Asian-American children treated in the mental health system: A comparison of parallel and mainstream outpatient service centers. *Journal of Clinical Child Psychology, 23,* 5–12.

Ying, Y. (1990). Explanatory models of major depression and implications for help-seeking among immigrant Chinese-American women. *Culture, Medicine and Psychiatry, 14*(3), 393–408.

Ying, Y., & Miller, L. S. (1992). Help-seeking behavior and attitude of Chinese Americans regarding psychological problems. *American Journal of Community Psychology, 20*(4), 549–556.

Yu, E., Murata, A. K., & Lin, C. (1982). *Bibliography of Pacific/Asian American materials in the Library of Congress* (Bibliography Series No. 3). Chicago: Pacific/Asian American Mental Health Research Center.

Zane, N., Hatanaka, H., Park, S., & Akutsu, P. D. (1994). Ethnic-specific mental health services: Evaluation of the parallel approach for Asian-American clients. *Journal of Community Psychology, 22,* 68–81.

Zane, N., & Sasao, T. (1992). Research on drug abuse among Asian Pacific Americans. *Drugs and Society, 6*(3–4), 181–209.

Zhou, H. H., Koshakji, R. P., Silberstein, D. J., Wilkinson, G. R., & Wood, A. J. J. (1989). Racial differences in drug response: Altered sensitivity to and clearance of propranolol in men of Chinese descent as compared with American Whites. *New England Journal of Medicine, 320*(9), 565–570.

32

Cross-Cultural Communication: Therapeutic Use of Interpreters

EVELYN LEE

In many professions, effective communication is essential for a successful provider–consumer interaction. In particular, in mental health counseling, clinicians rely on verbal and nonverbal communication as the primary tool for obtaining a thorough psychiatric and psychosocial history and forming a therapeutic relationship with the client. Language barriers can lead to miscommunication, which can further lead to under- or overdiagnosis and inappropriate treatment.

Overcoming language discrepancies between the patient and clinician is not an easy task. Both parties interpret cues based on a set of culturally determined beliefs and values. The cultural rules underlying how they respond to each other determine the course of their communication in the therapeutic encounter. Research demonstrates that considerable complexity can arise due to differences in social class, even when the patients and clinicians share a common language (Pendleton & Bochner, 1980) and gender (Felton, 1986). Few studies document how differences in culture and primary language affect the direct provision of counseling. Studies that do exist highlight several negative effects when a common language is not shared: diagnoses of more severe psychopathology, low ratings of clinicians' empathy and therapeutic rapport, and lack of patients' self-disclosure (Belton, 1984; Doolgin, Salazar, & Cruz, 1987; Erzinger, 1991; Marcos, 1979, 1988).

There are few studies documenting the positive effects on treatment outcomes if a common language between the clinician and patient is shared. One recent study indicated that when Asian clients and therapists shared either a common language or a common ethnic origin, there was a significant increase in the number of client sessions with the primary therapist (Flaskerud & Liu, 1991). If we assume that language match can bring more beneficial effects to treatment outcome, we need to have many more bilingual mental health professionals. In our current culturally diverse population with a dramatic increase of immigrants whose primary language is not English, it is next to impossible to staff an organization competent in so many languages and dialects. Therefore, the use of interpreters is necessary to bridge the language and cultural gap, even though it may not be the ideal communication medium. Although many organizations already use interpreters, at least three problem areas exist: (1) Most interpreters are not properly trained in the art of interpreting, particularly in the mental health setting; (2) most clinicians are not skilled in the use of interpreters; and (3) most patients are ill-informed as to their rights to receive services in their own language and often find it difficult to express themselves through interpreters.

The purpose of this chapter is to provide clinicians with knowledge and skills to develop their competency in working with interpreters. This chapter provides a practical guide to identifying common problems in interpreting, the role of the cultural interpreter, interpreting formats and stages, and effective communication skills in working with non-English-speaking patients. The therapeutic triad model is introduced as an effective tool in working with interpreters.

DEFINITIONS

The term "translation," in general, refers to written work. It is judged by its denotative accuracy. The translater must have excellent command of the two languages. The term "interpretation" refers to the transfer of connotative as well as denotative meaning and usually applies to dialogue rather than written materials (Westermeyer, 1989).

A "cultural interpreter" is an active participant in a cross-cultural/lingual interaction, assisting the provider in understanding the beliefs and practices of the client's culture and assisting the client in understanding the dominant culture, by providing cultural as well as linguistic links. This model of interpreting service was developed out of an awareness that communication is seriously impaired by insensitivity to the role of culture in the content and manner of communication, particularly in formal interactions (Cairncross, 1989).

INTERPRETATION MODELS

Institutions vary in their arrangements for meeting the needs of mono-lingual patients. Even in urban cities with large numbers of immigrants who do not speak English, many facilities have not dealt with language and cultural barriers in a formal operational sense and systematic way. Providing interpreters is not seen as an institutional responsibility. With the financial crisis facing many health care facilities, funding for formal interpreting services is not seen as a priority.

Models of interpretation currently being used in mental health settings broadly fall into five different categories:

1. *The "approximate-interpreting model"* applies when the responsibility for interpretation falls on the shoulders of the nearest person who is bilingual and convenient to the scene. This person is sometimes the relative of the patient or a stranger who happens to be in the vicinity (e.g., janitorial staff or bilingual worker in another department). In some hospitals, other patients are used as interpreters. There are major problems with this substitute for a trained interpreter. Persons put into this position usually do not have the level of dual fluency needed and it is unlikely that they have the necessary technical vocabulary. Another problem is the inability to adhere to the confidentiality ethic. The patient may not be willing to share many personal and often private thoughts with a stranger from the same ethnic community or with other family members. When children are used as interpreters, the conflicts resulting from the reversal of roles between the parent and the child can have a lasting negative effect on the family relationship (Cairncross, 1989).

2. *The "tele-active model"* uses the telephone dial to select from a menu offering different languages/dialects. The patient interacts with computer and software without human interaction. This mode of service may be used during emergencies or crises after hours when an interpreter is not available. Such machine contact should not replace face-to-face communication on a regular basis.

3. *The "bilingual worker/interpreter model"* works as a "clinician's assistant" who sees the patient alone under supervision or functions as an interpreter if needed. If the worker is not professionally trained, this model may present certain legal and ethical problems. If the worker is experienced and well trained, this model can be quite effective. Many refugee clinics and mental health clinics serving large number of mono-lingual patients are using this model.

4. *The "volunteer interpreter pool model"* recruits a pool of volunteers to provide services upon request. They usually have not received formal training in interpreting skills.

5. *The "staff interpreter model"* employs paid staff to provide interpretation. Most of them have received formal training.

Table 32.1 provides a listing of competency criteria for the interpreter.

TABLE 32.1. Competency Criteria for the Interpreter

Technical
Good command of English in both speech and reading
Proficiency in language of origin in both speech and reading
Ability to translate fine shades of meaning
Familiarity with and understanding of the terminology and procedures used in different organizational settings
Ability to translate not only verbal communication but also such nonverbal communication as body language, facial expressions, and speech patterns

Cultural
Intimate knowledge of his or her ethnic community, including migration history, cultural values, social and power structures, community healers, and cultural views of health and illness
Ability to make cultural connection and rapport with patient
Familiarity with U.S. culture
Ability to act as cultural broker—to interpret with linguistic and cultural perspective and to explain why a suggestion from the clinician may be unacceptable or unrealistic to patients
Ability to understand the culture of the organization

Interpersonal
Good awareness of personal values, attitudes, and personal biases
Good understanding of own communication style
Ability to assess areas of incompatibility with clinician or patient and to react appropriately
Ability to get along with peers and other staff members
Ability to deal with conflicts arising from role confusion or unrealistic expectations from clinician or patient

Ethical
A professional ethics code that includes confidentiality, impartiality, proficiency, and general rules with respect to conflicts of interest

Others
Ability to be an effective advocate for patient
A good memory
Careful attention to detail
Flexibility in handling different situations

Note. Adapted from Cairncross (1989).

STAGES OF INTERPRETING

Using interpreters correctly requires time, planning, and experience. Generally speaking, for the clinician, an ideal interpreting session should consist of four stages.

Language Assessment and Interpreter Assignment

The clinician makes an initial assessment of the patient's country of origin, language, and dialect and matches these characteristics with those of the interpreter. There are dialectical differences even for patients from the same country or same region. For example, a Chinese patient from Vietnam may not speak Vietnamese. Also, the Chinese speak many different dialects (Cantonese, Mandarin, Chiuchow, etc.). It is important to find an interpreter to match the exact dialect. For the patient who speaks "some English," it is advisable to provide an interpreter to avoid language and cultural misunderstandings. It is quite difficult for patients whose primary language is not English to express their emotional states in English. On the other hand, unless the monolingual provider is thoroughly effective and fluent in the patient's language, he or she should always use an interpreter. In addition to language match, it is also desirable to assign an interpreter of the same sex in some cases. Very often, an age match is useful.

It is also important to assess the interpreter's knowledge and understanding of the organization. The interpreter should know about the mission of the agency, range of services provided, terminology and institutional language used, legal forms required, roles of different professionals, and types of patients served.

Preinterview Meeting with the Interpreter

The clinician should take time to prepare the interpreter before the actual interview. Questions to consider include the following:

1. What are the objectives of the interview?
2. What topics are to be covered?
3. What is the patient like (background, symptoms, behavior)?
4. What are the particularly sensitive topics?
5. What are the interpreter's experiences with patients with emotional problems?
6. How much time will the interview require?
7. What are the preferred translation formats?

The preinterview meeting gives the clinician an opportunity to build a relationship of trust and team spirit with the interpreter and to get across to the interpreter the concept of "I need your help" or "I need your input." In the event the clinician finds that the patient's culture is unfamiliar, he or she might give the interpreter permission to bring up cultural issues.

Actual Interview with the Patient

During the actual interview, the clinician should be aware of translation problems, verbal and nonverbal communication styles of everyone in the interview, different types of translation formats, and cultural misunderstandings. More details will be covered later in the chapter.

Review of the Session

After the interview, the clinician and the interpreter should review the session to clarify any confusion that may have arisen, to discuss any cultural issues, to vent any feelings about working with each other, and to plan future sessions.

ROLE EXPECTATIONS

Clinicians have different role expectations for the interpreters, depending on the resources available in the organization and the training received by the providers. Generally speaking, there are three major types of relationships:

1. *Treating the interpreter as a "robot" or voice machine.* The only task of the interpreter is to pass the message verbatim from one person to the other. The interpreter is not expected to give any input, cultural or otherwise. This type of interaction may work well in court settings or in multilingual conferences but may not be the most effective model for mental health interviews.

2. *Treating the interpreter as a "clinician."* The clinician lacks confidence in working with the patient from a very different culture and hands over the clinical judgment to the interpreter.

3. *Treating the interpreter as a "team partner."* The clinician understands that he or she brings professional expertise and knowledge in the helping process. At the same time, the clinician recognizes and respects the interpreter's expertise in language, culture, and community resources.

THERAPEUTIC TRIAD MODEL

When three persons work together within a limited physical space, using two different languages in a structured task, three distinct interactions are occurring. What develops is a triangle with three sets of pairs, or dyads, each one operative at a given point in time (see Figure 32.1). The clinician, the interpreter, and the patient form a "therapeutic triad" with three interlocking sets of relationships. Unlike two-way communication, there is a shift of power balance within the triangle. The interpreter is the only one who knows the two different languages. In this situation, the only means of communication between the clinician and the patient is nonverbal communication. Although only one of these dyads is operative at any one time, nonverbal communication is taking place with each dyad at all times.

INTERPRETING FORMATS

1. *Word-for-word interpreting* gives verbatim or line-by-line translation. The interpreter is expected to act as the "messenger" to translate each word spoken by the provider. This format allows minimal participation by the interpreter, who attempts to be a neutral party whose primary task is to pass information between the patient and the provider. The clinician may find this format to be helpful in situations such as asking factual questions, giving information, and explaining technical procedures. However, this format is not the best if the subject being discussed needs to be expressed in a summary fashion without constant interruption. This

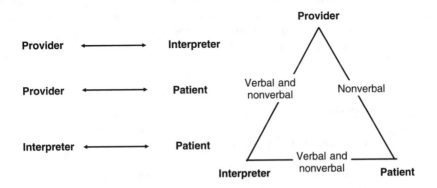

FIGURE 32.1. Therapeutic triad model.

format also does not allow room for untranslatable words or concepts. This process takes at least twice as long.

2. *Concurrent interpreting* consists of the interpreter translating and speaking while the clinician or patient is speaking. Although this method saves time, it can have many disadvantages (e.g., more chances for error, greater emphasis on denotative translation at the expense of connotative interpretation, and no room for the interpreter to assist with his or her cultural expertise).

3. *Summary interpreting* summarizes the important points without necessarily using the same word or sentence sequences. It is a much faster method than verbatim interpreting but less accurate in terms of reflecting the actual exchanges of the communication. This format is helpful when patients need to tell their stories on emotionally charged topics. This model requires high degree of trust between the clinician and the interpreter.

4. *Consecutive interpreting* requires accurate interpretation segment by segment as each party speaks.

5. *Cultural interpreting* gives permission to the interpreter to convey the parties' messages in a way appropriate to the cultural background and understanding of the speaker and the receiver. The interpreter acts as the "cultural broker" to minimize cultural misunderstanding.

COMMON PROBLEMS IN INTERPRETATION

There are many problems associated with the utilization of interpreters, especially in the fields of mental health and psychiatry. Interpreting requires three-way dyadic communication in two languages by three individuals (more in the case of family interviews or group interviews). Each member in the session is different in terms of dialect, accent, grammar, and linguistic style. Generally speaking, problems fall into two areas: technical difficulties, and role conflicts.

Technical Difficulties in Interpretation

The following common problems are drawn from both the literature (Putsch, 1985) and my personal experiences in working with interpreters. Any of these problems may prevent the clinician from obtaining accurate and pivotal information.

1. *Deletion/omission of information.* For example: Patient [in Vietnamese]: "I decided to escape by boat but I did not tell my mother about my plan. I did not want her to worry so much since my father was still in the educational camp." Interpreter: "Mr. L says he came by boat."

2. *Bad paraphrasing.* For example: Patient: "It is my right leg that's

bothering me for the past three weeks. My back hurts if I stand up too long." Interpreter: "Mr. Y has problems with both his leg and his back."

3. *Lack of translatable words or concepts.* For example: A psychiatrist asks a newly arrived woman from Laos during a mental status examination: "What does 'A rolling stone gathers no moss' mean to you?" Interpreter: "???"

4. *Inaccurate translation of words and concepts.* For example: Clinician: "Mrs. W, do you hear voices?" Interpreter: "The doctor asks you whether you hear any noises?" ("Voice" and "noise" are the same word in Chinese.) Patient: "Yes, I hear noises all the time. I live on a busy street."

5. *Blocked verbal communication.* For example: Mrs. C and the interpreter engaged in a 10-minute dialogue, and then the interpreter tells the doctor: "Mrs. C does not want to take the medication."

6. *Distortion of meaning.* For example: Physician: "Are you allergic to any medications?" Interpreter: "Does the Western drug make you vomit?" Patient [in Cantonese]: "No."

7. *Exaggeration/adding.* For example: Patient [in Cambodian]: "I am glad I have decided to come to this country." Interpreter: "Mr. B is excited that he and his family are in the United States. They are now receiving welfare and living in an apartment with a new television."

8. *Lack of familiarity with professional terminology.* For example: Clinician: "What kind of mood have you been in recently." Interpreter: "How have you been feeling?" Patient: "Well, you see my head used to ache all the time. . . . "

9. *Inability to interpret the cultural meaning of the symptoms and behavior.* For example: Patient [in Cantonese]: "I took the whole bottle of 60 *po chia* pills last night." The interpreter used word-for-word format to repeat the statement without giving a cultural explanation that this pill is a popular Chinese medicine that usually requires the user to take the whole bottle. Psychiatrist: "Mrs. D, were you trying to kill yourself last night?"

10. *Inability to detect paralinguistic or nonverbal behavior.* For example: A young medical student in a refugee clinic: "Mrs. P, are you having regular sexual intercourse with your husband?" The patient appears embarrassed and looks at the floor after the translation. The medical student consults the chart and repeats the same question.

Role Conflicts

In addition to problems arising from technical errors, the quality of interpretation is often affected by role conflicts and confusion. One common problem is the shifting of power from the professional to the interpreter. Some professionals may try to overcompensate for this relinquishment of power by becoming more rigid and controlling. The interpreter is also in an uneasy situation. It is difficult for the interpreter to be entirely neutral and nonpartisan. As the sole possessor and processor of both clients' views, the interpreter is in a position to manipulate not only the information exchange but also the situation (Putsch, 1985). Other common problems develop in the interpreter–provider–patient triangle, such as the following:

1. Overidentification of patient with the interpreter due to cultural and language bonds.
2. Overdependence of provider on the interpreter due to unfamiliarity of language and culture.
3. Rejection of the interpreter by the patient due to fear of breach of confidentiality.
4. Overexercising the power and authority by the interpreter in relating to patient due to social class difference.
5. Role conflict faced by the interpreter as community advocate and institutional employee. Over- or underexpectations by professional of interpreter lead to frustration for both parties.

ISSUES AND PROBLEMS IN CLINICAL ASSESSMENT

Using an interpreter for such clinical assessments as mental status examination poses more complications. Even the sophisticated interpreter and trained clinician face difficulties in pursuing topics such as hallucination, delusions, suicide, mood changes, sexual dysfunction, and so on. Presentations of psychiatric patients, such as flight of ideas, illogical thinking, poverty of speech, thought content, and pressured speech, are difficult to translate. In addition, when the clinician conducts a comprehensive evaluation, there is a constant shifting of contents between history gathering, problem solving, psychotherapy, and education.

In psychiatric settings, it is not uncommon that the interpreter attempts to "normalize" the patient's psychopathology to protect the patient from medical authorities. Interpreters may sometimes fall into the trap of trying their best to "make sense" of the patient's disorganized or illogical responses. These efforts to make sense out of nonsense may be motivated by a desire to be an advocate for the patient and trying to help the patient be understood by the interviewer. Interpreters' emotional responses to the questions being asked in the evaluation can add further complications. Many interpreters feel overwhelmed by the responsibility. They may feel embarrassed by some of the interviewer's questions or by some of the things the patient says. Some feel pressured to give more information to the interviewer than the patient actually gave. Some experience frustration about being asked to translate the same questions again and again, or some may feel offended by the "culturally incompetent" questions asked by the interviewer. Unfortunately, many interpreters do not share their feelings openly because of their lower job status and nonassertive communication style. Dynamics such as these interfere with the quality of the interpretation and affect the working relationship.

OVERCOMING THE LANGUAGE BARRIERS: EFFECTIVE COMMUNICATION WITH NON-ENGLISH-SPEAKING PATIENTS

1. Clinicians should be aware of their own verbal and nonverbal communication style.

2. The clinician should try to find an interpreter who can speak the patient's dialect and understand the patient's cultural background. Clinician and interpreter should convene briefly before meeting the patient to discuss the purpose of the interview, the translation formats, and other clinical information. It is also important to ask about the interpreter's previous experience in working with patients with emotional problems.

3. Clinicians must build a relationship of trust with the interpreter. They should interact with the interpreter in a respectful manner and project positive energy.

4. The clinician should try to conduct the interview in a comfortable, professional setting. It is helpful for clinicians to organize the seating arrangement in a way that will allow them to engage in face-to-face contact with both patient and interpreter. I recommend a 60-degree triangular arrangement.

5. The clinician should always talk to the patient, even if the patient does not understand the clinician's language. Questions should be addressed to the patient directly. Clinicians should address the patient as "Mrs. C" or "you" rather than through the interpreter as "she" or "her."

6. It is up to the clinician to explain his or her role and the interpreter's role clearly to the patient.

7. Clinicians must demonstrate that they understand the importance of confidentiality.

8. Clinicians should be aware of the ethnic/age/sex/class differences of the patient and interpreter.

9. Clinicians must be sensitive to and aware of the different cultural assumptions between themselves and the patient. They should use the interpreter as the "cultural broker" to avoid unnecessary cultural misunderstanding.

10. Clinicians should practice nonverbal communication skills throughout the interview. Actual spoken words account for only a small

portion of emotional expression, while the majority of emotional messages are received nonverbally.

11. It is imperative to be aware of the cultural meanings of body language—smiling, nodding, eye contact, touching, foot movement, and other facial expressions. The clinician must maintain "gentle" eye contact when the patient or the interpreter speaks.

12. The clinician must be a good listener and must not fake attention.

13. The clinician should not take excessive notes during the interview.

14. It is wise to use short, simple statements and stick to one topic at a time. When lengthy explanations are necessary, the clinician should break them up into several short sentences.

15. A clinician should speak clearly and should not raise his or her voice. Tone and volume should be compatible with the patient's.

16. The clinician should speak slowly throughout the session. He or she should conduct the interview in a quiet, unhurried manner and should try to sit down during the conversation.

17. The clinician should use words or examples the patient and interpreter are likely to know. He or she must avoid idioms, ambiguous statements, jargon, abstractions, and metaphors. Also, he or she should avoid indefinite phrases that use "would," "could," "if," and "maybe." These can be mistaken for actual approval of a course of action.

18. Clinicians must be alert to translation errors. In the event of obvious omission, the clinician should ask gently but persistently that the interpreter make a more complete translation.

19. The clinician must try to regulate the flow of the conversation. Clinicians must maintain a good balance between focus on self and on others. They should plan what they want to say ahead of time and avoid confusing the interpreter by backing up, rephrasing or hesitating.

20. Clinicians must encourage the interpreter to tell them when he or she is having difficulty. The clinician should ask the interpreter to comment on the patient's word content and emotions. He or she should conduct a postinterview meeting with the interpreter to review the session.

REFERENCES

Belton, M. A. (1984). The effect of therapist dialect upon the black English-speaking patient's perception of therapist empathy, warmth, genuineness and expertise. *Dissertation Abstracts International, 44*(8-B), 2547.

Cairncross, L. (1989). *Cultural interpreter training manual.* Ontario: Queen's Printer for Ontario.

Doolgin, D. L., Salazar, A., & Cruz, A. (1987). The Hispanic treatment program:

Principles of effective psychotherapy. *Journal of Contemporary Psychotherapy,* *17*(4), 285–299.

Erzinger, S. (1991). Communication between Spanish-speaking patients and their doctors in medical encounters. *Culture, Medicine and Psychiatry, 15,* 91–110.

Felton, J. R. (1986). Sex makes a differences: How gender affects the therapeutic relationship. *Clinical Social Work Journal, 14*(2), 127–138.

Flaskerud, J. H., & Liu, P. Y. (1991). Effects of an Asian client–therapist language, ethnicity and gender match on utilization and outcome of therapy. *Community Mental Health Journal, 27*(1), 31–42.

Marcos, L. R. (1979). Effects of interpreters on the evaluation of psychotherapy in non-English-speaking patients. *American Journal of Psychiatry, 136,* 171–174.

Marcos, L. R. (1988). Understanding ethnicity in psychotherapy with Hispanic patients. *American Journal of Psychoanalysis, 48*(1), 35–42.

Pendleton, D. A., & Bochner, S. (1980). The communication of medical information in general practice consultations as a function of patients' social class. *Social Science and Medicine, 14A,* 669–673.

Putsch, R. (1985). Cross-cultural communication—The special case of interpreters in health care. *Journal of the American Medical Association, 254*(23), 3344–3348.

Westermeyer, J. (1989). *Psychiatric care of migrants: A clinical guide.* Washington, DC: American Psychiatric Press.

Index

Abstinence from alcohol, 306
Academic pressures, adolescents, 187–190
Acculturation
  adolescent conflicts, 178
  Cambodian families, 39, 40
  differential levels in families, 253, 254
  East Indian families, 88, 89
  and help seeking, 235, 467
  Korean families, 129, 130
  Laotian families, 142
  rates of, 5
  and somatization, 466
  and stress assessment, 19, 20
  and therapeutic approach, 468
Adolescents, 175–195
  acculturation conflicts, 178, 184, 185
  case examples, 187–192
  cultural brokering in families, 189
  cultural value conflicts, 177
  ethnocultural assessment, 182–185
  family system, 183, 184
  generational status, 182
  identity formation, 176, 177
  immigration history assessment, 182, 183
  intergenerational conflicts, 178, 187–190
    case example, 187–190
  intervention, 187–192
  parallel assessments, 178–186
  racism issue, case example, 191, 192
  school system considerations, 185, 186
Adulthood, 196–206
  assessment issues, 202–204
  barriers to treatment, 204, 205
  career choice, 198
  conceptualization, 196–198
  "dual identity" in, 197
  life cycle stresses, 198–200

mental health problems, 201, 202
migration impact, 198–200
and negotiator/interpreter role, 199
social life, 198, 199
Affect
  assessment in adolescents, 180, 181
  cultural influences, 324–326, 429
Affective symptoms, 240
Aggression
  childrearing practices, 325
  Western cultural value, 329
Aging (see Elderly)
Agoraphobia, epidemiology, 310
AIDS (see HIV/AIDS)
Alcohol abuse, 295–308
  abstinence versus controlled drinking, 306
  assessment, 303–305
  disulfiram treatment, 299
  job skills training approach, 305
  Koreans, 131
  psychotherapeutic approaches, 299
  recruitment process, 303, 304
  service projects, 305, 306
  Twelve-Step program, 299, 300, 306
Alcoholics Anonymous, 299, 300
Alienation, adolescents, 177
Alprazolam
  ethnopharmacology, 391, 392
  in posttraumatic stress disorder, 282
"Americanized" families, 12
Amitabha Buddha, 461
Ancestor worship
  Chinese, 211
  Vietnamese, 154
Ancestral spirits, and mental illness, 232, 233